Praise for

THE PALEO C

"Chris Kresser is the most knowledgeable clinician in the Paleo/ancestral health scene. He has helped thousands of people, often with the most complex cases. *The Paleo Cure* condenses Chris's vast knowledge and clinical experience to help you look, feel, and perform your best."

—Robb Wolf, *New York Times* bestselling author of *The Paleo Solution*

"Chris Kresser is a leading voice within the Paleo nutrition community for his objective, balanced, and evidence-based approach. In *The Paleo Cure*, Chris has done the heavy lifting for you by pulling together all of his best advice in one place. Whether this is the first you're hearing of it or you already follow a Paleo type of diet, this book will support your deeper understanding of the approach and outline a clear-cut plan for your transition."

—Diane Sanfilippo, *New York Times* bestselling author of *Practical Paleo*

"If every physician memorized this book and used it as a major adjunct to their practice, the world would be a healthier, happier, and more productive place. I can't wait to implement everything I've learned from Chris. The book is yet another testament to how much he still has to teach me and other physicians."

—Kirk Parsley, MD, former Navy SEAL, physician for West Coast SEALs, Division Officer for SEAL Tactical Athlete Center

"We humans might all run on the same basic physiological equipment and follow the same laws of biochemistry, but our varied experiences and journeys and choices throughout life change our relationship to those foundations. With *The Paleo Cure*, Kresser heeds the evolutionary ties that bind us together while showing us how to design a healthy, personalized lifestyle that acknowledges our differences."

—Mark Sisson, author of *The Primal Blueprint*

"There is no 'one size fits all' approach to health, but how do you know what works best for you? Thanks to Chris Kresser's *The Paleo Cure* now your ideal health plan is easy to create and implement. Kresser's detailed step-by-step action plan will teach you how to eat better, sleep better, move more, and stress less—and help you tweak your approach until it's just right."

—Dallas and Melissa Hartwig, *New York Times* bestselling authors of *It Starts with Food*

THE PALEO CURE

Eat Right for Your Genes, Body Type,
and Personal Health Needs—Prevent
and Reverse Disease, Lose Weight Effortlessly,
and Look and Feel Better than Ever

CHRIS KRESSER

LITTLE, BROWN AND COMPANY
NEW YORK   BOSTON   LONDON

Little, Brown and Company
Hachette Book Group
1290 Avenue of the Americas, New York, NY 10104
littlebrown.com

Originally published in hardcover as *Your Personal Paleo Code* by Little, Brown and Company, December 2013
First Little, Brown and Company paperback edition, December 2014

Little, Brown and Company is a division of Hachette Book Group, Inc. The Little, Brown name and logo are trademarks of Hachette Book Group, Inc.

The publisher is not responsible for websites (or their content) that are not owned by the publisher.

The Hachette Speakers Bureau provides a wide range of authors for speaking events. To find out more, go to hachettespeakersbureau.com or call (866) 376-6591.

For detailed notes and references to studies cited throughout the book, see ChrisKresser.com/ppcnotes.

Library of Congress Cataloging-in-Publication Data
   Kresser, Chris.
   The paleo cure : eat right for your genes, body type, and personal health needs — prevent and reverse disease, lose weight effortlessly, and look and feel better than ever/Chris Kresser. — First paperback edition.
     pages cm
   Includes bibliographical references and index.
   ISBN 978-0-316-32289-8 (hc) / 978-0-316-32292-8 (pb)
   1. High-protein diet.   2. Low-carbohydrate diet.   3. Prehistoric peoples — Nutrition. I. Title.
   RM237.65.K74 2013
   613.2'833 — dc23   2013032951

10 9 8 7 6 5 4 3 2 1

RRD-C

Printed in the United States of America

To all who struggle with chronic illness:
may this book be a catalyst for healing and self-discovery

Contents

STEP 2:

REBUILD YOUR LIFE

STEP 3:

REVIVE YOUR HEALTH

Foreword

We live in extraordinary times. Human ingenuity has given us flight, space travel, lasers, the Internet, and amazing medical technologies that can help the deaf hear and the blind see. Biohackers and tech folks talk of uploading the consciousness before death, allowing the mind a second (and presumably very lengthy) existence as a program. So much is possible. Yet the highly modern *Homo sapiens* is struggling with debilitating and chronic health conditions: obesity, depression, diabetes, autoimmune disease, and cancer, among others.

A number of doctors, laypeople, and scientists have come to accept the mismatch hypothesis to explain much of modern chronic disease. Our species, having had only a few hundred generations to adapt to agriculture—and only decades to adjust to the lightbulb and the digital age—is simply not equipped to handle industrial processed food, endless artificial light, and a sedentary modern life. As a psychiatrist, a medical doctor specializing in mental illness, I deal with the emotional and neurological consequences of this mismatch all the time in my clinical practice. We might call the low mood, crying spells, anxiety, and insomnia depressive disorder, but in truth, it is a breakdown of resiliency. Members of our hardy species can take only so much stress before we begin to experience anxiety, depression, and other consequences of our frenetic lives. To go forward into the future, we have to come to terms with our biology and its limitations. We must rebuild our resiliency to recover our health.

The prescription seems simple enough: Eat wholesome, real foods. Get plenty of sleep along with appropriate play and activity. But as a physician and working mother, I know far too well how difficult it can be to handle the pace of modern life, meet the needs of your family, and find the time and patience to keep yourself truly healthy and functioning at your best. In addition, despite the fact that we are all members of the same species, we each have very individual needs based on current health conditions and activity.

Chris Kresser struggled with serious, disabling health problems that modern medicine seemed to have no solution for. He used science, wisdom, and trial and error to heal himself, and due to that experience, he decided to pursue integrative medicine. He chose a master's program in California that combined Western and Chinese medicine, because he felt the holistic model it offered gave him a better way to understand and help the ill than the fragmented, specialty model of conventional medicine. His clinical experience, curiosity, and scientific savvy helped him to become enormously successful. His private practice has thrived, and his website and podcasts reach hundreds of thousands of eager readers and listeners around the world.

With *The Paleo Cure*, Chris sets out the basic prescription for health and resiliency and then offers techniques so you can tailor the program for *your* needs and make it work on a personal level. He calls this your Personal Paleo Cure. His three-step program steers you to diet and lifestyle changes that will have you feeling better than you have in years—perhaps better than you've ever felt. Chris gives you everything you need—not just recipes but a recipe for living—to achieve that improvement in health and functioning, but then he takes that a step further and addresses the complexities of your personal situation. Everything is spelled out in this book, and in addition, his website offers bonus chapters, more details on the science behind the Paleo movement, and copious online tools to ease your transition to good health.

By uncovering your own Personal Paleo Cure, you can benefit from Chris's experience, clinical acumen, wisdom, and common sense to find that state of lasting health that can be so elusive in the modern world. Recover your natural human resiliency and thrive.

Emily Deans, MD
Board-Certified Psychiatrist
Clinical Instructor of Psychiatry, Harvard Medical School

JOIN THE PERSONAL PALEO CURE COMMUNITY

My website is an important extension of this book, an additional resource to enrich your quest for optimal health. Throughout the book I'll refer you to the website for further information on a particular topic, program-enhancing tools, helpful resources, ongoing education, and, perhaps most important, support. Making significant dietary and lifestyle changes can be challenging, and I've found over the years that community is essential to success.

Visit ChrisKresser.com/PPC to find:

- Bonus chapters with more than a hundred and fifty pages of additional information about customizing your diet and lifestyle to address common health conditions. I'll refer to these bonus chapters throughout the book.
- A user forum with people from around the world following the Personal Paleo Cure approach, moderated by my approved Paleo Ambassadors
- An additional three weeks of delicious meal plans and recipes, including snacks and side dishes
- Handy shopping lists
- A supplement guide with specific recommendations mentioned throughout the book, updated regularly so you can order the ones that meet my strictest guidelines for safety and efficacy
- Links to online sources of pasture-raised meats, wild-caught fish, Paleo-friendly snacks, and other essentials
- A guide to finding and working with a Paleo-oriented clinician
- And much more…

You'll also find links to over seven hundred original studies I cite in the book, as well as detailed chapter notes and references.

So head over to **ChrisKresser.com/PPC** now to connect with others who are creating their own Personal Paleo Cures and taking charge of their own health and well-being. I hope you'll love becoming part of this supportive community.

THE
PALEO
CURE

This Book Can Save Your Life

You may have picked up this book for several reasons.

You may want to lose weight, boost your energy, or improve your overall health. You may be looking for ways to naturally treat a particular health problem, such as irritable bowel syndrome, hypothyroidism, or high blood pressure. You may feel well already but want to optimize your athletic performance, feel sharper at work, or increase your longevity.

What if you could create your own personalized approach to nutrition, one that is designed exactly for your body? An approach that respects the wisdom of your genetic template but also acknowledges your own unique circumstances and needs? This is exactly what I'm going to teach you how to do in this book. I call it your Personal Paleo Cure — your unique prescription for optimal health.

WHAT'S A PERSONAL PALEO CURE?

Perhaps you've heard of the Paleo movement. Millions of people around the planet are joining this health revolution based on the latest cutting-edge science, seeking to eat and live in closer harmony with human genetics and biology. This development has come just in time. Throughout the industrialized world, humans are in a health crisis, getting sicker and fatter every year, dying from chronic diseases our ancestors never faced. We thrive when we eat and live a certain way, and our profound sickness stems directly from contemporary choices far different from that ideal way of living. We were never meant to eat the sugar, refined flour, and industrial seed oils that are the mainstay of the standard American diet (and what an apt acronym that makes!). We were never meant to work around the clock under the glare of artificial lights. Or spend half our lives sitting and staring at computer screens. Or live in relative isolation, with Facebook and Twitter standing in for genuine human contact.

Both the fossil record and studies of contemporary hunter-gatherer cultures suggest that our Paleolithic forebears enjoyed excellent health: they were lean, fit, and apparently free of chronic disease. The benefits of copying their lifestyle are undeniable. Those who walk the Paleo road report near-effortless weight loss, newfound vitality, and, often, miraculous resolution of the most dire health issues. However, even the most dedicated Paleo purists hit a wall. Weight loss stalls. Symptoms persist. Energy flags. People tire of restricted eating.

As a licensed clinician who practices functional medicine (different than conventional medicine; see page 342), I specialize in helping seriously ill patients figure out natural solutions to their health challenges. Through in-depth research, personal experience, and clinical investigation, I developed a three-step process to help them. The first step is the Thirty-Day Reset Diet, which follows the typical Paleo approach very closely. The results from Step 1 are amazing. "I'm medication-free after just thirty days," one patient told me. "I feel like a new man!" Another said, "I've never felt or looked better in my life." "Energy levels more even, tennis elbow inflammation disappeared, asthma improved, waistline shrunk," reported another. The testimonials speak for themselves. Paleo works.

However, as I tracked the experiences of people, including some of my patients, who adhered to the typical Paleo approach, I began to notice certain drawbacks. Sometimes the benefits don't go far enough — or they're not sustainable.

I don't stop after Step 1 with my patients for exactly this reason. I've discovered that Paleo functions best as a general template, not a rigid prescription. Think of it as a starting point, not a destination. Even though we all share much of the same DNA, we each have unique circumstances and needs. We need a program that addresses our specific health issues. A more flexible, dynamic approach that recognizes the joys of eating yet goes far beyond food and takes into account how each of us likes to move, live, love. My goal is to help people, individual by individual, discover what works for them and keep them from adhering to a dogmatic regimen just because it sounds authentic.

We don't live in the Paleolithic era anymore. We're not cavemen, so why should we follow a strict caveman diet? Why should we cut out foods we love and might thrive on simply because our ancestors didn't eat them? We've evolved, and we need a plan that's evolved to meet our individual needs and preferences. (Some of my patients are even vegetarians — anathema to hard-core meat-eating Paleo purists.) Why not combine the best of ancient wisdom and the best of modern nutrition?

That's why I created the three-step Personal Paleo Cure: an approach custom-made for your individual genetic blueprint, one that enables you to enjoy lifelong health and vitality.

ONE SIZE DOESN'T FIT ALL

If you're like most of my patients, you've tried a lot of diets over the years. Some did nothing at all, some made you worse, and some worked — for a little while. Or maybe they solved some problems (like being overweight), but caused others (you were exhausted all the time, your hair fell out, and your hands and feet felt like ice cubes).

Perhaps you've already tried a Paleo-style diet, eating the same kinds of natural foods our ancestors enjoyed. At first, you were ecstatic. You lost weight and felt so much better. But after a while, you noticed some of your old problems creeping back in. Or maybe you hit a plateau and just couldn't lose those last ten pounds no matter what you did. Or maybe you just got tired of special diets in general and wanted to find a better approach to nutrition that would be more sustainable over the long term.

So you set out to find some help. You search some of the popular health websites, post a few messages in discussion forums, and e-mail your friends who are trying the same thing.

Everyone is happy to help—you get a ton of advice. The problem is, it's all different!

A new study just proclaimed the Mediterranean diet as the best. "Very low-carb is the way to go," you hear on that morning talk show; didn't another expert on that same show say the exact same thing about vegan diets last week? "No, you've got to eliminate nightshades and eggs," a friend says. "Dr. Google" says that if you've got a thyroid problem, you need to eat a lot more starchy vegetables and fruit. One website says yogurt helps with digestion; another says you should avoid dairy entirely.

It's enough to make you crazy.

You want to feel better, lose weight, and fix your health problems—but how do you know you're making the right choices? And how do you ensure that the next diet you try doesn't end up being yet another failed experiment?

Here's the truth: There is no single formula to follow that will guarantee you perfect health in three weeks—or seven days, or any other arbitrary number you find on the bestseller list. As seductive as that sounds, it just doesn't work that way. The only formula I want to give you is the formula for figuring out how not to follow a formula! If my clinical experience treating patients has taught me one thing, it's this: there's no one-size-fits-all approach when it comes to diet and lifestyle. After all, the fossil record indicates that not all Paleolithic people ate the same way. So why should we expect a single program to be the perfect fit for everybody?

Personalization is the missing ingredient. I've found that even two people who come to my office with the exact same health condition might need different solutions. For example, I recently saw two patients with ulcerative colitis. Eating even a small amount of dairy sent one running to the bathroom in three seconds flat. For the other, fermented dairy (e.g., yogurt or kefir) was a crucial component of the healing process. This is why so many typical diets—even very good ones, like the Paleo diet—often fail in the long run, and it's why I teach all my clients how to discover their own unique Personal Paleo Cure. Because no two patients are alike, no two walk out of my office with the same plan.

For example, when Tina, age fifty-four, visited my office, she was almost forty-five pounds overweight and had high blood pressure and early-stage type 2 diabetes. She was fed up with feeling so sluggish and hated the way her clothes fit. "I tried every low-fat diet out there, but nothing works," she told me. I put her on a lower-carbohydrate version of my Step 1 Reset Diet, with a few additional tweaks because of her blood-sugar problems. She began to lose weight immediately while enjoying foods her doctors had forbidden, like red meat and butter. "I can't get over it," she said. "I'm never hungry, and I don't feel deprived!" After three months, Tina had lost thirty-five pounds; her skin glowed, her digestive system ran smoothly, and there was no sign of diabetes. "I've never felt better," she told me, "and my doctor is amazed by my test results."

When Mark, age thirty-three, came to see me, he was virtually crippled by Crohn's disease, spending much of his day in the bathroom. He was on a cocktail of medications, including steroids and mesalamine. "I'm scared," he told me. "My gastroenterologist wants to remove part of my colon." Mark was desperate to avoid surgery. I decided that his Personal Paleo Cure would include an intensive gut-healing diet, along with some stress-reducing measures. Mark felt dramatically better in just a week. Within a month, he felt like a new person. Six months later, Mark was in complete clinical remission, no surgery necessary!

At thirty-eight, Sam couldn't control his blood pressure. His doctor wanted him to go on medication to lower it. During my intake examination, I asked Sam about his diet. "It's funny," he told me, "but I went on one of those very low-carb diets to lose weight, and my blood pressure shot up." I suspected that Sam might be potassium deficient, which can worsen high blood pressure. His Personal Paleo Cure included potassium-rich foods like potatoes, plantains, and cold-water fish, along with two cups a day of hibiscus tea, which has been shown to decrease blood pressure. Three months later, Sam's blood pressure was normal—without medication.

In all these cases, and hundreds of others like them, I worked closely with these people to determine each one's unique formula for vibrant good health. Now I'm going to teach you how to do it for yourself. First, though, I'd like to give you some background on why I'm such an ardent believer in this lifestyle. My personal experience is what motivates me to share my knowledge with others, because finding my own Personal Paleo Cure changed—even saved—my life.

My Story: Cracking the Code for Health

My own journey into the Personal Paleo Cure lifestyle began with a devastating illness—one that dogged me for more than a decade.

In 1998, not long after I graduated from college, I quit my job, sold off my possessions, and took off to see the world. Thailand was the first stop on my trip. I studied traditional Thai massage, Kriya yoga, and Vipassana meditation, deepening the practice I'd begun as an eighteen-year-old.

The next stop on my trip was Indonesia. I'm a lifelong surfer, so I was drawn to this mecca for its perfect waves and warm water. Then one day I woke up delirious, with a high temperature, chills, vomiting, and severe diarrhea. (I later found out that I, along with several other surfers, had been sickened when some locals dug a trench that allowed stagnant water polluted with cow feces to drain into the surf break.) An Australian friend gradually nursed me back to health with some antibiotics in his medical kit.

After recuperating, I tried to continue my world tour, but my recurring illness forced me to head back to the States. The first doctor I saw, suspecting parasites, gave me powerful antibiotics that initially worked, but eventually I felt worse again: exhausted, listless, with nearly continuous digestive distress. Unfortunately, my illness lingered, and over the next few years I saw at least fifteen doctors; nobody could tell me what was wrong, and nothing they told me to do worked.

I decided to attend graduate school to study traditional Chinese medicine. Perhaps herbal medicine and dietary changes might help where conventional doctors and antibiotics had failed. I tried vegetarian and macrobiotic vegan diets and I consulted with several different professors at my school who had expertise in treating digestive problems. Nothing helped. After two years, determined to find a cure, I dropped out of school and moved to the Esalen Institute, a residential community and retreat center in Big Sur, California, that offers holistic educational and personal development programs. I'd begun to wonder whether there might be an emotional, a psychological, or even a spiritual element to my illness.

My time at Esalen was transformative, mind- and heart-opening, and healing at the deepest levels. My experiences there helped me to accept my illness and find peace in the midst of the intense struggles I was going through. But unfortunately, they didn't heal my body. I was still suffering from severe digestive distress and fatigue and developing new symptoms like muscle and joint pain, difficulty concentrating and memory issues, and insomnia.

The next few years were the most challenging of my life. With my savings exhausted, I moved back to Los Angeles and found myself working long hours in a stressful position at a start-up company. Within two years, I had a complete breakdown; I was utterly exhausted and demoralized after years of illness, pain, and unsuccessful searches for answers. I had seen world-renowned doctors, specialists in every field of alternative medicine, shamans, energy workers, psychotherapists, and spiritual teachers. I'd taken multiple courses of antibiotics, steroids, and anti-inflammatories. I'd tried every special diet under the sun; my "supplement graveyard" had more than a hundred bottles of herbs, potions, and pills I'd taken over the years. I was beginning to lose hope.

Then one day I walked into a bookstore and saw a book called *Nourishing Traditions* on display. It advocated a real-food, nutrient-dense approach to illness based on traditional diets. Something about this resonated deeply with me. Hey, I'd tried every other diet; why not give this one a shot? I started eating the foods the book recommended: bone-broth soups, sauerkraut, fermented dairy products, slow-cooked meats, eggs, and cold-water, fatty fish. I felt better almost immediately. However, even though I used the extensive preparation methods suggested in the book (including soaking and fermentation), the whole grains and legumes recommended irritated my gut—so I eliminated them, along with industrial seed oils (corn, soybean, cotton, sunflower, and safflower), sugar, and all processed and refined foods. I didn't know it at the time, but I was on a Paleo diet.

I couldn't get over the dramatic change in my energy level and gut health. I felt like a different person: vibrant, excited about my future, and ready for a fresh start. I continued my meditation practice and added techniques for stress management to reduce the physical and psychological symptoms associated with chronic pain and illness, and eventually I formulated a supplement regime that further improved my health. I didn't have the name for it yet, but I'd discovered my own Personal Paleo Cure, the individual prescription for my optimal health.

I felt a strong calling to use all of the knowledge and experience I had acquired in my own healing journey to help others with theirs, so I applied to the Acupuncture and Integrative Medicine College in Berkeley, California, to finish the degree in traditional Chinese medicine that I had started years before.

While there, I started a blog called *The Healthy Skeptic* (now it's at ChrisKresser.com), mainly as a journal to keep track of my research and study. My grandfather had died following complications after bypass surgery; I suspected he hadn't gotten the best treatment. The more I delved into the research about diet and cardiovascular disease, the more fascinated I became—why were Bapa's doctors following a medical model that was half a century old? What other research was being overlooked?

I became deeply interested in the scientific evidence for various medical approaches to illness and began to blog about my findings. I was quite surprised the first time someone left a comment on one of my posts. I hadn't told anyone about the blog, and to this day, I still don't know how people found it. Within a relatively short time, though, I had thousands of readers from all over the world. By the time I graduated and became licensed, I was fortunate to have a full and thriving private practice. Shortly thereafter, I was introduced to some members of the vibrant Paleo community. Now I had a name for the lifestyle I'd stumbled upon independently. I realized that I had found my tribe—a group of revolutionary individuals committed to helping people obtain optimal health.

Today, I'm blessed with excellent health, a loving family, and a flourishing practice. It's incredibly rewarding to help patients discover their own Personal Paleo Cure and recapture their health and vitality.

Beyond Diet: 360-Degree Wellness

The Personal Paleo Cure is a way of life, a process for helping you discover your own ideal way of eating and living. The food we eat is perhaps the single most important influence on health. But the ways we sleep, exercise, spend time outdoors, have fun, manage our stress, and connect with others really matter; I'd argue that they separate a life merely lived from a life worth living. Just as I'll help you customize the diet that works optimally for you, I'll help you find the unique Personal Paleo Cure that embraces every other part of your life so you can live healthfully and joyfully. Diet and lifestyle, taken together, form 360-degree wellness.

Everyone's path to health is unique. I can tell you from working with hundreds of patients in my practice and guiding thousands of others through my blog that it will take about thirty days of following the Reset Diet for you to experience dramatic relief from aggravating symptoms, lose your cravings for the foods that aren't good for you, see a pleasing weight loss, and probably feel better than you ever have! After that, you'll be powerfully motivated to follow the rest of my three-step plan to arrive at a recipe for living that works best for you. For some readers, it'll be a few more weeks. For others, I refuse to make an empty promise about what that timetable should be; that's for you to discover, with my guidance. That's what makes this program work — you!

You'll find some significant differences between the cure you develop and traditional Paleo/primal diets, because my plan will be customized to your needs. What's forbidden on those other diets may be a welcome addition to your table. Based on time-tested ancestral wisdom combined with the best of modern science, your Personal Paleo Cure is firmly grounded in your personal experience, which means you'll find it easy to follow, its benefits will be sustainable, and you'll thoroughly enjoy it.

WARNING: CONVENTIONAL WISDOM MAY BE HAZARDOUS TO YOUR HEALTH

I'm going to challenge a lot of conventional wisdom in this book—not because I'm a contrarian or want to generate attention, but because I've spent years poring over original research and major studies. I don't believe a health claim simply because I've seen it repeated multiple times. I look at the evidence—the size of the original study samples, the length of the studies, the quality of the research design, and other factors. I look for the difference between causation and correlation. If conventional wisdom holds that taking a certain medication will help people live longer or prevent a certain illness, I want to see the research that proves that. So that's what I do; I carefully investigate the evidence behind health claims.

And what I've found, based solely on the scientific evidence, is often very different from popular health claims. For example, I've found that saturated fat is not the evil nutrient we've been led to believe it is and that whole grains aren't nearly as healthy as we've been told they are. These ideas—and many similar ones—are so deeply ingrained in our collective psyche that few of us stop to question them. But the fact that a belief is widely accepted doesn't make it true.

When research, even gold-standard research, produces new information, there's often a significant amount of time before that information is accepted by the wider medical community, and sometimes even longer before the information is communicated to the public. I'm no conspiracy theorist; I dislike those screaming headlines that shout "Doctors Are Withholding Secrets That Could Save Your Life!" The way I see it, part of the problem is that once something is widely reported and becomes accepted as medical dogma, few people invest the work needed to study alternative theories, and those few researchers who do get minimal attention and funding.

Perhaps one of the best examples of dogma in medicine is the idea that eating foods that contain cholesterol raises cholesterol levels in the blood. Early studies suggested this was true, but more recent and better-designed trials have shown that dietary cholesterol doesn't increase blood cholesterol in the majority of people. Today, few researchers working in the field believe that eating eggs has a significant effect on cholesterol levels in the blood. Yet the public and much of the conventional medical establishment still think there's a connection. And millions of Americans continue to avoid nutrient-rich foods like eggs and red meat on the basis of this outdated science.

Admitting we don't have all the answers is the key to progress in science and medicine. I would invite you to keep an open mind as you read this book, especially when you encounter sections that challenge your beliefs. If you have scientific training or you're just the curious type, you can also scour the detailed chapter notes and references for this book (listed on the website) and read the original studies I cite.

Science is constantly evolving. We look back on the beliefs people held one hundred years ago and think them ignorant. What do you imagine people living one hundred years from now will think about our ideas?

Three Steps: Reset, Rebuild, and Revive

There are three steps to discovering your own Personal Paleo Cure: Reset, Rebuild, and Revive.

In **Step 1: Reset,** you'll begin the Thirty-Day Reset Diet. This quickstart eating plan presses the reset button on your diet, targeting and eliminating the modern foods that humans aren't genetically designed to eat—the foods that are the leading culprits in weight gain and health problems. I formulated this program so you'd feel better right away, and I think you'll be pleasantly surprised to discover how many of the foods you thought were off-limits you can enjoy. You'll experience improved digestion, reduced inflammation, fewer allergic reactions, more energy, and an evening out of your blood sugar and mood. You'll also burn fat and shed pounds. If you're like my patients, you'll feel better than you have in years!

In **Step 2: Rebuild,** you'll begin to customize your Personal Paleo Cure by reintroducing some foods you eliminated during the Thirty-Day Reset to see how they work for your body. A lot of Paleo purists believe humans shouldn't eat anything that wasn't around at the time of our Paleolithic ancestors. Therefore, they'd keep tomatoes, potatoes, peppers, and other nightshade vegetables off your table forever. They'd have you bid a permanent farewell to dairy products and all grains and legumes. But the science doesn't support this stance, so neither do I. Why rule out dairy, for example, if you thrive on it? I'll show you my proven method for testing gray-area foods so you can rebuild the repertoire of foods you love.

In **Step 3: Revive,** you'll take the final steps in creating your unique prescription for optimal health, tweaking your Personal Paleo Cure until it's a perfect fit. What's the ideal balance of proteins, carbohydrates, and fats for your unique needs? What makes you feel your best? Three meals a day? Six? Intermittent fasting? We'll figure out all this and more—including how to be flexible when you need to be (see "The 80/20 Rule," below)—so that you can follow your Personal Paleo Cure for life.

I'll help you get started on this exciting new way of eating with seven days of meal plans that include delicious fan-favorite recipes developed by a foodie/chef couple whose creations are big hits on my website and some brand-new culinary delights created by a French chef trained at Paris's renowned École de Cuisine La Varenne. On the website, you'll also find an additional three weeks of meal plans and recipes.

But life is about so much more than what we eat. You'll also learn other techniques to make your life more joyful; I'll show you how to manage your stress, find fun ways to move, sleep more deeply, emphasize pleasure and play, and reconnect with nature.

Do you have a particular health problem? I've got you covered. You'll learn specific diet and lifestyle tweaks to address conditions like weight gain; heart disease; high blood pressure; digestive problems; high or low blood sugar; anxiety and depression; thyroid disorders; difficulty concentrating and memory issues; and acne, psoriasis, and other skin problems. These natural approaches are sometimes all it takes to halt or even reverse symptoms that have plagued you for years.

THE 80/20 RULE

Once you have worked through the Thirty-Day Reset in Step 1 and have fully customized your Personal Paleo Cure, I recommend you follow it closely 80 percent of the time but loosen up the other 20 percent of the time and eat what you like. A truly healthy body is a resilient body, one that doesn't get sick if you have foods outside your Personal Paleo Cure.

In time, most people end up very happily eating more like 90/10 or 95/5 because they've lost the physical and psychological cravings for the Chips Ahoy! cookies or the can of soda. Why? Because after doing Step 1, they feel so much better *without* those foods, and they've filled out their diets with an array of new and delicious foods, as you will. They save their full-out 80/20 times for that Caribbean vacation or Super Bowl weekend.

I want you to nourish yourself at every level, including having the joy of eating foods outside your Personal Paleo Cure. Your mother's cherished Sunday dinners. The incredible buffet at the wedding. The chef's special at that fantastic new restaurant you and your friends are heading to on Saturday. Enjoy yourself! (For more on how to follow the 80/20 rule for life, see pages 324 to 327.)

HOW TO USE THIS BOOK

- **Feel better right away.** If you're new to the Paleo approach and eager to get started because you're feeling lousy or you want to lose weight, **start with Step 1.** Once you're on the Thirty-Day Reset Diet, you'll experience the benefits of the Personal Paleo Cure right away, and that will give you the motivation to continue with Steps 2 and 3. While you're going through your Thirty-Day Reset, read up on topics like nutrient density, minimizing toxins in your diet, and choosing the best possible foods; you'll realize why you feel so good. Continue with Step 2

(Rebuild Your Life) to find out how to improve your sleep, manage your stress, exercise more effectively, and more. Then move on to Step 3 (Revive Your Health) to help you customize your program further for any particular health conditions or goals you might have and for tips on following your Personal Paleo Cure for life.

- **Improve your results.** If you're already following a Paleo-style diet, but you're not getting the results you'd hoped for, you might want to **start with Step 2,** Rebuild, to focus on some of the important lifestyle factors you might have neglected until now. Then move on to Step 3, Revive, to learn how to personalize your diet and lifestyle according to your unique needs so they are even more effective. (I do suggest you take a look at Step 1, Reset, to make sure that the diet you're currently following tracks with my recommendations.)

Doing the Thirty-Day Reset Diet is the essential first step in discovering your Personal Paleo Cure, but in the same way that there's no one-size-fits-all approach to diet, there's no right or wrong way to read this book. Just choose what works best for you depending on your background, needs, and goals.

YOUR PERSONAL PALEO CURE, YOUR WAY

Throughout this book, I'm going to remind you to trust yourself. Of course, you should always partner with your health professional and learn all you can about health options from trusted resources, but no one is more motivated than you to create your optimal health.

I'm not doctrinaire. I don't think that all medications and surgery are evil or even avoidable. I refer my patients to physicians when I think a drug or surgery may be necessary. We live in amazing times, when we can pick and choose from many quarters to find the best options available to us. Stay curious, motivated, and involved. Learn all you can. Let this book be one of many powerful tools at your disposal.

I've helped hundreds of my patients and thousands of blog readers and podcast listeners overcome chronic health problems using the knowledge and experience I gained over my own ten-year healing journey as well as in my formal education as a practitioner of integrative medicine. But there's more work to be done. There are so many others out there still suffering from chronic illness or weight problems who haven't been able to find help anywhere else. Maybe you're one of them. If so, this book is for you. It will teach you how to heal yourself so your health won't stand in the way of your fulfilling your dreams. The methods I share in this book have changed my life and the lives of thousands of others. It is my deepest wish that they will also change yours.

So let's get started. In the next chapter, I'm going to give you a brief history lesson. (Don't worry; there's no pop quiz!) I'll lay out the scientific argument that explains why you can live longer into the future by eating the way our ancestors did tens of thousands of years in the past.

CHAPTER 1

Why Paleo? From Cave to Chronic Illness

Consider the following:

- Diabetes and obesity combined affect more than a billion people worldwide, including one hundred million Americans.
- More than half of Americans are overweight; a full third are clinically obese.
- Heart disease causes four out of every ten deaths in the United States.
- One-third of Americans have high blood pressure, which contributes to almost eight hundred thousand strokes every year—the leading cause of serious, long-term disability. Annually, there are 12.7 million strokes worldwide.
- More than thirty-six million people are now living with dementia.
- Depression is now the leading cause of disability, affecting more than 120 million people worldwide.

I could go on, but I think you get the point. We're getting fatter and sicker every year.

Notes for this chapter may be found at ChrisKresser.com/ppcnotes/#ch1.

Now imagine, for a moment, a world where:

- Modern, chronic diseases, like diabetes, obesity, some cancers, autoimmune disorders, and heart disease, are rare or nonexistent.
- The world population is naturally lean and fit.
- We all age gracefully with strong bones, sharp vision, and normal blood pressure.

While this might sound like pure fantasy today, anthropological evidence suggests that this is exactly how human beings lived for the vast majority of our species' evolutionary history.

Today, most people accept disorders like obesity, diabetes, and heart disease as normal. But while these problems may be common now, they're anything but normal. Our species evolved roughly two million years ago, and for more than sixty-six thousand generations, humans were free of the modern diseases that today kill millions of people each year and make countless others miserable. In fact, the world I asked you to imagine above was the natural state for humans' history on this planet up until the agricultural revolution occurred, about eleven thousand years (366 generations) ago—less than 0.5 percent of the time recognizably human beings have been here. It's a tiny blip on the evolutionary time scale.

What happened? What transformed healthy and vital people free of chronic diseases into sick, fat, and unhappy people?

In a word? *Mismatch.*

AGRICULTURE: THE WORST MISTAKE IN HUMAN HISTORY?

Like it or not, we humans are animals. And like all animals, we have a species-appropriate diet and way of life.

When animals eat and live in accordance with the environment to which they've adapted, they thrive. Cats, with their sharp teeth and short intestinal tracts, evolved to be carnivores, so when we feed them grain-rich kibble, they develop kidney trouble and other woes. Cows naturally graze on grass; when they eat too much grain, harmful bacteria proliferate and make them sick. We humans face a similar mismatch. Our biology and genes evolved in a particular environment. Then that environment changed far faster than humans could adapt, with a few important exceptions that I'll cover later in this chapter. The result? The modern epidemic of chronic disease.

For the vast majority of existence, humans lived as Paleolithic hunter-gatherers, eating the meat they hunted, the fish they caught, and the vegetables, fruits, and tubers they picked while on the move. The agricultural revolution dramatically altered humans' food supply and way of life. They learned to stay put, planting crops and domesticating cows, sheep, goats, and pigs. Early farmers consumed foods that their hunter-gatherer predecessors didn't eat, such as cereal grains, milk and meat from domesticated animals, and legumes and other cultivated plants.

While scientists have argued that these developments allowed our species to flourish socially and intellectually, the consequences of this shift from a Paleolithic to an agricultural diet and lifestyle were disastrous for human health. In evolutionary terms, eleven thousand years is the blink of an eye, not nearly long enough for humans to completely adapt to this new way of eating. This is why the influential scientist and author Jared Diamond called agriculture "the worst mistake in human history." He argued that hunter-gatherers "practiced the most successful and longest-lasting lifestyle in human history" and were all but guaranteed a healthy diet because of the diversity and nutrient density of the foods they consumed. Once humans switched diets and became more sedentary, our species' naturally robust health began to decline.

How do we know that agriculture has been so harmful to humanity? There are three main points of evidence:

- A decline in health among hunter-gatherer populations that adopted agriculture
- The robust health of contemporary hunter-gatherers
- The poor health of people who rely heavily on grains as a staple

Let's look at each of these in more detail.

What happened when hunter-gatherers became farmers?

Studying bones gives scientists a window into the health of our distant ancestors and offers insight into what an optimal human diet might be. Some archaeologists and anthropologists today may have a better understanding of human nutrition than the average health-care practitioner!

So what have these scientists learned from examining the bones of humans who shifted from a Paleolithic hunter-gatherer lifestyle to an agricultural one? The fossil record shows a rapid and clear decline in health in places where agriculture was adopted. Tooth decay and anemia due to iron deficiency became widespread, average bone density decreased, and infant mortality increased. These changes resulted in large part from the nutritional stress of eating a diet inappropriate for our species.

We also shrank. Skeletal remains from Greece and Turkey indicate that the average height of hunter-gatherers at the end of the ice age was five nine for men and five five for women. After agriculture was adopted in these areas, the average height fell to a low of five three for men and five feet for women. Archaeologists have found similar shrinkage in skeletons all over the world when populations shifted to agriculture.

Early farmers lost more than inches from their skeletons; they lost years from their lives. Anthropologist George Armelagos studied the American Indians living in the Ohio River Valley in approximately AD 1150. His team compared the skeletons of hunter-gatherers that lived in the same area with those of the early farmers who followed them. The farmers had 50 percent more tooth-enamel defects (suggestive of malnutrition), four times as much iron-deficiency anemia, three times more bone lesions, and an overall increase in degenerative conditions of the spine. Their life expectancy at birth also dropped, from twenty-six years to nineteen years.

In their book *The 10,000 Year Explosion*, anthropologists Gregory Cochran and Henry Harpending argued that these dramatic declines in health were brought on by a major shift in the human diet. When hunter-gatherers switched to farmers' diets, their average carbohydrate intake shot up while the amount of protein plummeted. The quality of that protein also decreased, since almost any type of meat has a desirable amino acid balance, whereas most plants do not. Vitamin shortages were common because the new diet was based on a limited set of crops and was lower in more nutrient-dense animal products. Evidence suggests that these early farmers, who depended on one or two starchy crops, like wheat or corn, may have developed vitamin-deficiency diseases such as beriberi, pellagra, rickets, and scurvy. Their hunter-gatherer ancestors, who ate a wide variety of foods rich in vitamins and minerals, rarely suffered from these diseases.

Because of "plentiful protein, vitamin D, and sunlight in early childhood," our Paleo ancestors were "extremely tall," had very good teeth, and larger skulls and pelvises, according to one group of archaeologists. Their farming descendants, by contrast, suffered skull deformities because of iron-deficiency anemia, had more tooth decay, were more prone to infectious diseases, and were much shorter, "apparently because subsistence by this time is characterized by a heavy emphasis on a few starchy food crops." Farming may have offered our ancestors a more stable and predictable food supply, but this stability came at a great price.

DIDN'T OUR PALEO ANCESTORS DIE YOUNG?

A common question I hear from Paleo skeptics is something along the lines of "Didn't Stone Age people die before their thirtieth birthday?"

It's true that, on average, our Paleo ancestors died younger than we do. However, these averages don't factor in challenges largely absent from modern American lives: high infant mortality, violence and accidents, infectious diseases, and lack of medical care. Hunter-gatherer populations had infant-mortality rates about thirty times higher than those in the United States today; early-childhood-mortality rates were more than one hundred times higher. These

(continued)

higher infant- and childhood-mortality rates were caused by accidents, trauma, exposure to the elements, violence, warfare, and untreated acute infectious diseases—issues that, fortunately, few of us in the developed world face. These untimely deaths had the net effect of dragging down average life expectancy. If, out of ten Paleo people, three died in infancy, two died during childhood from exposure to the elements, and two died as teenagers in warfare, then even if the remaining three lived long, healthy lives, the average life span in this hypothetical group would still be short.

Recent research that has taken the high infant-mortality rates of our Paleolithic ancestors into account suggests that if our Stone Age forebears survived childhood, they had life spans roughly equivalent to those of people living in industrialized societies today, with a range from sixty-eight to seventy-eight years. Even more important, they reached these ages without any signs of the chronic inflammatory and degenerative diseases that we consider to be normal in developed countries, including obesity, type 2 diabetes, gout, hypertension, cardiovascular disease, and some cancers. Sure, those of us living in modern industrialized societies might live a little longer than hunter-gatherers, on average. But most of our elderly people now suffer from painful and debilitating diseases, take several medications a day, and have an unsatisfactory quality of life.

Fortunately, we don't have to choose between eating like our ancestors and reaping the benefits of modern medicine. We can combine them to get the best of both worlds and enjoy long life spans without the degenerative diseases that are so common in the industrialized world.

Contemporary hunter-gatherers: A study in good health

Modern studies of contemporary hunter-gatherers—people who have had minimal exposure to industrial civilization and follow a traditional diet and lifestyle—suggest they are largely free of the chronic inflammatory diseases that have become epidemic in the industrialized world.

Anthropological and medical reports of these contemporary hunter-gatherers show they have far fewer modern illnesses, such as metabolic syndrome, cardiovascular disease, obesity, some cancers, and autoimmune disorders, than Westernized populations. In their study "The Western Diet and Lifestyle and Diseases of Civilization," nutrition researcher Pedro Carrera-Bastos and his colleagues compared the health of traditional populations with the health of people living in industrialized societies. The contemporary hunter-gatherers were superior in every measure of health and physical fitness. They had:

- Lower blood pressure
- Excellent insulin sensitivity and lower fasting insulin levels (meaning they were less likely to develop type 2 diabetes)
- Lower fasting leptin levels (leptin is a hormone that regulates body fat)
- Lower body mass indexes and waist-to-height ratios (one way of measuring optimal weight)
- Greater maximum oxygen consumption (a measure of physical fitness)
- Better vision
- Stronger bones

Let's look at some examples of contemporary hunter-gatherer populations around the world that, at least until a short time ago, followed the traditional diet and lifestyle.

The Kitavans

Kitava is a small island in the Trobriand Islands archipelago in Papua New Guinea. Though not technically hunter-gatherers (they are horticulturalists), the Kitavans were, until recently, one of the last populations on earth still following a traditional diet similar in composition to Paleolithic diets. According to Dr. Staffan Lindeberg in his 1989 book *Food and Western Disease*, residents of Kitava subsisted "exclusively on root vegetables (yam, sweet potato, taro, tapioca), fruits (banana, papaya, pineapple, mango, guava, watermelon, pumpkin), vegetables, fish and coconuts."

The Kitavans enjoyed excellent health. Dr. Lindeberg's study of 2,300 Kitavans found that:

- None had ever experienced heart disease or a stroke (which was particularly remarkable because most Kitavans smoked, and smoking is one of the biggest risk factors for heart disease).
- They were very lean, with an average body mass index (BMI) of 20 in men and 18 in women. (By contrast, in 2010, the average BMI of Americans—both men and women—was 27, which is considered overweight and is only three points away from the obese category.)
- Compared to Westernized populations, Kitavans had very low levels of leptin and insulin, the hormones that regulate food intake and energy balance. Low levels of each are associated with leanness and overall metabolic health.

Most significant, Kitavans rarely suffered the diseases of aging that are so common in developed countries. Lindeberg noted, "The elderly residents of Kitava generally remain quite active up until the very end, when they begin to suffer fatigue for a few days and then die from what appears to be an infection or some type of rapid degeneration. Although this is seen in Western societies, it is relatively rare in elderly vital people. The quality of life among the oldest residents thus appeared to be good in the Trobriand Islands."

A long, healthy life followed by an easy, quick death. Don't we all want that?

The Inuit

The Inuit are a group of hunter-gatherers who live in the Arctic regions of Alaska, Canada, and Greenland. They eat primarily fish, seals, whale, caribou, walrus, birds, and eggs: a diet very high in fat and protein, with very few vegetables or fruits. They live in a harsh environment that is marginal at best for human habitation. Yet early explorers, physicians, and scientists unanimously reported that the Inuit they encountered enjoyed excellent health and vitality.

Dr. John Simpson studied the Inuit in the mid-1850s. He noted that the Inuit were "robust, muscular and active, inclining rather to spareness, rather than corpulence, presenting a markedly healthy appearance. The expression of the countenance is one of habitual good humor. The physical constitution of both sexes is strong." This is especially remarkable considering the inhospitable environment the Inuit lived in, and it's a testament to the nutrient density of the animal foods that made up the majority of their diet.

Nearly a hundred years later, an American dentist named Weston A. Price noticed an alarming increase in tooth decay and other problems in his patients, and he set out to determine whether traditional peoples who had not adopted a Western diet suffered from the same problems. In 1933, he took a trip to the Arctic to visit the Inuit, one of many cultures he studied, and he was deeply impressed by what he found. He praised the Inuit's "magnificent dental development" and "freedom from dental caries" (that is, they had no cavities).

It's especially impressive that the Inuit enjoyed such robust good health when you consider that their diets were 80 to 85 percent fat, a percentage that would surely horrify the American Medical Association!

Aboriginal Australians

Aboriginal Australians, or Indigenous Australians, were the original inhabitants of the Australian continent and surrounding islands. They traditionally lived as hunter-gatherers, consuming mostly animal products — including land mammals, birds, reptiles, sea creatures, and insects — along with a variety of plants. The quality of their diet depended in large part on where they lived: the subtropical, coastal areas were lush and provided abundant food; the harsh desert interior offered less in terms of both diversity and amounts of food.

Nevertheless, numerous studies suggest that even those Aboriginal Australians living in marginal environments were free of modern diseases like obesity, diabetes, and heart disease. Weston Price described them as "a living museum preserved from the dawn of animal life on the earth."

Even today, contemporary Aboriginal Australians who maintain a traditional lifestyle are lean and fit and show no evidence of obesity, insulin resistance, type 2 diabetes, or cardiovascular disease. A study published in 1991 found that this population had optimal blood pressure, fasting-glucose levels (high levels indicate diabetes), and cholesterol levels, with an average body mass index well below that of Australians living in urban environments.

Aboriginal Australians who make the transition from their traditional hunter-gatherer lifestyle to a Westernized lifestyle develop unusually high rates of diabetes, cardiovascular disease, and obesity, according to the same study, and Westernized Aboriginal Australians experience a dramatic improvement in metabolic and cardiovascular health when they return to their traditional ways.

These three groups of hunter-gatherers have enjoyed good health with their traditional lifestyles into the twenty-first century, although each eats a very different diet. This may indicate that what we don't eat might be just as important as what we do.

Are people who eat more grains less healthy?

Another way to evaluate whether traditional Paleolithic diets are healthier than modern diets is to look at cultures and groups that consume large amounts of grains. Are they more likely to have health problems? There's a great deal of research that says yes. Whole grains, legumes, nuts, and seeds contain compounds called phytates that bind to minerals such as calcium, iron, zinc, and manganese, making them more difficult to absorb. If a food contains nutrients that you can't absorb, you're not going to reap their benefits.

Studies show that children on vegetarian macrobiotic diets— "healthy" diets composed of whole grains (especially brown rice), legumes, vegetables, and some fruits—are deficient in vitamins and minerals and are more likely to develop rickets than their meat-eating peers. Breast-fed babies of macrobiotic mothers may be getting lower levels of vitamin B_{12}, calcium, and magnesium, according to some research, which may result in these babies having delayed physical and cognitive growth.

Cultures that are heavily dependent on grains often show signs of severe vitamin A and protein deficiencies, which make them more susceptible to infectious diseases. Dr. Edward Mellanby, the discoverer of vitamin D, compared the agricultural Kikuyu tribe with the pastoralist (livestock-raising) Masai tribe, who consume primarily the milk, blood, and flesh of the cows they raise. Dr. Mellanby discovered that the Kikuyu, who lived mainly on cereals, had a far higher incidence of bronchitis, pneumonia, tropical ulcers, and tuberculosis.

We've been raised to believe that healthy whole grains are nutritional marvels, but cereal grains like corn, wheat, and rice don't deserve the label *healthy*. They're inferior to animal products as a source of protein because they're incomplete, meaning that they are missing one or more essential amino acids. (Essential amino acids are those that we can't synthesize and therefore have to get from our diets.) They're also lower in vitamins and minerals compared to meat and the variety of wild fruits and vegetables consumed by our ancestors.

The evidence suggests that when we eat grains at the expense of more nutritious foods—especially when those grains are not properly prepared to reduce phytates and toxins—our health suffers.

HOW MEAT MADE US HUMAN

Eating meat and cooking food is quite literally what made us human. The transition from a raw, exclusively plant-based diet to one that included meat and cooked food (as well as starchy tubers) is what enabled the brains of our pre-human ancestors to grow so rapidly.

Humans have exceptionally large, neuron-rich brains relative to body size compared to nonhuman primates. For example, gorillas have bodies that are three times larger than ours, but they have smaller brains with only about a third the number of neurons that we have. So why is it that the largest primates don't also have the largest brains?

(continued)

The answer is that the brain competes with other organs for resources in the body. Gorillas require a large, metabolically expensive digestive tract to process the high-fiber, low-calorie plant matter they consume. This doesn't leave enough resources for larger, higher-performance brains (like ours). The human brain is an expensive metabolic tissue: it consumes 20 percent of total body energy even though it represents only 2 percent of body mass.

The larger you are, the more you need to eat. The more you need to eat, the more time you have to spend feeding yourself. Gorillas, who are vegetarians, already spend as much as 9.6 hours of a twelve-hour day eating, in part because the fibrous plant matter they consume takes so long for their bodies to break down and absorb. In order to provide enough energy for a human-like brain, a gorilla would have to eat for an extra two hours a day! Likewise, early humans eating only raw vegetation would have needed to eat for more than nine hours a day to get enough calories to support their large brains.

Gathering food was both dangerous and time-consuming, so it is unlikely that our ancestors had a completely vegetarian raw diet. When they cooked their meat, it became easier for them to chew and therefore to digest and absorb, which increased both the calories available and the nutritional density of their diet.

As you'll see in chapter 3 (which focuses on nutrient density), meat provides an ideal mix of amino acids, fats, and vitamins and minerals for brain growth and maintenance. Vitamin B_{12}—available only in animal foods—is particularly important for developing brains.

It's possible to survive on these vegan or vegetarian diets today, but they're far from optimal or normal for our species. People choose not to eat meat for many reasons, including concerns about the ethical treatment of animals, the amount of resources depleted in raising animals for consumption, and religious beliefs. Those are complex issues beyond the scope of this book. My point is simply that we may not have become the humans we are without this nutritious food source.

THE INDUSTRIAL REVOLUTION: OUT OF THE FRYING PAN AND INTO THE FIRE

The agricultural revolution began humans' transition away from sixty-six thousand generations of good health. But this shift wasn't really complete until about six generations ago, when humans reached another milestone: the Industrial Revolution, which ushered in a new age of mass production, transportation, urbanization, and economic development.

Although the beginning of the Industrial Revolution dates back to the eighteenth century, its dietary effects didn't become evident until the late 1800s. Improved transportation meant greater access to food for more people. Mass-production methods meant that items like white flour, table sugar, vegetable oil, dairy products, and alcohol could become fixtures at every table. White flour, for example, became widespread in the United States after 1850, but it didn't reach the saturation point until the 1890s. People living in England in the mid-Victorian period, between 1850 and 1890, generally enjoyed great health and still ate a fairly preindustrial diet. With falling prices and improved transportation, however, by around 1900, modern foods made up about 70 percent of the total calories the average person consumed each day—a remarkable change when you consider that none of them was available for the vast majority of human history.

Another significant change that came with the Industrial Revolution was a decrease in the diversity of the human diet around the world. Paleolithic hunter-gatherers consumed a large variety of plant species, primarily fruits, tubers, and vegetables, as do their modern counterparts. (For example, the Alyawarra tribe in Central Australia consume ninety-two different plant species, and the Tlokwa tribe in Botswana a hundred and twenty-six.) Thanks to improved railways, roads, and canals, a limited number of crops could be grown and shipped cheaply to every corner of the planet. Today, 80 percent of the world's population lives on only *four* principal staple plants: wheat, rice, corn, and potatoes.

The food introduced on a large scale by the Industrial Revolution (and grown with newly invented pesticides containing toxins) may be cheaper for us, but it isn't better. A hundred grams of sweet potato (about half a potato) contains only about 90 calories, and a hundred grams (one small serving) of wild-game meat contains about 150 calories, but both of these foods contain a wide spectrum of beneficial micronutrients. By contrast, a hundred grams (less than a cup) of refined wheat flour contains 361 calories, the same amount of sugar contains 387 calories, and both have virtually no beneficial nutrients. A hundred grams of corn oil (about seven tablespoons), a staple of modern diets, contains a whopping 881 calories and has essentially no nutritional value.

Even worse, industrialization completely changed the way humans lived. In 1800, 90 to 95 percent of Americans lived in rural areas or in small villages. In 1900, about half the population resided in nonurban environments. Today, less than 16 percent of all Americans live in rural areas. People who moved to cities to work became more sedentary. Longer work hours meant less time in the sun and less sleep. Stress—chronic, unrelenting—became a fixture in everyday life. While the Industrial Revolution undoubtedly improved human health in many ways (e.g., greater protection against infectious disease and better emergency medical care), these benefits did not come without significant cost. We have the Industrial Revolution to thank for new diseases of civilization that were rare or virtually nonexistent in preindustrial cultures:

- In the early 1950s in Uganda, only 0.7 percent of people above the age of forty showed evidence of having had heart attacks, according to an autopsy study. Today in Uganda, a country where the Western-style diet has taken hold, heart disease is the fourth-leading cause of death.
- In Papua New Guinea, heart attacks were unknown prior to urbanization. Today, the rate of heart attacks is skyrocketing, with upward of 400,000 heart attacks a year in a population of 5.4 million people.
- Among the Pima Indians in Arizona, the first confirmed case of diabetes was reported in 1908. Thirty years later, there were twenty-one cases, and by 1967, the number had risen to five hundred. Today, half of all adult Pima Indians have diabetes.

- When some of the South Pacific people of Tokelau migrated to nearby New Zealand and switched to a Western diet, they developed diabetes at three times the rate of those who had remained in Tokelau.

As study after study shows, the more Westernized a traditional culture becomes, the more disease it experiences. Today obesity, diabetes, heart disease, and other chronic degenerative conditions affect well over a billion people worldwide and kill millions of people each year. It may be nearly impossible for you to imagine life without these disorders. Yet they've been common for only the past two hundred or so years, a tiny fraction of the time humans have existed on the planet.

WE'RE STILL EVOLVING

I've argued that humans are mismatched with an agricultural diet because the environment changed faster than our species' genes and biology could adapt. But this doesn't mean that we haven't developed *any* adaptations to agriculture or that human evolution stopped in the Paleolithic era.

In fact, the pace of genetic change in humans has actually increased during the past few thousand years. Evolutionary biologist Scott Williamson suggests that evolution is occurring one hundred times faster than its previous average over the six million years of hominid evolution and that as much as 10 percent of the genome shows evidence of recent evolution in European Americans, African Americans, and Chinese.

This rapid increase in genetic change has been driven by two factors, say anthropologists Gregory Cochran and Henry Harpending in their book *The 10,000 Year Explosion:*

- A significant change in environment, which increased the selective pressure to adapt to it
- A dramatic increase in population, which increased the likelihood that adaptive mutations would arise by chance

If there's a new source of slightly indigestible food available to a population that lacks abundant food sources, there will be a lot of selective pressure for the species to adapt so they are able to consume that food. That's exactly what happened with milk. For most of our species' history, humans produced lactase, the enzyme that helps digest the milk sugar, only during infancy and early childhood. Since mother's milk was the only lactose-containing food in the human diet at that time, there was simply no need for children to continue making lactase after they stopped breast-feeding, which was at about age four for most hunter-gatherers.

However, this all changed with the dawn of the agricultural revolution and the domestication of cattle, which made cow's milk a readily available food source. Early farmers who relied heavily on grains were prone to mineral, especially calcium, deficiencies. Their skeletons, shorter than their hunter-gatherer predecessors', indicated they also probably lacked vitamin D, which plays a role in skeletal development. Milk is rich in calcium, contains some vitamin D, is a complete protein, and may promote growth during childhood. It also provided hydration and sustenance during periods of drought. Individuals who carried a genetic mutation allowing them to digest milk beyond their breast-feeding years would have been favored by natural selection, and their genes would have spread rapidly through farming populations.

In fact, archaeological evidence and gene-mapping studies suggest that a genetic mutation that allowed the continued production of lactase into adulthood originated about eight thousand years ago somewhere in Europe and spread rapidly thereafter. Today, approximately one-third of the global population produces lactase into adulthood. In cattle-herding tribes in East Africa, like the Tutsi, the rate is up to 90 percent. In some Northern European countries, like Denmark and Sweden, the genes are present in up to 95 percent of people.

There are several other relatively recent changes—genetic and otherwise—that have influenced our response to modern foods. For example:

- Populations with historically high starch intake produce more amylase in their saliva than populations with lower starch intake. Amylase is an enzyme that helps digest starch and glucose, both of which are forms of carbohydrates.
- New versions of genes that affect insulin and blood-sugar regulation have also arisen in the relatively recent past. These mutations appear to increase carbohydrate tolerance and reduce the likelihood that a higher-carbohydrate diet will lead to problems like diabetes.
- Changes in the *expression* of certain genes (which can happen much faster than changes to the underlying genes themselves) may help some populations that rely on grains as staples to process them more effectively.
- Finally, changes in the gut microbiota — the beneficial microorganisms that live in our digestive tracts — can directly affect one's ability to assimilate certain nutrients. Researchers have identified a type of bacteria in the colon of Japanese people that produces an enzyme that helps them digest seaweed (nori in particular). And some studies suggest that lactose intolerance can be eliminated simply by eating increasing amounts of yogurt containing live bacteria, which can naturally metabolize lactose.

So, our bodies have adapted in some ways to the challenges of an agricultural diet. Human innovation has also helped. As I mentioned in the previous section, cereal grains and legumes contain phytates, which bond with zinc, iron, calcium, and other minerals. The human gut is unable to break these bonds, which means that it's difficult for us to absorb the minerals from grains. But traditional cultures soaked grains and grain flours in an acid medium (such as whey or lemon juice), fermented them, germinated (sprouted) them, or leavened them (for example, baking bread with natural sourdough starter), which significantly reduced their phytate content and thus made the minerals they contained more bioavailable (that is, easier to absorb).

WILL EVOLUTION CATCH UP TO
WESTERN DIETS?

Humans, it would seem, are well adapted to Paleolithic foods like meat, vegetables, fruits, and tubers because our species has been eating them for millennia, and the evidence shows human health declined with the introduction of agricultural foods. However, the fact that a food wasn't available during the Paleolithic era doesn't *necessarily* mean we should avoid it entirely today. The genetic and cultural changes I've described above occurred (at least in part) to help humans adapt to an agricultural diet, and they *do* influence how individuals tolerate Neolithic foods. This explains why some people are able to include moderate amounts of dairy, grains, and/or legumes in their diets—especially when these foods are predigested by fermenting, soaking, sprouting, or leavening—without ill effect. (I'll have more to say on this topic later in the book.)

But these genetic changes *don't* mean we can eat a diet high in cereal grains and low in animal protein without adverse health consequences. These adaptations are often simple mutations of single genes and can be relatively crude. For example, the mutation that enables people to digest milk beyond childhood simply breaks the genetic switch that is supposed to turn off lactase production after infancy. This rather haphazard fix reflects the short time frame in which it took place; it's much easier for the body to break something that already exists than to create something new.

Eventually, it's at least *possible* that humans could evolve a more complex adaptation (involving the coordinated action of several different genes) to a grain-heavy diet. This might include changes in the gastrointestinal tract that would allow better absorption of the nutrients in grains. But even if such an adaptation occurred, it wouldn't change the fact that grains are far less nutrient dense than meats, fish, and vegetables—the staple foods of our Paleolithic ancestors. This is especially true when you take into account the bioavailability of nutrients, which is high in animal products and low in grains.

For these reasons, the best approach is to make the Paleolithic foods our species evolved to eat the foundation of your diet and then personalize it from there depending on your own unique combination of genetics, health status, activity level, life circumstances, and goals. That's exactly what I'm going to show you how to do, starting in the very next chapter.

Obviously, a lot has changed since our Paleo ancestors roamed the earth, and most of us aren't living like the contemporary hunter-gatherer populations I've mentioned in this section. How do we know their lifestyle is our best option today? Beyond the considerable anthropological record, there are several lines of modern, clinical evidence supporting the health benefits of a Paleo-template diet and lifestyle. These include:

- The high nutrient density of Paleo foods
- The minimal presence of toxins and antinutrients in Paleo foods
- The superior balance of fats in a Paleo diet
- The beneficial effects of the Paleo diet on gut bacteria
- The benefits of integrating physical activity throughout the day and minimizing sedentary time, the way our Paleo ancestors did
- The benefits of sleeping at least seven to eight hours a night and minimizing exposure to artificial light (although the latter was something our Paleo ancestors never had to contend with)
- The benefits of sun exposure (which go beyond vitamin D) and spending time outdoors
- The importance of pleasure, play, and social connection

I'll cover each of these — and much more — in Steps 1 and 2. Again, the good news is that we don't have to live in caves or roam the earth for food to enjoy the benefits of a Paleo-style diet. And there's no need to run to a geneticist to see if you have the right alleles to digest milk or wheat. Your Personal Paleo Cure will lead you to the perfect diet. For now, I hope I've convinced you that a Paleo template is the right place to begin.

Ready? Let's get started!

RESET YOUR DIET

CHAPTER 2

Reset to Feel Better Fast

When your computer starts running slowly, applications are crashing left and right, and you can't even move the cursor anymore, what do you do?

You press the reset button. You hit Control-Alt-Delete.

Sometimes we need to do the same thing with our bodies. They're under constant assault in the modern world. Refined, processed food, environmental toxins, stress, sleep deprivation, and chronic infections can all wreak havoc on our health.

We're simply not designed to live this way. With a few exceptions (which I'll cover later), we're still hardwired to eat the foods our hunter-gatherer ancestors ate. When we follow that two-million-year-old genetic template, as humans did for thousands of generations, we're naturally healthy and vital. But when we stray from it, as we have in the recent past, we suffer. If you want to feel better fast, the best thing to do is get back to basics.

So: How do you hit the reset button?

With Step 1's **Thirty-Day Reset Diet.** You commit to a thirty-day period where you eliminate the modern foods that contribute to disease as well as the foods people are most often allergic to or intolerant of and focus on the safe, nourishing foods our ancestors thrived on for more than sixty-six-thousand generations.

After you've hit the reset button and returned to that basic template,

---

Notes for this chapter may be found at ChrisKresser.com/ppcnotes/#ch2.

you can customize it to find the approach that works best for you over the long term (as you'll see later in Steps 2 and 3).

THE THIRTY-DAY RESET DIET

The Reset Diet is designed to reduce inflammation, improve digestion, burn fat, identify food sensitivities, reduce allergic reactions, boost energy, regulate blood sugar, and stabilize your mood.

It seems almost too good to be true. But I've done this myself, and I've guided thousands of people through it. And I can tell you this: it works! No other therapy—natural or otherwise—can come even remotely close to accomplishing all of these goals in such a short period.

Why thirty days? Because that's how long, on average, it takes my patients to experience the full benefits of the reset. It's absolutely essential that you commit to making these changes for at least thirty days—without cheating. Later on in the program, you'll have more leeway, and you'll be able to go off the rails every now and then. After all, there's more to life than food! But the Reset phase is not one of those times. This is where you gather your strength and buckle down. I know you can do it, because thousands of other people just like you already have.

In Step 2 of the program, you'll reintroduce some of the foods you eliminated during the Thirty-Day Reset Diet to see if you tolerate them. In Step 3, you'll learn how to make them part of a flexible lifestyle. But for now, the only way to find out if these foods are causing problems is to avoid them entirely.

As with any new diet or exercise program, check with your health-care professional before you begin.

WHAT FOODS CAN YOU EAT?

I've broken it down into three categories to make it as easy as possible: Eat Liberally, Eat in Moderation, and Avoid Completely.

- **Eat Liberally:** You can enjoy as much of these foods as you like. No counting calories or calculating ratios of proteins, fats, and carbohydrates. This isn't a cleanse or a fast. If a food is on this list, you're free to eat it.
- **Eat in Moderation:** You can eat these foods, but don't go wild. I've indicated how often or how much of them I think is safe, but in general you want to limit consumption of these foods compared with those in the Eat Liberally category.
- **Avoid Completely:** Yes, completely. The success (or failure) of the program hinges on your ability to steer clear of these foods during the Thirty-Day Reset.

As you'll see in later chapters, there are convincing reasons for choosing or avoiding specific foods in each of these categories. For now, however, let's look at what's on—or off—the list during the Reset.

Eat Liberally:

- **Meat and poultry.** Emphasize beef, lamb, and mutton, as well as pork, chicken, turkey, duck, goat, and wild game (like venison and ostrich). Organic and free-range meat is always preferable, but it is especially important during this part of the program, when you're trying to minimize all toxins in your diet. However, if those options are not available, don't let that get in the way of your Reset.
- **Organ meats (especially liver).** Liver is the most nutrient-dense food on the planet, rich in vitamin A, iron, and all the essential amino acids. If you don't like its taste, chop fresh liver into half-inch cubes, freeze them in an ice-cube tray, then pop out the liver cubes and store them in a freezer bag. When you're making any meat dish, defrost a cube, chop it finely, and mix it in. You won't notice the taste but you'll get all the nutrients. If you're adventurous, try heart, kidneys, spleen, tongue, and brains. (Note: If you have iron overload, a condition of excess iron storage in the body,

you should not eat organ meats. See pages 156–157 for more information.)

- **Bone-broth soups.** It's essential to balance your intake of muscle meats and organ meats with homemade bone broths. Bone broths differ from stocks in that they're simmered for a long time—up to forty-eight hours—to get the maximum nutrition from the bones. The broths are not only delicious but rich in glycine, an amino acid found in collagen, which is a protein important in maintaining a healthy gut lining.

- **Fish.** Especially fatty fish, like salmon, sardines, mackerel, anchovies, and herring. Wild is preferable. Eat three six-ounce servings of fatty fish per week to get enough of the omega-3 fats EPA and DHA, which I'll discuss in chapter 5.

- **Eggs.** Preferably free-range and organic. And, yes, yolks are allowed—I even encourage them, because they're an excellent source of vitamin D, selenium, and other important nutrients.

- **Starchy plants.** Yams, sweet potatoes, tapioca, yuca (also sold as cassava or manioc), taro, lotus root, plantains (ripe and unripe), and breadfruit. (Boil the yuca first for thirty minutes, then roast or mash it before eating to remove toxic goitrogens, compounds that can impair thyroid function in susceptible individuals.) No white potatoes allowed during Reset, but don't worry, you can see whether they belong back on your plate during Step 2.

- **Nonstarchy vegetables.** Cooked or raw. These include artichoke, asparagus, beets, broccoli, broccoli rabe, Brussels sprouts, cabbage, carrots, cauliflower, celery, chilies, cucumber, eggplant, garlic, green onions, greens (beet, collard, dandelion, kale, mustard, turnip), jicama, leeks, lettuce (endive, escarole, iceberg, leafy varieties, radicchio, romaine), mushrooms, okra, onions, parsley, parsnips, peppers, pumpkin, radishes, rutabaga, scallions, spinach, summer squash, Swiss chard, tomato, turnips, and zucchini.

- **Fermented vegetables and fruits.** Sauerkraut, kimchi, curtido, beet kvass, coconut kefir, and so on. Loaded with good bacteria, fermented foods are excellent for gut health.

- **Traditional fats.** Coconut oil, ghee, red palm oil, palm kernel oil, macadamia oil, lard (rendered from free-range pigs if possible), duck fat, beef tallow (from free-range cows if possible), and olive oil (preferably extra virgin).
- **Olives, avocados, and coconuts** (including coconut milk).
- **Sea salt and spices.** Avoid sugar and artificial flavorings.

Eat in Moderation:

- **Processed meat.** Sausage, bacon (both cured and uncured), salami, pepperoni, and jerky. Make sure they're gluten-, sugar-, and soy-free, and organic and/or free-range meat is preferable. Two to four servings a week is fine.
- **Whole fruit.** Up to four servings per day, depending on your blood-sugar balance (see below) and the type of fruit. Choose a wide variety of colors: green, red, orange, and yellow. All fruit is permitted, but favor low-sugar fruits, like berries, grapefruit, oranges, and peaches, over tropical fruits, apples, grapes, and pears. Watch out for dried fruit; it's easy to consume a lot of sugar with a single handful. (See NutritionData.com to find the amount of sugar in fruits, along with nutrient values for other foods.)
- **Nuts and seeds.** Allowed nuts include almonds, Brazil nuts, cashews, hazelnuts (filberts), macadamias, pecans, pine nuts, pistachios, and walnuts. (Note: peanuts are actually legumes, not nuts, and they're not allowed during the Thirty-Day Reset Diet.) Favor nuts lower in omega-6, like hazelnuts and macadamias, and minimize nuts high in omega-6, like Brazil nuts and almonds. Allowed seeds include chia, flax, pumpkin, sesame, and sunflower. It is easy to overeat nuts and seeds, but limit yourself to a handful per day. (See chapter 3 for important information on how to prepare nuts to make them easier to digest and more nutritious.) Sesame oil should be used only sparingly, since it contains relatively high levels of omega-6 linoleic acid, which is not good. I'll explain more in chapter 5.

- **Green beans, sugar peas, and snap peas.** Though technically legumes, they are usually well tolerated. You may eat four to six servings of these per week.
- **Coffee and black tea.** All teas and coffee are permitted; you can drink them black or with coconut milk. Limit these caffeinated beverages to one eight-ounce cup a day (not one triple espresso — one cup of brewed coffee or tea), and only before noon. However, if you experience fatigue, insomnia, anxiety, hypoglycemia, mood swings, or depression, you should eliminate *all* caffeine entirely. (Check labels; you'll find caffeine lurking in many headache and cold preparations.) Caffeine stimulates the adrenals and can worsen all of these conditions. Once your adrenal issues have been addressed — see chapter 20 — you may be able to add caffeine back, in moderation.
- **Vinegar.** Apple cider, balsamic, red wine, and other varieties. Apple cider vinegar is especially well tolerated. Vinegar may be used in small amounts every day as part of a salad dressing or sauce.
- **Restaurant food.** Restaurants cook with industrial seed and vegetable oils (on the Avoid Completely list, below), which can wreak havoc on your health. Also, it's hard to escape grains (hidden in various dishes) and some of the other foods on the Avoid Completely list. For these reasons, limit restaurant food as much as possible during the Thirty-Day Reset. I'd suggest eating out no more than twice a week (lunch included). In chapter 19, I'll offer tips on how to order in restaurants.

Avoid Completely:

- **Dairy.** Including butter, cheese, yogurt, milk, cream, and any dairy product that comes from a cow, goat, sheep, or other mammal. Ghee (aka "butter oil") is permitted because it contains only trace amounts of dairy proteins (e.g., casein) and lactose, and is well tolerated by all but the most sensitive individuals.

- **Grains.** Including wheat, rice, cereal, oats, pseudograins, and nongluten grains like sorghum, teff, quinoa, amaranth, buckwheat, spelt, rye, barley, couscous, malt, graham flour, and so on. No bread, pasta, cereal, or pizza. And for now, don't go shopping for gluten-free substitutes.
- **Legumes.** Including beans of all kinds (soy, black, kidney, pinto), peas, lentils, and peanuts. (Read labels: soy lurks in miso, tofu, bean curd, natto, tamari, tempeh, texturized vegetable protein, edamame, and elsewhere.)
- **Sweeteners, real and artificial.** Including sugar, high-fructose corn syrup, dextrose, coconut sugar, molasses, maple syrup, honey, agave, brown-rice syrup, Splenda, Equal, NutraSweet, xylitol, mannitol, and stevia.
- **Chocolate.** Milk chocolate contains both dairy and sugar and therefore should be avoided. There's nothing wrong with dark chocolate (with greater than 75 percent cacao content); in fact, it's one of the most nutrient-dense foods available, as you'll learn in chapter 3. However, many people who are intolerant of gluten are (unfortunately!) also intolerant of proteins in chocolate, so it should be avoided during the Step 1 Reset. You can reintroduce it during Step 2.
- **Processed or refined foods.** As a rule, if it comes in a bag or a box, don't eat it. This also includes highly processed "health foods" like protein powder, energy bars, dairy-free creamers, and so on.
- **Industrial seed and vegetable oils.** Soybean, corn, safflower, sunflower, rapeseed, peanut, cottonseed, canola, and so forth. Read labels — seed oils are in almost all processed, packaged, and refined foods (which you should be mostly avoiding during this phase anyway).
- **Sodas, including diet sodas, and fruit juice.** All forms, including "natural" varieties. Avoid fruit juice during the Reset because it's high in sugar and easy to overconsume. Coconut water is fine, but limit yourself to half a cup a day; it's quite sweet. Plain soda water or mineral water is fine.

- **Alcohol.** In any form. (Don't freak out. You'll be adding this back in in Step 2.)
- **Processed sauces and seasonings.** Soy sauce, tamari, and other processed sauces and seasonings (which often have sugar, soy, gluten, or all of the above).

DOES RED MEAT CAUSE HEART DISEASE?

You might be surprised that red meat is included in the Eat Liberally category. After all, haven't we been told for years that red meat contributes to heart disease? It's true that some studies show an association between red-meat consumption and heart disease. Yet others—especially those that separate fresh-red-meat consumption from processed-meat consumption—have found none. A large review of studies covering more than 1.2 million participants found that consumption of fresh, unprocessed red meat was not associated with an increased risk of coronary heart disease (CHD), stroke, or diabetes. In addition, it's hard to draw conclusions from observational studies on red meat and disease owing to something known as the healthy-user bias; that is, because red meat has been viewed as unhealthy for so long, those who consume more of it are also more likely to engage in other behaviors perceived (correctly, in these cases) as unhealthy, like smoking, eating processed and refined food, and not getting enough exercise.

If eating red meat causes heart disease, then we'd expect to see lower rates of heart disease in vegetarians and vegans. Again, early studies suggested this was true. But they suffered from the same healthy-user bias as the red-meat studies (meaning that since vegetarians tend to be more health conscious than the general population, their lower incidence of heart disease could be explained by other factors, such as their exercising more and smoking less). Newer, higher-quality studies that have controlled for these confounding factors haven't found any difference in rates of heart disease between omnivores and vegetarians. For example, one study compared the risk of death from heart disease of people who shopped in health-food stores (both vegetarians and omnivores) to the risk of death from heart disease in people in the general population. They found that vegetarians and omnivores in the health-food-store group had a lower risk of death from heart disease than people in the general population, but there was no difference in risk between the health-food-store omnivores and the vegetarians.

So there's no reason to feel guilty or frightened about digging into that juicy steak or beef stew!

HOW TO BE A FOOD DETECTIVE

Before you begin your Thirty-Day Reset, police your pantry and get rid of foods that are off-limits. Dairy, sugar, and fat lurk in many products, so read the ingredient labels; you won't believe where culprits are hiding!

Where Dairy Hides: Anything containing casein, whey, malt, or an ingredient with the prefix *lacto-* is off-limits during the Reset, as are foods with the word *curd, pudding,* or *custard* on the packaging. Many artificial flavors and colorings also have dairy.

Where Sugar Hides: You expect to find sugar in cereal and drinks, but did you know it's frequently in salad dressing, canned soup, peanut butter, beef jerky, and tomato sauce? In "healthy" granola bars and yogurt? Dried fruit may also contain added sugar. *Fat-free* is often code for "We snuck a lot of sugar into this so you won't miss the fat." You'll also find sugar hidden inside other words commonly found on food labels: Watch out for fruit-juice concentrate, corn sweetener, malt syrup, malto-dextrin, evaporated cane juice or syrup, and any words ending in *-ose,* such as *sucrose, dextrose, galactose,* and *maltose.* Sugar is sugar, no matter where it comes from or what form it takes.

Where Industrial Seed Oils Hide: Read the labels to make sure that your healthy nuts aren't roasted in unhealthy fats. Also, if a product has been processed to be shelf stable, it probably has industrial seed oils and artificial trans fats (watch for the words *partially hydrogenated*) — another reason for you to avoid boxes and bags, especially during the Reset phase.

CAVEATS AND TWEAKS FOR
SPECIAL CONDITIONS

If you've been diagnosed with certain health conditions, you'll need to modify the Thirty-Day Reset Diet. If you're not sure if you have a particular condition, take the Reset Diet symptom quiz below. Add up the total number of points in each section for the symptoms you experience, then proceed to the answer key to determine which diet you should follow.

Reset Diet Symptom Quiz

BLOOD SUGAR AND WEIGHT REGULATION	POINTS
Diagnosed with diabetes, impaired glucose tolerance, or hypoglycemia	50
Feel fatigued directly after meals	5
Crave sweets during the day	5
Eating sweets doesn't relieve cravings for sugar	5
Must have sweets after meals	5
Feel agitated if you don't eat frequently	5
Irritable or light-headed between meals	5
Eating relieves fatigue	5
Feel shaky or jittery, especially between meals	5
Need caffeine to get yourself started in the morning	5
Easily upset or nervous	5
Poor memory or forgetful	5
Waist circumference equal to or larger than hip circumference	5
Difficulty losing weight	5
Increased thirst or appetite	5

BLOOD SUGAR AND WEIGHT REGULATION	POINTS
Frequent urination	5
Blurred vision	5
TOTAL	

Answer key

SCORE	BLOOD SUGAR AND WEIGHT REGULATION
0–40	Follow the normal Thirty-Day Reset.
>40	Follow the Thirty-Day Reset with blood sugar and weight regulation modifications (listed below).

AUTOIMMUNE PROBLEMS	POINTS
Diagnosed with autoimmune disease	50
High C-reactive protein and other inflammatory markers on lab tests	5
Muscle or joint aches and pains	5
Persistent fever	5
Extreme fatigue	5
Swollen glands	5
Abdominal pain, digestive problems, constipation, or diarrhea	5
Itchy skin or skin rashes	5
Tingling in hands and/or feet	5
Sudden, unexplained weight loss or weight gain	5
Changes in skin color	5
Food allergies or multiple food sensitivities	5
TOTAL	

Answer key

SCORE	AUTOIMMUNE PROBLEMS
0–40	Follow the normal Thirty-Day Reset.
>40	Follow the Thirty-Day Reset with autoimmune modifications (listed below).

If you scored over 40 on each of the quizzes, you should follow the modifications for both blood-sugar and autoimmune problems during the Thirty-Day Reset and consult with your health-care provider.

Tweaks for problems with blood sugar or weight regulation

If you scored 50 points or more in this category and/or you're trying to lose weight, you should limit fruit and starchy vegetables during your Thirty-Day Reset. Eat all the nonstarchy vegetables you want, but restrict your fruit and starchy vegetables to roughly 10 to 15 percent of calories from carbohydrates. This amounts to roughly 65 to 100 grams daily for a moderately active male and 50 to 75 grams daily for a moderately active female. To give you a general idea of what this looks like in terms of food, 50 grams of carbohydrates is equal to one large sweet potato and 1/2 cup of blueberries; 100 grams of carbohydrates is equal to 1/2 cup of blueberries, 1/2 cup of strawberries, and two large sweet potatoes. You can search online databases like the ones from the USDA to determine the carbohydrate content of foods.

Tweaks for autoimmune problems

If you scored 40 points or higher in this category, please follow the Thirty-Day Reset, but also avoid the following:

- Eggs (both whites and yolks). Eggs contain proteins that are common allergens, particularly in susceptible people.
- Nightshades (potatoes, tomatoes, sweet and hot peppers, eggplant, tomatillos, pepinos, pimentos, paprika, and cayenne

pepper). Nightshades have compounds called alkaloids that can cause inflammation and worsen joint pain in susceptible people.

Not everyone with an autoimmune condition needs to be on the protocol forever—you'll experiment with adding these foods back in Step 2.

FREQUENTLY ASKED QUESTIONS ABOUT STEP 1: THE THIRTY-DAY RESET DIET

If you're completely new to this way of eating, you might be feeling pretty overwhelmed right now. "I thought saturated fats were bad," you say. "Aren't whole grains healthy?" I'll take up these questions and others in the chapters that follow. For now, let's tackle some of the more immediate concerns you might have.

How do I do it?

I recognize this will be a dramatic change for many of you. The best way to do it is to just dive right in. Begin right now. If you procrastinate or delay, it only gets harder.

Use the meal plans and recipes in chapter 21 to work out what you're going to eat for the first week. (You can find additional meal plans, recipes, and shopping lists on the website.) Then head out to the grocery store, farmers' market, butcher, or wherever you shop and stock up for the next week. All you have to think about is what to eat and what not to eat. There are no calories to count. Just eat the foods that are allowed, and don't eat the ones that aren't.

When will I get results?

The first few days can be hard. Your body will be going through withdrawal from everyday substances like sugar and wheat; you may notice symptoms like mood swings, strong cravings, irritability, and fatigue as your body adjusts to life without them. If you've been drinking four cups of coffee every day for twenty years, cutting back to one cup will be tough. Does that mean you shouldn't do it? That it won't benefit your health in the long run? No. It just means you're probably going to need some support along the way.

If you've been eating a poor diet with a lot of processed food as well as smoking, drinking too much alcohol, and leading a sedentary life filled with chronic stress, I truly understand that the transition to a healthy diet will be a big challenge.

But at some point, you will recover and start feeling better than you did before you began the program. Most of my patients say that the first four to seven days are the hardest. After that, you'll start having a lot more energy; those familiar dips in energy in the afternoon may well disappear completely, and without the hit of that afternoon coffee and candy bar. In fact, your cravings may disappear altogether; you'll find yourself eyeing that pizza or pasta and saying, "No, thanks." Your skin will clear up, the breakouts and redness disappearing. Your digestion will be smoother. You'll sleep more deeply and wake feeling more rested. Those up-and-down mood swings will stabilize. You'll start shedding some pounds (only if you need to, usually). Even if the scale doesn't budge, you may find that muffin top melting. Aches, pains, and mysterious symptoms you've had for ages will—seemingly miraculously—begin to improve.

This program has the potential to change your life. I realize that it's difficult; I know how much work it is, and I remember what it was like to cut out all of these foods. I've been there myself, although I can hardly remember why I used to love some of that junky food so much (cold cereal was a particular weakness). But I also know from my own experience and from supervising many people through this transition that the results are worth the effort.

I thought fat was bad for me and I should limit my intake, but some of the foods on the okay-to-eat list are fatty.

The biggest mistake people make on this program is not eating enough fat. You're eliminating a lot of foods from your diet (bread, grains, beans, etc.), and you have to replace those lost calories with something. Healthy fat is that something. If you're concerned about your weight, take comfort in the knowledge that the vast majority of my patients and readers shed pounds on the Thirty-Day Reset. Fat is the preferred fuel source of the body and should constitute about 40 to 70 percent of the calories in your diet, depending on individual needs. (My only caveat is chicken fat. Although it's delicious, it often comes from chickens that are fed grains, so the ratio of healthy omega-3 fat to not-so-healthy omega-6 fat isn't great; in a later chapter, you'll see why that ratio matters. If you can find chicken fat from pastured chickens, go for it.) You can exchange that dry, boneless, skinless chicken breast for a luscious pork chop or a nice juicy steak.

A little cheat here and there can't hurt, right?

Once you've figured out your ideal diet, I'd agree with that. But as I said above, this isn't the time to cheat. Don't do it. It's not worth it.

By removing the foods that most commonly cause problems, you allow your body to rest and recover from whatever symptoms those foods have been provoking. Just one cheat could trigger a whole new cascade of reactions. A single piece of bread or one glass of milk could restart the inflammatory process and throw your body back into the chaos that led you to the Personal Paleo Cure program in the first place. Some of the greatest benefits of the Reset Diet don't kick in until the third week — right when the finish line is in sight. At some point, you won't even miss those foods you think you can't live without now. So don't cheat. It could set you way back. If you go thirty days, it will get easier. I promise.

Shouldn't I be counting calories and calculating macronutrient ratios?

Relax—no calculators. (The only exceptions here are for people with specific health conditions; see below.) In Step 3, I'll discuss how to determine the optimal amount of fats, carbohydrates, and proteins to eat based on your individual circumstances. In the Step 1 Reset, we're focusing more on the *quality* of macronutrient than the quantity. That said, you can use the following ranges as a starting point during the Reset:

- Fats: 40 to 70 percent of your total daily calories (that's 115 to 200 grams for a moderately active male eating 2,600 calories per day, and 100 to 155 grams for a moderately active female eating 2,000 calories per day)
- Carbohydrates: 15 to 30 percent of your total daily calories (that's 100 to 200 grams for a moderately active male eating 2,600 calories per day, and 75 to 150 grams for a moderately active female eating 2,000 calories per day)
- Proteins: 10 to 20 percent of your total daily calories (that's 65 to 130 grams for a moderately active male eating 2,600 calories per day, and 50 to 100 grams for a moderately active female eating 2,000 calories per day)

Don't overanalyze what you're eating. Enjoy your food. Make cooking fun and leave time to savor your creations. You'll find recipes and meal plans in chapter 21. There are also more recipes on the website. You've got real, delicious, nutrient-dense foods to choose from.

Can I juice?

If you juice with whole fruits or veggies with water, unsweetened nut milk, or half a cup of coconut water with no sugar added, you should be fine, although some of my patients say that they tend to feel hungrier when they drink their meals. Focus on the veggies and the lower-sugar fruits, like berries. And avoid prepared juices or smoothies, which often contain large amounts of natural sugar or processed sugars like high-fructose corn syrup, which you should avoid completely on the Reset.

This is too hard. How can I make it easier?

No man (or woman) is an island. Change is hard, and the more support you have in doing this, the easier it will go. Try enlisting your spouse, your significant other, or a good friend to do this with you. (People may not be eager, but they'll thank you later.) Have a Personal Paleo Cure potluck. Invite friends over to cook with you. Connect online with others who are following this approach. Be sure to check out my website's online forum, where you can discuss your dietary changes with fellow adventurers. Ask questions. Get help.

Instead of thinking about what you can't have on the Thirty-Day Reset Diet, focus on what you're getting: That looser waistband. Not feeling exhausted in the middle of the afternoon. Seeing a clearer complexion in the mirror. Your knees not being so achy anymore. Feeling sharper, less moody. Your digestion running more smoothly. Knowing that you're on your way to feeling better than you have in years—or maybe ever!

I'm really physically active. Should I eat more?

If you're an athlete or very physically active, you will generally need more calories and a higher carbohydrate intake, especially after working out. As a rough idea, if you're seeking to maintain your current weight or gain muscle, you should aim to get about 25 to 60 percent of your calories from carbohydrates; if you're trying to lose fat, aim to get between 7 and 20 percent of calories from carbohydrates. For protein, most athletes should aim for 0.8 to 1.0 grams of protein per pound of body weight per day if they're trying to lose fat or maintain weight, and 1.0 to 1.25 grams per pound of body weight per day if they're trying to gain muscle or increase performance. See chapter 18 for detailed recommendations for those with high activity levels.

I'm going out to eat. What do I do?

If you're dining out, choose a place that can accommodate your needs. Call ahead and ask if there are gluten-free items on the menu. Pick a restaurant that offers meat and vegetable dishes, and order a side salad. (Skip the dressing, since it may have sugar, and ask for vinegar and olive oil on the side instead.) If you don't plan in advance, you could find yourself in a situation where you're starving, and then you might end up eating a big plate of pasta because that's all that's available. The same rules apply when you're traveling, and make sure you stock up on Personal Paleo Cure–friendly snacks, such as nuts and veggies. See chapter 19 for more tips and tricks for sticking to your Thirty-Day Reset Diet when you're eating out or on the road. Advance planning makes it possible!

I'm taking a lot of supplements.
Should I continue taking them during Step 1?

This one's a little harder to answer. Always check with your health-care provider before starting or stopping any prescription medication or supplement. If you know the supplement helps you or you're taking it for a specific purpose (for example, iodine for thyroid function), by all means, continue. If you can't remember why you're taking a certain supplement or if you're uncertain about whether it's helping you, I suggest stopping it during Step 1. Not all supplements are beneficial, and some may even cause harm. (I'll discuss which supplements are mostly likely to help and which cause harm in more detail in chapter 18.)

How can I stay organized and motivated?
Will your website help?

Go to ChrisKresser.com/PPC to register for the free Personal Paleo Cure resources I mention throughout the book, including additional meal plans, recipes, and shopping lists; a Paleo troubleshooting guide; and other resources to take all of the guesswork out of it for you. Take a look around the website and familiarize yourself with what's available. Print out charts or whatever you need, put them up on your refrigerator, and take them with you to the store if you get stuck. Don't forget to get involved with the forum, where you can get support from other Personal Paleo Cure users who may be dealing with similar issues and who may have helpful recommendations to get you through each phase of the program.

If you're having some difficulty beyond the usual adjustment period, don't be alarmed. It doesn't mean the Personal Paleo Cure won't work or isn't a good choice for you. Not all damage done to the body is quickly reversible; sometimes the Thirty-Day Reset Diet isn't enough to heal that damage without additional help. You may need to tweak things a bit, and add a few things to your program.

INFLAMMATION: WHY YOUR PERSONAL PALEO CURE WILL PROTECT YOU

Throughout this book, I'll be discussing foods and nutrients that may have inflammatory or anti-inflammatory properties. It's important to note which of these can trigger inflammation or alleviate it, as this condition is the cause of so many modern, chronic diseases.

When health-care professionals and scientists talk about inflammation, you may automatically think of conditions like joint pain—most notably arthritis—which can involve swelling that you can often see. However, while swelling can be a symptom of inflammation, inflammation itself is actually the body's response to infection or other threats, which it deals with through the production of white blood cells and other substances.

In many cases, this inflammation is invisible to you, because it's occurring inside the body—but that doesn't mean it's any less harmful than the kind you can see. In fact, just about all of the modern diseases that plague us today are caused, at least in part, by inflammation, including bowel diseases like Crohn's and ulcerative colitis, autoimmune diseases like Hashimoto's thyroiditis and rheumatoid arthritis, cardiovascular disease, obesity, type 2 diabetes, Alzheimer's, and even depression. The good news is that when you follow a diet that aligns with your Personal Paleo Cure, you naturally reduce the risk of inflammation and protect yourself from related illness.

"I'M SO GLAD I STUCK WITH IT"

The Thirty-Day Reset Diet can be a big adjustment, but it offers big rewards! I hope you'll be inspired by these reports from people who took the plunge:

- "My acid reflux went away after one week and my knee stopped swelling after two weeks. Imagine jumping into a time machine and traveling back in time twenty years! Imagine fitting into the clothes you wore when you were twenty-five years old! Imagine shocking your doctor and watching his double take when he reviews your new blood work! I am fifty-one years old and I feel as if I was thirty years old again."

- "No more hemorrhoids, no more pimples, no more dry skin, no more acidity in my mouth, no more farting, more energy. No post-lunch fatigue, better sleep, less sugar cravings."

- "After about a week, I started noticing moles that were raised were now flat as a pancake and starting to disappear. I stayed with it for forty-five days just because I was feeling so much better. Also dropped twelve pounds with no effort. What a difference. Leg cramping, that 'heavy' feeling, lethargic issues are all gone. Fingernails started to grow faster and stronger."

- "On the fifth night, I started sleeping deeply for the first time in my life, I lost weight for the first time since being diagnosed with hypothyroidism three years ago and have maintained a thirty-pound weight loss. I have more energy than I have ever had before. Also my digestion is solid."

- "Energy levels more even, tennis elbow inflammation disappeared, asthma improved, waistline shrunk. Definitely glad I stuck with it."

- "There were a couple of days with the flu-ish feeling as my body adjusted to the lack of sugar and salt. Within days, though, my digestion was improved. Dropped twenty-five points on both sides of my blood pressure and dropped cholesterol from a starting 280 to 147 about six months later. I avoided statins and dropped my blood pressure meds that I'd been on for five years."

- "I feel the best ever. No insulin anymore and no three big drugs for blood pressure."

- "My blood chemistry improved greatly, especially my triglyceride count (from 378 to 45 in thirty days). I lost about fifteen pounds in the first month. I got my health back, and my family's health back. Once you learn the truth about anything, diet included, you can never go back."

- "After thirty days, my IBS was gone and acne cleared up. I had tons of energy at the gym and slept great."
- "I kept wondering when the magic was going to happen, then digestion, sleep, energy, hunger, skin tone and weight all seemed to improve as quickly as if I had passed through a doorway. I am so glad I stuck with it. My mental and physical health have improved ten-fold. It is amazing how much your body can heal in only thirty days."

HOW DO I KNOW WHEN TO MOVE ON TO STEP 2?

Follow the Step 1 Reset Diet for a minimum of thirty days—even if you're feeling significantly better or most of your symptoms improve sooner. As mentioned, I've found that thirty days is the minimum amount of time it takes to establish a new pattern in the body. If you move on too quickly, you risk sabotaging your hard-won improvement.

After thirty days, if you feel you're still making progress and want to give yourself more time to reap the benefits of the Reset, then continue for as long as you'd like. The Reset Diet is completely safe to follow for a lifetime. (As a reminder, check with your health-care professional before you start the program.) When you feel ready to reintroduce some foods or if you begin to feel like your improvements are leveling off, that's an indication that you're ready for Step 2.

If you stay on the Reset Diet for more than thirty days and your progress plateaus for more than two weeks, it's unlikely you will see further improvement by continuing with Step 1, so I recommend moving on to Step 2. In many cases, adding foods back in during Step 2 can kick-start the improvement again.

Feeling better fast is a powerful motivation to move on to Step 2. In the following chapters, I'm going to explain the core principles behind the Personal Paleo Cure, which will give you even more motivation while you are doing the Reset.

CHAPTER 3

Nutrient Know-How: Maximizing Nutrient Density in Every Bite

Aurora, age sixty-five, came to see me complaining of numbness, tingling, and weakness in her legs, reduced mobility, and decreased balance and coordination. She also had what I call brain fog—difficulty focusing, solving problems, even spelling common words—and her memory sometimes failed her. "I have suffered for years from these symptoms," she said, "but I always thought they were just a normal part of getting older." When her symptoms worsened, she sought help. Two doctors she visited both suspected multiple sclerosis, but Aurora was skeptical of this diagnosis and came to see me for another opinion.

In discussing her medical history with her and asking about her diet, I learned that Aurora had been a vegetarian for the past twenty-five years but had never had her B_{12} levels tested. Vitamin B_{12} deficiency can mimic many of the symptoms of MS—peripheral neuropathy (numbness and tingling in the arms and legs), cognitive decline, and poor coordination and balance—and it is extremely common among long-term vegetarians. Sure enough, after I ran a full blood panel for her, I found that her B_{12} levels were dangerously low. I immediately started her on intensive B_{12} supplementation, and within a matter of weeks, her symptoms had vastly

Notes for this chapter may be found at ChrisKresser.com/ppcnotes/#ch3.

improved. Unfortunately, her recovery was not complete because some damage caused by B_{12} deficiency is irreversible. This highlights the importance of this essential vitamin.

"I can't believe something so simple to diagnose and treat could cause so many problems," she told me upon learning of her B_{12} deficiency. "I only wish I would have known this sooner." Though she'd been a vegetarian for more than two decades, Aurora decided to start incorporating meat and fish back into her diet to give her body the B_{12} it so desperately needed.

There are many reasons why people choose to eat a vegetarian diet, and I respect individual choice. However, Aurora's story is a good example of what happens when we don't choose a *nutrient-dense* diet, and it highlights one of the greatest benefits of the Personal Paleo Cure approach: it contains the full spectrum of nutrients that humans require for optimal health.

WHY NUTRIENT DENSITY MATTERS

There are two types of nutrients in food: *macronutrients*, which include protein, carbohydrates, and fat, and *micronutrients*, which are vitamins, minerals, and other compounds required in small amounts for normal metabolic function.

The nutrient density of foods refers primarily to micronutrients and amino acids (the building blocks of protein). Carbohydrates and fats are important to health, but, with the exception of two fatty acids — which we'll discuss in chapter 5 — they can be provided by the human body for a short amount of time if dietary intake is insufficient. The same cannot be said for micronutrients and the essential amino acids found in protein, which must be obtained from the diet.

Your body needs about forty different micronutrients for proper physiological function; suboptimal intake of any of them will contribute to disease and shorten life span. Unfortunately, nutrient deficiency is widespread in people following an industrialized diet that is energy but not nutrient dense. *Energy density* is the number of calories in a given amount of food; *nutrient density* is the concentration of nutrients in a given amount of food. With that in mind, you can understand why a large sugary soda has high energy density (lots of calories) but virtually no nutritional density.

Vegetable oils and sugar contribute about 36 percent of the calories in a typical American's diet, yet they are essentially devoid of micronutrients. Not surprisingly, studies have shown that the more energy-dense, nutrient-poor foods someone consumes, the more likely he or she is to have nutrient deficiencies. More than half of Americans are deficient in zinc, calcium, magnesium, vitamin A, vitamin B_6, and vitamin E, according to a 1997 survey. Approximately one-third are also deficient in riboflavin, thiamine, folate, vitamin C, and iron. In many cases, these aren't mild nutrient deficiencies; up to 50 percent of Americans consume less than half of the recommended daily allowance (RDA) for several micronutrients.

This is especially alarming when you consider the fact that the RDA is based on the amount of a nutrient required to avoid acute deficiency symptoms. It does not reflect the amount required to avoid deficiency symptoms over an extended period. This amount is not known for most micronutrients, but it is almost certainly higher than the RDA, which means that an even larger percentage of Americans than the number given above are not getting enough of these vitamins and minerals. Aurora, my patient with the B_{12} deficiency, is hardly alone!

THE CONSEQUENCES OF NUTRIENT DEFICIENCY

You've already read about the precipitous decline in health among hunter-gatherers when they adopted agriculture; those effects were in large part due to nutrient deficiencies caused by their new grain-based diet. Unfortunately, 366 generations later, many people are still taking in an inadequate amount of micronutrients and suffering the multiple problems that causes.

It starts at a subcellular level in the body, where nutrient deficiency can mimic the effects of radiation and chemicals on DNA, causing single- and double-strand breaks, oxidative lesions, or both. Simply put, nutrient deficiency threatens your body's ability to function normally and can shorten your life span. Here are just some of the conditions triggered by nutrient deficiency.

Immune function is adversely affected by poor intake of nearly every essential vitamin and mineral, which compromises our ability to fight infections. And antioxidant vitamins, carotenoids, and minerals are required to prevent **premature aging** and protect against **cellular damage.**

Cardiovascular disease affects more than sixty-five million Americans and is the leading cause of death in this country each year (responsible for almost four out of ten deaths). In the United States, 65 percent of adults are **overweight,** and 34 percent meet the criteria for **metabolic syndrome,** a constellation of disorders including low HDL cholesterol, high triglycerides, high fasting blood sugar, high blood pressure, and abdominal obesity. **Diabesity**—a term coined by Dr. Mark Hyman that refers to the continuum of metabolic disorders from mild blood-sugar imbalance to full-blown type 2 diabetes—affects one in two Americans.

Micronutrient deficiency may contribute in part to all of these conditions. For example, magnesium deficiency is associated with an increased risk of metabolic syndrome and cardiovascular disease. Vitamin K_2 deficiency is associated with heart disease and coronary calcification. Deficiency of folate leads to increased levels of a compound that damages the fragile lining of blood vessels and is thought to contribute to heart disease. Folate deficiency also impairs a process called methylation, which in turn can lead to altered expression and suppression of genes and increase the risk of cancer.

WHOLE FOODS VS. SUPPLEMENTS

You might be thinking a multivitamin can prevent nutrient deficiency, but supplemental nutrients do not have the same effect on the body as nutrients gotten from food. Humans have evolved to get their nutrients from whole foods—not supplements. Most nutrients require specific enzymes and other substances to be properly absorbed. While these are naturally present in foods, they are often not included in synthetic vitamins with isolated nutrients. This may explain why several trials have shown that adding antioxidant supplements to a typical American diet not only doesn't prevent people from getting heart disease and cancer but may actually increase their risk. While supplements can (and should) be used for therapeutic effect in specific health conditions or to replace certain nutrients that are difficult to obtain from food, they should never be used to replace nutrients that can be found in a nutrient-dense diet.

ARE VEGETARIAN OR VEGAN DIETS HEALTHIER THAN OMNIVORE DIETS?

Many vegetarians and vegans choose not to eat meat or animal products for ethical reasons, and I respect that choice. That said, from a nutritional perspective, I find it difficult to justify a diet that results in deficiencies of several nutrients critical to human function. While it may be possible to address this through targeted supplementation (an issue that is still debated), it makes far more sense to get your nutrients from food. Human bodies have evolved to obtain nutrients from food, and some evidence suggests that supplemental nutrients don't have the same effect on the body that nutrients in foods do. For more on my thoughts regarding vegetarianism versus omnivorous eating, as well as for detailed information on B_{12} deficiency and other nutritional challenges posed by following a plant-based diet, please see the notes for this chapter on my website.

YOU ARE WHAT YOU ABSORB: THE IMPORTANCE OF BIOAVAILABILITY

Now you understand the importance of eating nutrient-dense food. But even the most nutrient-dense food on the planet is worthless unless the nutrients it contains are bioavailable. Bioavailability refers to the portion of a nutrient that is absorbed by the body. The amount of bioavailable nutrients in a food is almost always lower than the absolute amount of nutrients the food contains.

The grass on your front lawn is a perfect example. Grass contains several vitamins and minerals, but they are largely inaccessible to humans because of grass's cellulose content. Cellulose is a fiber that forms the walls of cells in most green plants. Ruminants, such as cows and sheep, have a specialized compartment in the stomach called a rumen; it produces an enzyme that breaks down cellulose, allowing the nutrients in the grass to be absorbed. Ruminants also have other chambers in their stomachs to help them assimilate the nutrients from grass.

Humans don't have rumens, multiple stomach chambers, or the enzymes to break down cellulose, so we can't extract any nutrients from grass if we eat it. Fortunately, there is a solution to this problem: rather than eating the grass, humans can let animals do the hard work of assimilating the nutrients from grass, and then we can eat the animals.

There are three primary factors that affect the bioavailability of a food.

The first is the form that the minerals and other nutrients take. The classic example is iron, which appears in food in two forms: heme and nonheme. Heme iron comes from the iron in red blood cells and is found only in animal products, like meat, fish, poultry, and egg yolks; nonheme iron is found in both plant and animal foods. Only about 2 to 20 percent of nonheme iron is absorbed by the human body, compared to 15 to 35 percent of heme iron. In addition, the absorption of nonheme iron is reduced by several different compounds, such as phytates (found in whole grains and other foods), tannins (found in tea and coffee), and oxalates (found in spinach, sweet potatoes, and Swiss chard).

Second, the absorption of most nutrients is dependent on or influenced by the presence of other nutrients. Nutrient enhancers can keep a nutrient soluble or protect it from nutrient inhibitors. For example, beta-carotene, lutein, and lycopene are fat soluble, which means they require fat for optimal assimilation, so adding an avocado to a green salad (increasing its fat content by 47 percent) can help you absorb seven times more lutein and eighteen times more beta-carotene. Another example is heme iron. Heme iron is better absorbed than nonheme iron, and, in addition, it actually improves nonheme-iron absorption. Vitamin C also has been shown to increase iron absorption by as much as three times.

Third, nutrient inhibitors and antinutrients can decrease nutrient bioavailability. They can do this in several different ways: by binding the nutrient into a form not recognized by the digestive tract's uptake systems; by rendering the nutrient insoluble and so unavailable for absorption; and by competing for the same uptake system used by that nutrient. Phytate is an example of an antinutrient; it binds to minerals such as calcium, iron, and zinc and makes new compounds that the body can't absorb. Most cereal grains and legumes contain significant amounts of phytates, which is one of the reasons early humans developed nutritional deficiencies after adopting agriculture.

Even beneficial nutrients can inhibit the absorption of other nutrients. For example, both calcium and nonheme iron bind to a transporter in the intestines, but whereas nonheme iron is absorbed this way, calcium basically stays in that doorway and blocks the entry of iron into the bloodstream. This is why calcium supplements are sometimes used to impair iron absorption in patients with hemochromatosis, a genetic disorder that causes dangerously high iron levels.

Focusing on the nutrient density of foods alone is not enough. We need to maximize the intake of foods that are high in *bioavailable* nutrients and substances that improve nutrient absorption, and minimize the intake of foods that are poor in nutrients and have substances that impair nutrient absorption. The Personal Paleo Cure allows you to do just that.

MEASURING NUTRIENT DENSITY

There are several issues involved in measuring the nutrient density of foods, including:

- **Deciding which nutrients to measure.** Experts don't entirely agree on which nutrients are the most essential to human health and which are detrimental. However, there are several nutrients that are universally accepted to be beneficial, and these should be included in any nutrient-density scale. Likewise, nutrients that have not yet been conclusively shown to be important should not take the place of these essential nutrients.

- **Outdated science.** Many nutrient scales penalize foods that are high in saturated fat and cholesterol, though recently completed long-term studies show that eating saturated fat and cholesterol does not raise cholesterol in the blood for most people. The same is true for sodium. Early studies suggested that sodium raises blood pressure, but later studies have shown that this is true in only a small group of people, known as sodium hyper-responders. In addition, many scales don't include nutrients now known to be important for human health, such as the omega-3 fats EPA and DHA and vitamin K_2.

- **Bioavailability.** As I explained in the previous section, it doesn't matter how many nutrients a food contains; what matters is what we absorb when we eat that food. If bioavailability were taken into consideration on nutrient-density scales, foods like cereal grains, legumes, and nuts and seeds (which are high in phytates) would score much lower than foods with highly absorbable forms of nutrients, like meat and dairy.

- **Distribution of nutrients in the food supply.** Some nutrients, such as vitamin D, vitamin A (retinol), and magnesium, are difficult to find in food in bioavailable forms, whereas others, like protein and many minerals, are relatively easy to obtain. Ideally, the difficult-to-obtain nutrients should be weighted more heavily on a nutrient-density scale.

- **Combining calorie density with energy density.** Many nutrient-density scales give lower scores to foods with higher calorie content. While it's true that some calorically dense foods (e.g., processed and refined foods) promote overeating and weight gain, that is not always true for unprocessed high-calorie foods (like dairy products and animal fats). Nutrient density and calorie density should be considered separately.

In order to address the shortcomings of existing nutrient-density scales, Harvard University chemist Dr. Mat Lalonde created a new scale that he presented at the Ancestral Health Symposium in August of 2012. Using the USDA National Nutrient Database for Standard Reference, Dr. Lalonde ranked foods according to the following qualifying nutrients:

QUALIFYING NUTRIENTS FOR CHARACTERIZING NUTRIENT DENSITY (ADAPTED FROM LALONDE)		
Vitamin A (RAE)	Choline	Thiamine (**B**$_1$)
Riboflavin (B$_2$)	Niacin (B$_3$)	Pantothenic acid (B$_5$)
Pyridoxine (B$_6$)	Folate (B$_9$)	Vitamin B$_{12}$
Vitamin C	Vitamin D	Vitamin E
Calcium	Copper	Iron
Magnesium	Manganese	Phosphorus
Potassium	Selenium	Vitamin K
Zinc	Sodium*	

*While sodium is an essential nutrient, it was excluded from the calculation to prevent foods high in sodium from being penalized.

The results of Dr. Lalonde's analysis are below.

AVERAGE NUTRIENT-DENSITY SCORE OF SELECTED FOOD CATEGORIES (ADAPTED FROM LALONDE)	
CATEGORY	**AVERAGE NUTRIENT-DENSITY SCORE**
Organ meats	21.3
Herbs and spices	12.3

CATEGORY	AVERAGE NUTRIENT-DENSITY SCORE
Nuts and seeds	7.5
Cacao	6.4
Fish and seafood	6.0
Beef	4.3
Lamb, veal, and wild game	4.0
Vegetables (raw)	3.8
Pork	3.7
Eggs and dairy	3.1
Poultry	3.1
Processed meat	2.8
Legumes	2.3
Vegetables (cooked or canned)	2.0
Fruit	1.5
Plant fats and oils	1.4
Grains and pseudograins	1.2
Animal fats and oils	1.0
Canned grains	0.8

On the Lalonde scale, **organ meats are the most nutrient-dense foods by far, followed by nuts and seeds. Seafood, red meat, and wild game are more nutrient dense than raw vegetables; all forms of meat, fish, fruit, and vegetables (raw and cooked) are more nutrient dense than grains and pseudograins.**

Unfortunately, the USDA National Nutrient Database does not have data on bioavailability, so Dr. Lalonde was not able to take it into account in his analysis. However, had bioavailability been considered, given what we know about the antinutrients in legumes and grains, these foods would have been even lower on the scale when compared to organ meats, meats, dairy products, and fruits and vegetables. With this in mind, let's look at each category in more detail, using Dr. Lalonde's scale as the reference.

Organ meats

Calorie for calorie, organ meats are one of the most nutrient-dense foods on the planet according to Lalonde's scale. This is even more true when bioavailability is taken into account, since the amino acids, iron, zinc, and other vitamins and minerals organ meats contain are in highly absorbable forms. Even without taking that into consideration, Lalonde found that organ meats were nearly eighteen times more nutrient dense than whole grains and almost eleven times more nutrient dense than cooked vegetables. (This isn't a criticism of cooked vegetables as much as it is praise for organ meats! I will have much more to say about organ meats in chapter 9.)

Herbs and spices

Herbs and spices were second only to organ meats on the nutrient-density scale, with approximately half the score. But while it makes sense to consume a variety of herbs and spices for their nutrient value, they are unlikely to make a significant contribution to overall nutrient intake because of how little of them we eat.

Nuts and seeds

Nuts and seeds were third on the nutrient-density scale, with about one-third the score of organ meats. However, most nuts and seeds contain phytates, antinutrients that reduce the bioavailability of some of the minerals nuts and seeds contain. Fortunately, soaking nuts overnight and either dehydrating them (with a food dehydrator) or roasting them at low temperatures (150 to 170 degrees Fahrenheit) in an oven for four to eight hours breaks down much of this phytic acid and improves bioavailability. These methods also make nuts easier to digest, which is of particular benefit for those with sensitive digestive systems.

Cacao

Chocolate lovers will be happy to see that cacao was listed as the fourth-most-nutrient-dense food. Like nuts and seeds, cacao contains high levels of phytates; however, in the process of making chocolate, cacao is fermented, which is likely to break down some of the phytates and make the nutrients more bioavailable.

Fish and shellfish

On the nutrient-density scale, shellfish and fatty fish were the most nutrient-dense animal foods other than organ meats. Shellfish and fatty fish are indeed rich in several vitamins and minerals, but they're also the only significant source of DHA in the diet. As you'll learn in chapter 5, DHA is crucial to human health, and most Americans do not get enough.

Red meat

Beef, lamb, and wild game came just after seafood on the scale. This may surprise many of you, since red meat has been demonized for decades by the mainstream media and the medical establishment. (See page 48, "Does Red Meat Cause Heart Disease?," as well as the box below.) Yet one serving of beef (about 3.5 ounces) typically contains more B_{12}, niacin, vitamin E, vitamin D, retinol, zinc, iron, potassium, phosphorus, and EPA and DHA than the same amount of blueberries or kale, which are two of the most nutrient-dense plant foods. In addition, as is the case with organ meats, the nutrients in red meat are highly bioavailable when compared to foods like cereal grains, nuts and seeds, and legumes. Studies have shown that the bioavailability of zinc, for example, is four times higher in meat than it is in grains.

Vegetables (raw)

The placement of vegetables (both raw and cooked) on the ranking scale will likely come as the biggest surprise to most of you. Vegetables are a good source of many of the vitamins and minerals that were measured on this scale. They're also rich in some nutrients that weren't included in this nutrient-density scale but that an increasing number of studies suggest are beneficial, such as bioflavonoids and polyphenols. They are an important part of the diet for this reason. Note that raw vegetables would likely have scored lower if bioavailability had been considered because a portion of their nutrients are bound to compounds that are either difficult or impossible for humans to digest.

Pork

Pork is another meat that we are often told to avoid because of its high fat content. Yet it was more nutrient dense on this scale than legumes, cooked vegetables, fruit, and grains.

Eggs and dairy

One egg provides thirteen essential nutrients, all in the yolk (contrary to popular belief, the egg's yolk is far higher in nutrients than the white). Eggs are an excellent source of B vitamins, which are needed for vital functions in the body, and also provide good quantities of vitamin A, essential for normal growth and development. The vitamin E in eggs protects against heart disease and some cancers. Eggs from pasture-raised (but not conventionally raised) chickens contain significant amounts of vitamin D, which promotes mineral absorption and good bone health. Finally, eggs are one of the few significant dietary sources of choline, which helps maintain healthy cell membranes, nervous system function, immune balance, and cognitive function. Many people unnecessarily limit egg consumption because of concerns about cholesterol and heart disease, a misconception I will address in the bonus chapter on high cholesterol and heart disease available on my website.

The dairy category on the scale included yogurt, cheese, and milk. Dairy is one of the few good sources of retinol and calcium, which are difficult to obtain elsewhere in the diet. Dairy protein is also highly absorbable, which I'll explain in chapter 9.

Poultry

Poultry was found to be less nutrient dense than organ meat, red meat, and any type of seafood. That said, it's still a good source of bioavailable protein and other nutrients, especially niacin and selenium.

Processed meats

Processed meats were more nutrient dense than legumes, cooked vegetables, fruits, and grains. This is in large part because processed meats are made from red meat and pork, both of which scored highly on the nutrient-density scale. Some studies have shown an association between processed-red-meat consumption and cardiovascular disease and premature death, but people who eat more processed meat are also more likely to engage in other unhealthy behaviors that could increase their risks. Moderate consumption of processed meats within the context of a nutrient-dense, whole-foods diet is unlikely to cause problems.

Legumes

Legumes scored higher than cooked vegetables and fruit but lower than most animal foods. Like grains, nuts, and seeds, legumes contain significant amounts of phytates. This means that many of the minerals found in legumes will not be absorbed unless they are soaked, sprouted, or fermented prior to consumption. Most traditional societies that included legumes in their diet did this, but people living in Western industrialized societies rarely do. If you go to a Mexican restaurant and eat a bean burrito, for example, it's almost certain that the beans were not prepared in a way that reduced the phytates.

Vegetables (cooked)

Cooked vegetables scored lower than raw vegetables for three reasons. First, some of the cooked vegetables contained more water, which diluted the nutrient concentration. Second, the water used to boil vegetables washed away nutrients. Third, heat destroyed some of the nutrients that were included in the analysis. However, the nutrients in cooked vegetables are more bioavailable than those in raw vegetables because cooking breaks down some of the compounds in raw vegetables that limit nutrient absorption. This makes up for at least some of the nutrients lost in the process of cooking.

Fruit

Though fruit placed below all forms of meat and fish, eggs, dairy, legumes, and vegetables in terms of nutrient density, it remains a nutritious addition to the diet, and an especially important source of vitamin C.

Plant fats and oils

This category includes oils from olives, nuts, seeds, avocados, and coconuts. In general, fats — whether from animals or plants — are not significant sources of micronutrients. However, it's important to note that many nutrients in vegetables are fat soluble, which means they require the presence of fat for optimal assimilation. Eating steamed vegetables with butter, or salad greens with olive oil and avocado, will markedly improve your absorption of the nutrients in those vegetables.

The suitability of fats for human nutrition depends more on the specific fatty acids they contain. For example, many plant oils are high in omega-6 linoleic acid, which can promote inflammation when consumed in excess. I'll discuss this in more detail in chapters 4 and 5.

Cooked grains and pseudocereals

Cooked grains and pseudocereals were close to the bottom of the list, ahead of only animal fats and canned grains. (Pseudocereals produce cereal-like grains but, unlike true cereals, are not classified as grasses; some examples are quinoa, millet, and amaranth.) Since most grains and pseudocereals contain phytates, they would have scored even lower had bioavailability been taken into account. Though Dr. Lalonde didn't test whole and refined grains separately, refined grains would certainly have a lower score than whole grains. This is significant because 85 percent of the grain consumed in the United States is in the highly refined form, and refined flour accounts for approximately 20 percent of calories consumed by the average American.

Animal fats and oils

As I mentioned above, fats and oils aren't a significant source of micronutrients. But they are required to absorb fat-soluble vitamins, which are crucial to health, and along with glucose, they are the main source of energy for the body. In addition, some animal fats do contain modest amounts of uncommon nutrients like retinol and vitamin K_2 (in butter from pastured cows) and vitamin D (in lard).

Canned grains

The canned-grains category is made up primarily of cooked and creamed corn. As I explained above, even fresh, cooked whole grains and pseudo-cereals are low in nutrient density, so it's not surprising that canned grains are even lower on the scale.

Dr. Lalonde's scale, which utilized a wide-ranging and exhaustive amount of nutritional data and science, suggests that a diet based on fish, meat, eggs, dairy, vegetables, nuts and seeds, fruits, and herbs and spices provides all of the essential nutrients we require and in sufficient quantities, an approach that is consistent with the Personal Paleo Cure. Despite some nutrition experts' claims to the contrary, there is absolutely no need for grains or legumes in the human diet—these foods have been part of our species' diet for only a tiny fraction of our evolutionary history.

DOES RED MEAT CAUSE CANCER?

Some studies suggest that red meat increases the risk of cancer, especially colon cancer. Is that true?

One of the fundamental tenets of scientific research is that correlation does not imply causation. In other words, just because two things are correlated—that is, appear together—doesn't mean that one caused the other. In some observational studies, people who ate more

(continued)

red meat tended to die earlier and get more cancer than people who ate less. However, it's possible that it's not red meat but some other lifestyle factor that's causing the increased mortality and cancer.

In the majority of the red-meat studies, people who ate the most red meat were also the most likely to smoke, the least physically active, and the least likely to take multivitamins (the health effects of which are unknown, though it is a proxy marker in our culture of how health conscious someone is). Those who ate red meat frequently also had higher body mass indexes and alcohol intake; were more likely to eat processed food, sugar, and other less healthy foods; and had higher rates of diabetes. Perhaps it's not the hamburger that's increasing cancer and mortality risk but the highly refined flour bun or sugary chocolate milk shake on the side?

When all of this is taken into account, the case against red meat falls apart. In 2011, a research group published a study in the prestigious journal *Obesity Reviews* criticizing the epidemiological studies linking red meat and colorectal cancer. They performed a critical analysis of thirty-five studies that claimed to associate red meat with cancer and concluded that "the currently available epidemiological evidence is not sufficient to support an independent positive association between red meat consumption and colorectal cancer."

So rest easy. You can safely return steaks and hamburgers to your plate.

MAXIMIZING NUTRIENTS: YOUR PERSONAL PALEO CURE

- Build your diet around foods that are highest on the nutrient-density scale, like organ meats, meat, fish, poultry, dairy, eggs, nuts and seeds, vegetables, fruits, and herbs and spices. (And don't forget dark chocolate!)
- Avoid or significantly reduce your intake of foods that are lowest on the nutrient-density scale, like grains, pseudograins, and legumes.

CHAPTER 4

Three Foods to Avoid: Minimizing Toxicity in Your Diet

If exchanging the standard American diet for a full-scale Paleo diet feels overwhelming, you can still take a major step toward hitting the reset button by eliminating three toxins that contribute significantly to modern disease. Here they are:

- Gluten (grains aren't superfoods)
- Industrial seed oils (anything but heart-healthy)
- Refined sugar (in a word, *toxic*)

At the simplest level, a toxin is something capable of causing disease or damaging tissue when it enters the body. When most people hear the word *toxin*, they think of pesticides, heavy metals, and industrial pollutants. But even beneficial substances, like water, which is necessary to sustain life, are toxic at high doses.

The body has a built-in detoxification system that was designed to process and excrete toxins in small amounts. However, the detox system evolved over millions of years in an environment that was relatively pristine in comparison to the modern environment; earlier humans were simply not exposed to the range or volume of toxins we face today.

Notes for this chapter may be found at ChrisKresser.com/ppcnotes/#ch4.

This is important to understand as we examine the role of dietary toxins in contributing to modern disease. Most people won't get sick from eating a small amount of the foods I discuss in this section. But if we eat them in excessive quantities, the risk of developing modern diseases rises significantly.

That's exactly what's happening today. These three food toxins — gluten-containing grains, industrial seed oils, and refined sugar — make up the bulk of the modern diet. Bread, pastries, muffins, crackers, cookies, soda, fruit juice, and fast food and other convenience foods are all loaded with these toxins. In the United States, vegetable oils, grain flour, and table sugar (along with dairy and alcohol) make up 70 percent of the total calories Americans consume each day. When the majority of what most people eat on a daily basis is toxic, it's not hard to understand why their health is failing.

Let's look at each of these food toxins in more detail.

GLUTEN

Plants, like animals, have a biological imperative to survive and reproduce. But unlike animals, plants can't run away from predators (like humans). They have had to evolve other mechanisms for protecting themselves. These include:

- Producing toxins that damage the lining of the gut
- Producing toxins that bind essential minerals, making them unavailable to the body
- Producing toxins that inhibit digestion and absorption of essential nutrients, including protein

One of these toxic compounds is the protein gluten, which makes up 80 percent of the protein found in wheat, barley, and rye. Due to modern food-processing techniques, gluten can often be found in trace amounts in products containing other grains, such as oats and corn.

Celiac disease (CD) was initially described in the first century by a Greek physician named Aretaeus of Cappadocia. But neither Aretaeus nor anyone else knew that CD was caused by an autoimmune reaction to gluten, a protein in wheat. That didn't become clear until 1950—almost two millennia later—when Willem Dicke, a Dutch pediatrician, conclusively proved that gluten was the culprit. Dicke's discovery saved millions of people from the dangers of untreated celiac disease, which include malnutrition, stunted growth, cancer, severe neurological and psychiatric illness, and even death.

Since then, the mainstream view of gluten intolerance has been relatively black and white: Either you have celiac disease, in which case even a small amount of gluten will send you running to the bathroom in three seconds flat, or you don't, and you can chug down beer and munch bagels without fear. This all-or-nothing view has led some doctors to tell patients who suspect they're sensitive to gluten but who test negative for CD that they're simply imagining the affliction.

It turns out those doctors are wrong. We now know that *it's possible to have gluten intolerance without having celiac disease*—a condition known as non-celiac gluten sensitivity (NCGS)—and that gluten intolerance is more a spectrum of conditions than a single condition, with full-blown CD on one end, complete tolerance on the other, and NCGS in the middle. Let's discuss each of these three possible reactions to gluten in more detail.

(1) Celiac disease

Celiac disease is an autoimmune disease characterized by an inflammatory response to gluten and damage to the tissue in the small intestine. Signs and symptoms typically include diarrhea, bloating, abdominal pain, fatigue, lethargy, and malnutrition. But CD can also manifest with atypical signs and symptoms, ranging from chronic headaches to dermatitis to joint pain to insomnia.

Celiac disease has become dramatically more common over the past half a century. According to a study that compared blood samples from U.S. Air Force recruits sixty years ago with more recent samples, CD has increased by 400 percent during that period. Today, official statistics indicate that celiac disease affects between 0.7 percent and 1 percent of the U.S. population, but many experts in the field of gluten intolerance believe the actual prevalence is higher. Why the spike in CD? We don't know for certain, but many scientists believe that changes in gut micro-biota as well as changes in the way wheat is cultivated play roles.

Contrary to popular belief, celiac disease is not simply a digestive dis-order. One in two new patients diagnosed with CD does not have gut symptoms. For every diagnosed case of CD, there are 6.4 cases that remain undiagnosed—the majority of which are atypical or silent forms with no damage to the gut. This silent form of CD is far from harmless, however; it is associated with a nearly fourfold increase in the risk of death from all causes.

These findings surprised many researchers and physicians, because it was long believed that the damage done by CD was limited to the gastro-intestinal tract. But research over the past few decades has revealed that gluten intolerance can affect almost every other tissue and system in the body, including (but not limited to) the brain, endocrine system, stom-ach, liver, blood vessels, smooth muscle, and even the nuclei of cells.

This explains why CD is associated with numerous diseases. The fol-lowing is only a partial list of them:

- Type 1 diabetes
- Multiple sclerosis
- Dermatitis herpetiformis
- Autoimmune thyroid disease
- Osteoporosis
- Heart failure
- Depression
- ADHD
- Arthritis
- Migraine
- Allergies
- Asthma
- Obesity

How could a single condition be associated with such an astonishing array of diseases? CD causes the gut barrier to become permeable. As

I explain in chapter 10, when this happens, large proteins and gut microbes leak across the gut barrier and provoke a chronic, low-grade inflammatory response. But this response isn't limited to the gut; it can affect nearly every tissue in the body, as the list of conditions above suggests.

"REMOVING GLUTEN PUT MY HASHIMOTO'S INTO REMISSION"

Elise, age twenty-nine, came to me complaining of symptoms of Hashimoto's disease, an autoimmune condition in which the immune system attacks the thyroid gland and eventually causes hypothyroidism. Elise had several symptoms related to poor thyroid function, including difficulty concentrating and memory issues, constipation, hair loss, cold hands and feet, and crushing fatigue. Hashimoto's is diagnosed by measuring levels of antibodies to thyroperoxidase (TPO), an enzyme required to make thyroid hormones, and to thyroglobulin (TG), a protein in the thyroid gland. "I have high levels of thyroid antibodies," she said, "but the doctors told me there's nothing I can do about it."

I explained to Elise that the key to treating her thyroid condition was to balance and regulate her immune system. I also explained that there's a strong association between both celiac disease and non-celiac gluten sensitivity and Hashimoto's. I suggested she remove gluten (and all grains) from her diet for a period of ninety days. "I couldn't believe what happened," she said. "I felt so much better that I was able to go off Synthroid [prescription thyroid medication] completely. But if I ever fall off the wagon and eat gluten, my thyroid symptoms come back almost immediately." Gluten was aggravating Elise's immune system, which in turn exacerbated her Hashimoto's disease. When she removed gluten from her diet, her immune system settled down—and so did the attacks against her thyroid gland, which is what enabled her to get off her medication.

(2) Non-celiac gluten sensitivity

There's no consensus on the exact definition of non-celiac gluten sensitivity yet, but the most common understanding is that it's a reaction to gluten that is not autoimmune (like CD) or allergic (like wheat allergy). Another way of defining it is a reaction to gluten that resolves when gluten is removed from the diet and after CD and a gluten allergy have been ruled out. It's difficult to estimate the prevalence of NCGS because there is no definitive diagnostic test for it (see the "Testing for Celiac Disease and Gluten Intolerance" sidebar below for more on this). Another problem is that the symptoms associated with NCGS are so broad and non-specific (meaning they could be attributed to any number of causes) that many patients and doctors don't suspect it, and thus doctors don't order the necessary testing.

Even with these limitations, some estimates suggest NCGS may occur in as many as one in ten people, or approximately thirty million Americans.

While some mainstream medical professionals continue to insist that NCGS doesn't exist, scientists have validated it as a distinct clinical condition. In one major study, researchers reviewed the charts of 276 patients with irritable bowel syndrome (IBS) who had been diagnosed with NCGS using a double-blind, placebo-controlled wheat challenge (patients were put on a gluten-free diet and then given capsules containing either wheat or an inert substance). As a whole, the NCGS group had a higher frequency of anemia, weight loss, self-reported wheat intolerance, and a history of childhood food allergies than those in the IBS without NCGS group. The authors concluded that their data "confirm the existence of non-celiac wheat sensitivity as a distinct clinical condition."

As with celiac disease, NCGS can affect almost every cell, tissue, and system in the body. The list of documented signs and symptoms is diverse (and far too long to give in its entirety here!) but includes primarily:

- IBS-like symptoms, including abdominal pain, bloating, changes in stool frequency

- Difficulty concentrating and memory issues
- Headache
- Fatigue
- Joint and muscle pain
- Numbness and tingling in the arms and legs
- Dermatitis (eczema or skin rash)
- Depression
- Anemia

There is a particularly strong connection between NCGS and neurological and psychiatric diseases, including schizophrenia, autism, and even depression. For example, studies suggest up to 40 percent of patients with ataxia (problems with balance and coordination) and 25 percent of schizophrenic patients produce antibodies to gluten. And while the relationship to autism is less clear in the scientific literature, anecdotal evidence from the autism community indicates that gluten-free diets are very effective in some cases.

TESTING FOR CELIAC DISEASE AND GLUTEN INTOLERANCE

Dr. Alessio Fasano, a pioneer in the field of gluten intolerance, has proposed that a positive diagnosis for CD can be made if any four of the five factors below are present:

- The patient has typical symptoms of CD (diarrhea, bloating, abdominal pain, fatigue, lethargy, and malnutrition).
- The patient has elevated antibodies to alpha-gliadin (a type of gluten protein) or tissue transglutaminase-2 (an enzyme found in the gut and other organs).
- The patient improves on a gluten-free diet.
- The patient has a positive small-intestine biopsy (that is, there are indications of intestinal damage).

(continued)

- The patient has the genes that predispose him or her to CD (known as HLA-DQ2 and HLA-DQ8).

What about diagnosing NCGS? This turns out to be far more complicated because of the current limitations of laboratory testing: many people can react to parts of the wheat compound that are not screened for during most gluten-intolerance tests. That's why most experts on gluten sensitivity agree that the only reliable test for NCGS is a gluten challenge. This involves removing gluten from the diet completely for a period of at least thirty days (though preferably three months) and then adding it back in. If symptoms improve during the elimination period and return when gluten is reintroduced, a diagnosis of NCGS can be made.

However, for many people, a gluten-free diet isn't enough. Some grains that don't contain gluten, such as corn, oats, and rice, contain proteins that are similar enough in structure to gluten to elicit an immune response in people with CD or NCGS. Moreover, about 50 percent of patients with CD show signs of intolerance to casein (a protein in milk), and up to 30 percent of CD patients continue to have symptoms or clinical signs after adopting a gluten-free diet. This is one reason why the Step 1 Reset forbids all grains and dairy.

For detailed information on issues surrounding laboratory testing for NCGS as well as for information on a new NCGS lab test that may be helpful for some, please see ChrisKresser.com.

(3) Tolerance

The final category of response to gluten is tolerance. Dr. Weston Price, the American dentist who studied the health of traditional peoples (see pages 27–28), documented cultures that maintained excellent health while also consuming gluten-containing grains, such as the people of the Loetschental Valley in Switzerland. If gluten can make so many ill, why did these people remain so healthy? We don't currently understand all of the factors that contribute to gluten sensitivity, but genetics certainly plays a strong role in CD, and it probably does in NCGS as well. Researchers believe that patients who test negative for the two main genes associated with celiac disease — HLA-DQ2 and HLA-DQ8 — are significantly less likely to have NCGS. Diet, the gut flora, immune status, and other factors we don't yet understand all influence susceptibility to NCGS and CD.

The problem is it's difficult to know what category of gluten response you're in. Fewer than one in six people who have CD are aware they have it, and the percentage is almost certainly lower in the case of NCGS. The testing is flawed, and the symptoms are so broad and nonspecific that many doctors and patients with symptoms not typically associated with gluten sensitivity will overlook the possibility of NCGS or CD. Another issue is that we don't currently understand what moves someone from tolerance to intolerance or sensitivity.

Considering the seriousness of the conditions that gluten sensitivity can cause, the fact that there is no need for gluten in the human diet, and the low nutrient density and bioavailability of gluten-containing grains, I recommend that everyone perform a gluten challenge to determine whether he or she is intolerant. If you have a reaction to gluten when you add it back into your diet after the three-month period without it, it's crucial that you strictly avoid gluten indefinitely. If you do not react to gluten, I still recommend avoiding it for the most part because of its potential to cause harm and our uncertain understanding of what shifts people from tolerance to intolerance. That said, if you don't have an obvious reaction to gluten, an occasional piece of bread or gluten-containing food when you're out with friends or traveling is unlikely to cause problems.

THE MYTH OF HEALTHY WHOLE GRAINS

At this point you may be asking yourself, *If the nutrient-density scores for grains are so low, even without taking bioavailability into account, and gluten is so potentially toxic, why are these grains constantly referred to as healthy?* That's a great question, and it's not easy to answer quickly. There are many reasons for the emphasis on grains in the American diet, including their low price and ease of storage, a

(continued)

widespread lack of understanding of the nutrient inhibitors they contain, and the misguided fear of animal foods that has swept our nation over the past sixty or so years.

But the low nutrient scores of grains and their potential toxicity should make you question the American Heart Association's recommendation that you consume six to eight servings of grains a day. Following this advice will almost certainly result in your eating a less nutrient-dense diet, especially if the grains are in refined form (which is by far the most common way they are consumed in the industrialized world).

In addition to their generally low nutrient density, grains have significant nutritional shortcomings. For example, they contain no retinol (active vitamin A) at all and, with the exception of yellow corn, no beta-carotene (retinol's precursor) either. Nor do grains contain vitamin C or vitamin B_{12}. In the context of a mixed diet containing fish, meat, and fruits and vegetables, these shortcomings aren't particularly problematic. But in people following grain-heavy vegetarian and vegan diets, they can be serious problems.

Poor nutrient content is not the only thing to be concerned about when it comes to grains. As I've explained in this chapter, many grains contain proteins capable of provoking an immune response or allergic reaction. Gluten, which is found in wheat, barley, rye, and (sometimes) oats, is the best example of this.

Overall, the evidence indicates that grains are a suboptimal food source when compared to meat, fish, vegetables, fruits, and nuts. Does that mean you should strictly avoid them 100 percent of the time? Not necessarily. In my clinical practice, I've found that most people feel better without any grains or legumes in their diets. However, if you're fundamentally healthy, and you're following a nutrient-dense diet, you may be able to tolerate them in moderation. If you do choose to include grains and legumes in your diet, they should be prepared properly (soaked, sprouted, or fermented) to improve nutrient bioavailability and inactivate food toxins, and they should never replace more nutrient-dense foods like animal products, vegetables, and fruits. See my website for links to resources on how to properly prepare grains and legumes.

INDUSTRIAL SEED OILS

Industrial seed oils are oils made from the seeds of plants such as corn, soybean, cotton, sunflower, and safflower. Historically they've been used in a variety of applications, ranging from manufactured products (e.g., soaps, candles, perfumes, cosmetic products, and insulators) to lubricants to pet-food additives to fuel (e.g., biodiesel). (Their use in the preparation and manufacturing of so many products is why they're referred to as "industrial" seed oils.) But today they're marketed primarily as heart-healthy oils and used in just about all processed, packaged, and refined foods, as well as in most restaurant kitchens. This has led to a dramatic increase in the consumption of these oils. For example, intake of soybean oil has increased by more than a thousandfold since the early 1900s, and consumption of linoleic acid, the primary fatty acid in seed oils, has risen by more than threefold.

We're only beginning to understand the consequences of such a dramatic increase in seed-oil consumption, but based on current evidence, I believe they should be minimized in the diet for three reasons:

- They contain high amounts of linoleic acid (LA), which some research suggests is harmful when consumed in excess.
- They are easily oxidized (damaged), and oxidative damage is associated with numerous modern inflammatory diseases.
- There's no strong evidence that they protect against heart disease in humans, and there is some evidence that they may increase the risk.

Let's look at each of these reasons in more detail.

Excess linoleic acid

Linoleic acid (LA) is an essential fatty acid, which means the body requires it for proper function but can't synthesize it and must obtain it from the diet. However, the actual requirement for LA is very small: as little as 0.1 percent of total calories consumed per day. Studies show that intake of LA in the modern diet averages between 4 and 10 percent of total calories per day (mostly from highly processed seed oils), which means we're getting up to one hundred times the amount required.

In contrast, most traditional cultures had very low intakes of LA, and what they got came exclusively from whole foods like vegetables, nuts and seeds, and meat. As you'll see below, LA from industrial seed oils has a different effect on the body than LA from whole foods, because it is more likely to oxidize.

Oxidative damage

Linoleic acid is highly vulnerable to oxidation when exposed to heat (during food processing or cooking). It promotes the formation of compounds called OXLAMs, which are by-products of LA associated with a variety of diseases ranging from Alzheimer's to fibromyalgia to nonalcoholic fatty liver disease (NAFLD). OXLAMs are a major component of oxidized LDL and atherosclerotic plaques, and play a central role in development of heart disease. Oxidized linoleic acid causes atherosclerosis in animal studies, and at least one human study has shown that higher intake of LA in the presence of risk factors for oxidative damage (like smoking) increases the risk of heart disease. Reducing linoleic acid intake has been shown to decrease circulating OXLAM levels.

High intakes of linoleic acid are particularly problematic when the long-chain omega-3 fat DHA, found exclusively in seafood, is absent from the diet. This creates a pro-inflammatory environment in the body and may also interfere with neurological function because of the important role DHA plays in the brain and nervous system. Unfortunately, the combination of high LA intake and low DHA consumption is a common scenario in the typical modern diet, which is high in processed and refined foods and low in cold-water, fatty fish.

Heart disease

For years we've been taught that saturated fats found in such foods as red meat and butter will clog arteries and cause heart attacks and that vegetable oils are a heart-healthy alternative. As of 2013 the American Heart Association still recommended using liquid vegetable oils (like corn, safflower, sunflower, soybean, and canola oils) or nonfat sprays for cooking and drastically limiting use of coconut oil, butter, palm oil, and other saturated fats.

Yet these recommendations are based on outdated evidence that is decades old. While it's true that some early studies suggested that vegetable oils were heart-healthy, those studies did not distinguish between the effects of omega-3 and omega-6 polyunsaturated fats (which I'll cover in the next chapter) found in these oils. More recent research that studied the effects of omega-3s and omega-6s separately found that vegetable oils high in omega-6 linoleic acid did not prevent heart disease and in fact may actually increase the risk. One study demonstrated that, compared to control subjects, patients who increased their intake of linoleic acid and reduced their saturated-fat intake had a higher risk of death from cardiovascular disease and all other causes. This occurred despite a reduction in LDL and total cholesterol in these patients. An analysis of other randomized controlled trials—considered the gold standard of medical evidence—also found that higher intakes of linoleic acid increased the risk of heart disease and death.

Finally, it's important to note that industrial seed oil has almost no nutritional value: it is a calorie-dense but nutrient-poor substance. Given the serious health problems it can contribute to and the fact that it was entirely absent from the diets of healthy, traditional cultures, I think it's wise to avoid industrial seed oils as much as possible.

REFINED SUGAR

Studies going back more than forty years have shown that naturally occurring sugars in fruits and vegetables are beneficial to health and do not promote weight gain. Traditional cultures like the Hadza of north-central Tanzania and the Kuna of Panama obtain a large percentage of their total calories from foods that are high in natural sugars, such as fruit, starchy tubers, and honey. Yet they are remarkably lean, fit, and free of modern disease.

However, excess refined sugar—in the form of table sugar and high-fructose corn syrup—is a different story. Added sugars are harmful primarily because they promote overeating and weight gain. When people add fat to their diets, they tend to eat less of something else (usually carbohydrates), and if they eat more carbs, they'll usually eat less fat. However, the same kind of swap is not true for increased sugar intake—especially when the sugar is in liquid form (e.g., soft drinks and other sugar-sweetened beverages). Most people fail to reduce their caloric intake to compensate for the extra calories they're consuming in sweetened drinks. For example, a study of 323 adults found that subjects who increased the number of calories they obtained from sugar-sweetened beverages didn't then decrease the amount of calories they got from other foods and thus had greater calorie intake overall. Another study showed that total calorie intake among sixteen patients was greater on the days that sugar-sweetened beverages were given at lunch than on the days they weren't. Added sugar causes weight gain whether it's eaten in the form of glucose or fructose; contrary to popular belief, excess fructose is no more fattening than excess glucose.

Excess weight isn't just a cosmetic problem—it contributes directly to metabolic and cardiovascular disease. Studies consistently show that overeating and fat gain cause insulin resistance. Insulin resistance, in turn, is associated with diseases ranging from diabetes to heart disease to Alzheimer's.

Added sugar can also cause problems in the digestive tract, where it promotes bacterial overgrowth in the small intestine and may cause gas, bloating, and constipation or diarrhea. Excess fructose may be particularly harmful for the gut; it's poorly absorbed and leads to bacterial fermentation and excess gas production, particularly in people with digestive problems. In fact, there's almost no end to the list of problems too much refined sugar in the diet can cause. About twenty years ago, Nancy Appleton, PhD, began researching all the ways in which sugar destroys health. Over the years, the list has continuously expanded, and it now includes 141 points. Here's just a small sampling (the entire list can be found on her blog). Excess sugar:

- Suppresses the immune system
- Causes imbalances of essential minerals like copper and zinc
- Decreases tissue elasticity and function

- Interferes with nutrient absorption
- Causes tooth decay
- Decreases growth hormone levels
- Contributes to depression and other mood disorders
- Increases the risk of breast cancer

There's a lot more to the Paleo diet than removing food toxins from your diet. That said, if everyone on a standard American diet stopped eating cereal grains, industrial seed oils, and excess sugar tomorrow, I'm willing to bet that the rates of obesity, diabetes, heart disease, and just about every chronic inflammatory disease would plummet over the next decade. As I said at the start of this chapter, if going on a full-scale Paleo diet seems overwhelming or if you're not prepared to do it for whatever reason, begin with eliminating (or at least greatly reducing) these toxins in your diet. If you're like most of the people I've worked with, you'll feel like a different person. And that will give you the motivation and energy you need to take the next steps toward feeling even better.

MINIMIZING TOXINS:
YOUR PERSONAL PALEO CURE

- Avoid gluten completely during the Step 1 Reset and for at least two months afterward (for a total of ninety days). Then reintroduce and see how your body reacts.
- If you feel better without gluten and worse when you reintroduce it, you are gluten-intolerant and should strictly avoid it. If you don't react adversely, I still recommend avoiding or minimizing gluten, but you may choose to have it occasionally as part of your 80/20 rule (a slice of birthday cake, Mom's lasagna, or a piece of bread when you're dining out).
- Avoid industrial seed oils and refined sugar. They are high in calories, low in nutrients, and may contribute to inflammation and other health problems. As with gluten (assuming you're not gluten-intolerant), you may choose to have small amounts of them infrequently as part of your 80/20 rule.

CHAPTER 5

Fats as Fuel:
Give Yourself an Oil Change

Fats are a primary energy source for the body. They also play a role in maintaining healthy skin and hair, regulating body temperature, supporting immune function, insulating internal organs, and aiding in the absorption of the fat-soluble vitamins (A, D, E, and K).

But fats, in general, get a bad rap in our heart-healthy and fat-obsessed diet culture, partly because we're trained to put fat in the foods-to-avoid category. A food that is described as high-fat sets off alarm bells for most of us. But, as you're about to see, not all fats affect the body in the same way, and while some are harmful, many have beneficial, life-extending properties. When you follow your Personal Paleo Cure, you'll find that it's easy to select the right variety and combination of fats.

THE FACTS ON FAT

Gasoline and diesel are both fuel that cars can run on. If you put gasoline in a diesel engine, or vice versa, the engine may run but it won't run well — or for very long. In a similar way, the human body can run on the entire range of fats (combined with carbohydrates and proteins). But it runs much better on the types it was designed to run on, and if you eat too much of the other kinds, the body will eventually break down.

Notes for this chapter may be found at ChrisKresser.com/ppcnotes/#ch5.

Let's begin by examining the different types of fat to determine which are the preferred fuels for the human body.

The main fats we encounter in foods are:

- Saturated fats (long- and medium-chain)
- Monounsaturated fats
- Trans fats (natural and artificial)
- Polyunsaturated fats

During the Step 1 Reset, it's best not to worry too much about macronutrient ratios. That said, as a starting place, choose a rough target for carbohydrate intake based on your individual circumstances (see chapter 18 for more on this) and eat that amount. Your remaining calories will come from protein and fat, and since most people naturally eat the amount of protein their bodies need, you also won't have to think about how much fat to eat; that will fall into place without any calculations on your part. For example, say you decide to shoot for 30 percent of calories from carbohydrates. In the United States, most people get about 15 percent of their calories from protein. That means your fat intake would be about 55 percent of calories. This may be much more fat than you're accustomed to eating, especially if you've been following a low-fat, high-carbohydrate diet. But remember that the *quality* of fat you eat is often more important than the *quantity* when it comes to health and even weight regulation.

With this in mind, let's take a closer look at the various types of fat and their effects in the body.

SATURATED FATS

All fats are made up of molecular chains of carbon, hydrogen, and oxygen atoms. They are classified as short, medium, or long, based on the length of the molecular chain.

Long-chain saturated fats (such as myristic, palmitic, and stearic acid) are found mostly in the milk and meat of ruminant animals like cattle and sheep. They form the core structural fats in the human body, making up 75 to 80 percent of fatty acids in most cells, and they're the primary storage form of energy. In other words, when the body stores excess energy from food for later use, it stores it primarily as long-chain saturated fat. Unlike polyunsaturated fats and carbohydrates, like glucose and fructose, saturated fats have no known toxicity—even at very high doses—if insulin levels are in a normal range. Long-chain saturated fats are more easily burned as energy than polyunsaturated fats, and the process of converting saturated fat into energy leaves no toxic by-products. In fact, it leaves nothing but carbon dioxide and water.

Saturated fats have many other benefits. They:

- Play an important role in bone health by helping to incorporate calcium into the skeletal system
- Protect the liver from damage by alcohol, medications such as acetaminophen, and toxins
- Have beneficial effects on cardiovascular function, including reducing levels of lipoprotein(a)—also known as Lp(a)—an inflammatory substance in the blood that promotes heart disease, which subsequently reduces mortality caused by stroke. They also improve lipid profiles by increasing HDL (which you probably know as the good cholesterol, as opposed to the bad cholesterol, LDL), decreasing triglycerides, and making LDL particles larger and more buoyant, which means they are less likely to cause harm.
- Support healthy immune function
- Deliver the fat-soluble vitamins A, D, K, and E to the cells and tissues of the body
- Regulate the availability of beneficial polyunsaturated fatty acids like DHA

Main dietary sources

Fattier cuts of beef, lamb, and pork; cream, whole milk, butter, ghee. They are found in smaller amounts in coconut products and egg yolks.

FOODS AND OILS RICH IN SATURATED FAT	
FOOD	**SATURATED FAT, %**
Coconut oil	87%
Dairy products	64%
Tallow (beef)	50%
Palm oil	49%
Beef, chuck roast	40%
Lard*	39%
Beef, brisket	39%
Beef, ground (20% fat)	38%
Duck fat	33%
Chicken fat	30%
Egg yolks	30%

*Lard from conventional, grain-fed pigs is also very high in omega-6 linoleic acid, which is harmful in excess quantities. Look for lard from pastured pigs.

Verdict: Eat liberally

Along with monounsaturated fats (which we'll discuss shortly), saturated fats should make up the bulk of your fat intake.

If you're worried about saturated fat causing heart disease, it's true there are certain situations where saturated-fat intake should be moderated, and I'll explain those in later chapters. However, for most healthy people, the evidence that saturated fat leads to heart disease is weak at best. For decades we've been told that eating saturated fat increases cholesterol levels in the blood and that high cholesterol levels clog arteries and cause heart disease. But does the research actually support that theory?

Some studies do show that increased saturated-fat intake raises blood cholesterol levels. But these studies are almost all short-term, lasting only a few weeks. Longer-term studies have not shown an association between saturated-fat intake and blood cholesterol levels. In fact, of all of the long-term studies examining this issue, only one of them showed a clear association between saturated-fat intake and cholesterol levels, and even that association was weak. Perhaps saturated fat contributes to heart disease by some mechanism other than raising cholesterol? Not according to the research. A large review of twenty-one studies covering almost 350,000 participants found no association between saturated-fat intake and cardio-vascular disease. Moreover, studies on low-carbohydrate diets (which tend to be high in saturated fat) suggest that they not only don't raise blood cholesterol but have several beneficial impacts on cardiovascular-disease risk markers. (For detailed information on these studies and other findings, please see the notes for this chapter on my website.)

Medium-chain saturated fats (and medium-chain triglycerides) are found in coconut milk and breast milk, and they have unusual properties. They're metabolized differently than long-chain saturated fats: they don't require bile acids for digestion and they pass directly to the liver via the portal vein. This makes medium-chain saturated fats a great source of easily digestible energy. They're so easy to digest, in fact, that they're used in the liquid hospital formulas fed to patients who have had sections of their intestine removed and aren't able to digest solid food.

In addition to being a good energy source, medium-chain saturated fats have therapeutic properties:

- They're high in lauric acid, a fat found in mother's milk that has antibacterial, antiviral, and antioxidant properties.
- They promote weight loss. They have a lower calorie content than other fats; they are not stored in fat deposits as much as other fats; and they enhance fat burning (by thermogenesis).
- They promote the development of ketones, one of two substances (along with glucose) the brain can use as fuel. Ketones and

ketone-generating diets have been shown to benefit several neuro-logical conditions, including seizure disorders, Parkinson's, and Alzheimer's.

Main dietary sources:

Coconut: its flesh, oil, milk, and butter

Verdict: Eat liberally

Coconut oil is an especially good cooking fat, because it's not as vulnerable to the oxidative damage that occurs with high-heat cooking using other fats.

HOW TRADITIONAL FATS HELPED KARA GET PREGNANT

Kara was thirty-six years old and had been trying to get pregnant for two years when she came to see me. When I reviewed her diet I noticed that she was drinking skim milk and severely limiting other traditional saturated fats like butter, ghee, lard, and coconut oil.

This isn't unusual, of course; people have been told for decades that saturated fat will clog arteries and cause heart disease. Yet many traditional cultures emphasize the importance of these fats in pro-moting optimal health, and this is especially true during the precon-ception period. For example, the Masai tribe in Africa allowed women to become pregnant only after they'd spent several months drinking full-fat cow's milk in the wet season, when the grass is lush and the nutrient content of the milk is especially high.

Modern research has confirmed that saturated fats may promote fertility. A study at the Harvard School of Public Health found that women who ate two or more servings of low-fat dairy foods per day, particularly skim milk and yogurt, increased their risk of infertility by more than 85 percent compared with women who ate less than one serving of low-fat dairy food per week. I instructed Kara to reincor-porate traditional saturated fats into her diet and switch from nonfat to full-fat dairy products. After just three months on this new dietary

(continued)

regime, Kara e-mailed me with the news: she was pregnant! Kara continued eating this way throughout her pregnancy (gaining a normal amount of pregnancy-related weight) and delivered a healthy eight-pound, two-ounce baby girl.

MONOUNSATURATED FATS

Monounsaturated fats, such as oleic acid, are found primarily in olives, avocados, some meats, and certain nuts, like macadamias. Like saturated fats, monounsaturated fats form the core structural fats of the body and are nontoxic even at high doses. Interestingly, monounsaturated fats seem to be the only fats that typically fat-phobic groups, like the American Heart Association, and fat-friendly groups, like the Atkins diet organization and other low-carbers, can agree are completely healthy.

Monounsaturated fats are also known for their beneficial effects on cardiovascular-disease risk markers. They reduce LDL and triglycerides and increase HDL, decrease oxidized LDL, reduce oxidation and inflammation, lower blood pressure, decrease thrombosis (the formation of blood clots), and may reduce the incidence of heart disease. Some studies also suggest that monounsaturated fats promote healthy immune function.

Main dietary sources:

Olives, olive oil, avocados, lard (pork fat), duck, chicken, egg yolk, macadamia nuts, almonds.

DIETARY SOURCES OF MONOUNSATURATED FAT	
FOOD	**MONOUNSATURATED FAT, %**
Macadamia nuts	77%
Olives and olive oil	74%
Avocado	64%

FOOD	MONOUNSATURATED FAT, %
Almonds	62%
Duck fat	49%
Egg yolks	46%
Lard	45%
Chicken fat	45%
Tallow (beef)	42%
Butter	26%

Verdict: Eat liberally

But be aware that certain foods that are high in monounsaturated fats, like nuts and avocados, can contain significant amounts of linoleic acid, an omega-6 polyunsaturated fat. As I'll explain below, linoleic acid is pro-inflammatory if consumed in high amounts when intake of EPA and DHA are low.

TRANS FATS

There are two types of trans fats: **natural** and **artificial.**

Naturally occurring trans fats are formed when bacteria in the stomachs of grazing animals, such as cows or sheep, digest the grass the animal has eaten. Conjugated linoleic acid, or CLA, is a natural trans fat found in moderate amounts (between 2 and 9 percent of total fat) in grass-fed-animal meat and dairy products, and to a lesser degree in grain-fed-animal products. It is also produced in our bodies from the conversion of other naturally occurring trans fats in those same animal products.

Research over the last two decades suggests that CLA may protect against several different diseases. For example:

- CLA is inversely associated with heart disease. In other words, those who eat higher amounts of CLA have a lower risk of heart disease, and vice versa.

- CLA may help prevent and manage type 2 diabetes by improving glucose tolerance and insulin sensitivity, and observational studies show an inverse association between CLA levels in fat tissue and diabetes risk.
- CLA has been shown to reduce the risk of cancer, primarily by blocking the growth and metastatic spread of tumors, controlling the cell cycle, and by reducing inflammation.
- Some research suggests that CLA can help reduce body fat and promote weight loss in those who are overweight or obese.

Artificial trans fats have slightly different chemical structures than the natural trans fats found in beef and butter. But these minor differences in structure lead to dramatically different effects in the body. While natural trans fats may reduce the risk of cancer, heart disease, obesity, and inflammatory conditions, artificial trans fats have been shown to *increase* the risk of those diseases — even at relatively low doses.

Their effects on cardiovascular health are particularly harmful. They promote inflammation, damage the fragile linings of the blood vessels, increase the number of LDL particles, reduce HDL cholesterol, and reduce the conversion of shorter-chain omega-3 fats into DHA. Artificial trans fats are the quintessential junk food because they provide no benefit, have no role in human physiology, and cause significant harm.

Main dietary sources:

- **Natural trans fats:** Dairy and meat from pastured animals are the best sources of CLA and other natural trans fats. In fact, products from 100 percent grass-fed animals contain three to five times more CLA than products from grain-fed animals. And since CLA is in the fat, the best sources will be fattier cuts of meat, bone marrow, high-fat dairy products like butter and whole milk, and full-fat cheeses.
- **Artificial trans fats:** These are found in highly processed, refined, and fried foods (doughnuts, margarine, fast food, frozen food, chips, cookies, crackers, candy, and so on); packaged foods (for

example, instant soups, cake mixes, microwave popcorn, and fla-vored rice and pasta mixes).

FOODS HIGH IN NATURALLY OCCURRING CLA	
FOOD	CLA, MG/G FAT*
Cow's milk	3.4–23.6
Beef	3.7–17
Lamb	5.6–14.9
Butter	4.7–14.1
Goat's milk	5.8–10.5
Yogurt (cow's milk)	2.8–10.5
Cheese (cow's milk)	2.9–9.8
Cheese (goat's milk)	2.7–6.3

*Milligrams of CLA per gram of fat. The large range of values dis-played is due to the fact that the amount of CLA in a product largely depends on whether the animals were grass fed (higher val-ues) or grain fed (lower values), though altitude, the bacteria in the grazing animal's stomach, and other factors may play roles.

FOODS HIGH IN ARTIFICIAL TRANS FAT*	
FOOD	TRANS FAT, G/SERVING
White Castle Haas chocolate frosted doughnuts	9 g
Long John Silver's breaded clam strips	7 g
Celeste Pizza for 1	5 g

(continued)

FOOD	TRANS FAT, G/SERVING
Marie Callender's lattice apple pie	5 g
Pop Secret popcorn (butter flavor)	5 g
Pillsbury Grands! biscuits	3.5 g
Safeway Creme Wafer Cookies (vanilla)	3.5 g
Jimmy Dean croissant sandwiches	3 g
Sara Lee Chocolate Mint Creme Pie	3 g
Land O'Lakes margarine	2.5 g
Betty Crocker pie-crust mix	2.5 g

*Artificial trans fats are found exclusively in processed foods. Note that food manufacturers are not required to list trans fats on nutrition labels if the per-serving portion contains less than 0.5 grams; however, if you eat more than one serving of a food such as potato chips (many brands list 0 g of trans fat), you may be getting several grams of trans fat.

Verdict:

- **Conjugated linoleic acid (CLA): Eat pastured-animal meat and dairy products (if you tolerate them) to obtain CLA.** Note that CLA supplements do not have the same benefits as naturally occurring CLA. Most CLA supplements are derived from linoleic acid in safflower oil, and some studies have shown that CLA supplementation in humans can cause fatty liver disease, inflammation, unfavorable changes in lipid profiles (high LDL cholesterol and triglycerides and low HDL cholesterol), and insulin resistance. Furthermore, CLA supplements have not demonstrated the beneficial effects seen from dietary intake of CLA in human trials.
- **Artificial trans fats: Avoid like the plague.**

POLYUNSATURATED FATS

Polyunsaturated fats can be divided into two categories: **omega-6** and **omega-3**. Omega-3 fats are present in green leaves and algae (and the animals that eat them), and omega-6 fats are found primarily in seeds (as well as in the animals that eat them).

Polyunsaturated fats play both a structural and regulatory role in the body. They help form cell membranes, regulate gene expression, and aid in cell function. Omega-3 and omega-6 fatty acids have specific effects on the cells close to where they are formed, including both pro-inflammatory and anti-inflammatory effects. In general, both too much omega-6 and too little omega-3 cause inflammation, while restricting omega-6 and getting adequate omega-3 will prevent inflammation.

Polyunsaturated fats are a complex subject involving a lot of biochemistry. I'm going to spare you the unnecessary details, but there are a few basic concepts you'll need to understand about them before we proceed.

- Like all fats, polyunsaturated fats are chains of carbon, hydrogen, and oxygen atoms.
- There are **six different omega-6 fats** and **six different omega-3 fats.** They are classified by the length of their chains (that is, the number of carbon atoms each chain has) and the number of carbon-carbon double bonds.
- Essential fatty acids are the shortest-chain polyunsaturated fats. They are called essential fatty acids because they're required for the body's proper function but can't be produced by the body and thus must be obtained from the diet. There is **one essential omega-6 fat (linoleic acid)** and **one essential omega-3 fat (alpha-linolenic acid).**
- Linoleic acid (LA) and alpha-linolenic acid (ALA) are converted into longer-chain derivatives in our bodies. **The most important long-chain omega-6 fat is arachidonic acid (ARA), and the most important long-chain omega-3 fats are EPA and DHA.**

- Though linoleic acid and alpha-linolenic acid are considered essential because they can't be manufactured in the body, the **longer-chain derivatives (ARA, EPA, and DHA) are primarily responsible for the health benefits** we get from polyunsaturated fats.

With that in mind, let's take a closer look at omega-6 and omega-3 fats.

Omega-6

Linoleic acid (LA) is the essential omega-6 fatty acid. It is found in small or moderate amounts in a wide variety of foods, including fruits, vegetables, cereal grains, and meat. But it is present in large amounts in industrial processed and refined oils, like soybean, cottonseed, corn, safflower, and sunflower. These oils are ubiquitous in the modern diet, present in everything from salad dressing to chips and crackers to restaurant food. LA is also relatively high in most nuts and in all poultry, especially in dark meat with skin.

The evidence suggests that a moderate intake of linoleic acid from whole foods like poultry, vegetables, and nuts and seeds is unlikely to cause problems in the context of a diet containing sufficient amounts of long-chain omega-3 fats like EPA and DHA. But when linoleic acid is consumed in excess amounts—especially in the form of industrial seed oils (which have a tendency to oxidize)—and when intake of EPA and DHA is low, LA has a pro-inflammatory effect and may contribute to modern chronic diseases.

Arachidonic acid (ARA) is a longer-chain omega-6 fat that can be produced in our bodies using linoleic acid. It is also found in animal foods like chicken, eggs, beef, and pork, because animals are also capable of making this conversion. ARA is present in cell membranes, involved in cellular signaling (aiding cells in exchanging information), and can also act as a vasodilator (relaxing the blood vessels). It is necessary for the growth and repair of skeletal muscle tissue, and, along with DHA, it is one of the most abundant fatty acids in the brain. You may have seen stories in the media claiming that eating meat and other animal products causes inflammation in the body. This is based on the idea that ARA leads to the production of inflammatory compounds. Animal products are high in ARA, so it stands to reason that eating animal products would increase inflammation. Right?

Not so fast. While it's true that the compounds derived from ARA can be pro-inflammatory, recent evidence suggests that they may have important anti-inflammatory actions as well. Moreover, it's now clear that ARA serves as a precursor for a potent group of compounds that help reduce and resolve inflammation. (A precursor is a substance — in this case, ARA — from which another substance can be formed.) ARA is needed to make a class of molecules called lipoxins, which trigger the release of anti-inflammatory compounds synthesized from EPA and DHA. In epidemiological studies, higher plasma levels of ARA, EPA, and DHA were associated with the lowest levels of inflammatory markers. And clinical studies have found that adding up to 1,700 milligrams of ARA per day to the diet (an amount far greater than the average U.S. intake of 100 to 500 milligrams per day) does not promote inflammation.

Main dietary sources:

- **Omega-6 linoleic acid:** Found in whole foods like nuts, seeds, poultry, and avocados; also present (in large amounts) in industrial seed oils like corn, soybean, cottonseed, safflower, and sunflower. These oils are ubiquitous in processed and refined foods, and most restaurant kitchens cook with them (because they're so cheap).
- **Omega-6 arachidonic acid:** Found primarily in animal foods such as meat, poultry, and eggs.

INDUSTRIAL SEED OILS WITH HIGH OMEGA-6 CONTENT	
OIL	OMEGA-6, %
Safflower oil	72%
Sunflower oil	63%
Corn oil	52%
Wheat germ oil	53%
Soybean oil	49%
Cottonseed oil	50%
Peanut oil	31%
Canola oil	18%

FOODS WITH HIGH OMEGA-6 CONTENT	
OIL	OMEGA-6, %
Chicken leg	19%
Chicken breast w/skin	18%
Chicken breast w/o skin	17%
Ham	13%
Duck, roasted	12%
Tilapia	11%
Eggs*	11%
Bacon	10%

*Eggs are low in total fat, so the relatively high percentage of omega-6 is not a concern. Also, eggs from pastured chickens that are not grain-fed are likely to have a lower percentage of omega-6 than eggs from conventionally raised chickens. See chapter 8 for more on this.

Verdict:

- **Omega-6 linoleic acid (LA): Limit** LA intake to moderate consumption of whole foods like nuts, avocados, and poultry. Avoid industrial seed oils as much as possible.
- **Omega-6 arachidonic acid (ARA): Eat liberally** in animal foods such as meat, poultry, and eggs. Intake of more than five times the average has been shown to be safe.

Omega-3

Alpha-linolenic acid (ALA), the essential omega-3 fat, is found in plant foods such as walnut and flax. Eicosapentaenoic acid (EPA) and docosahexaenoic acid (DHA) are the most important long-chain omega-3 fats (and now you know why it's easier to refer to them as EPA and DHA!). They are found in seafood and, to a lesser extent, in the meat and fat of ruminant animals.

While ALA is considered essential, it's really EPA and DHA that are responsible for the benefits we get from eating omega-3 fats. (Some researchers have even proposed that DHA be considered an essential fatty acid, because, like ALA and LA, it's essential for human health and must be obtained from the diet to ensure adequate levels.)

A common misconception is that we can meet our omega-3 needs by taking flax oil or eating plant foods containing ALA. It's true that the body can convert *some* ALA to EPA and DHA. But that conversion is extremely inefficient in most people. On average, less than 5 percent of ALA gets converted into EPA, and less than 0.5 percent of ALA gets converted into DHA. Since this conversion depends on adequate levels of nutrients such as B_6, zinc, and iron, these numbers are likely to be even lower in vegetarians, the chronically ill, and the elderly. During the Paleolithic era, consumption of EPA and DHA averaged between 450 and 500 milligrams per day—a figure that greatly exceeds current intakes, which average around 90 to 160 milligrams per day for most Americans. This finding, along with the research indicating extremely poor conversion of ALA to DHA, suggests that we evolved to eat *preformed* EPA and DHA — in other words, readily available EPA and DHA that does not have to be converted from ALA. Research suggests that the ALA-to-EPA/DHA conversion pathway may not have been used at all by our ancestors.

The complete absence of preformed, ready-to-eat DHA in plant foods other than marine algae (which isn't exactly a staple in Western cuisine) is one of the primary reasons I believe vegetarian and vegan diets are not optimal for health.

How too much omega-6 and not enough omega-3 is making us sick

One of the most profound differences between traditional, ancestral diets and the modern, industrialized diet is the balance of essential fatty acids consumed. Anthropological research suggests that human intake of omega-6 and omega-3 fats was relatively low throughout most of our history (around 4 percent of total calories), with a ratio of omega-6 to omega-3 of between 1:1 and 2:1.

Today, Americans' intake of omega-6 fat is far higher than the evolutionary norm, primarily due to increased consumption of industrial seed oils. In addition, we're eating much less omega-3 than our ancestors used to. Despite a slight increase in fish consumption in recent years (fish being a primary dietary source for omega-3), intake is still far below historical levels. These changes have shifted the range of omega-6-to-omega-3 ratios in the modern diet to between 10:1 and 20:1, with a ratio as high as 30:1 in some individuals! This is between five and thirty times higher than the ratio has been for most of human history. Many scientists believe that this increase in total polyunsaturated fat intake, as well as the dramatic rise in omega-6 consumption relative to omega-3, is at least in part to blame for the rise of chronic conditions like obesity, type 2 diabetes, metabolic syndrome, autoimmune disease, and cardiovascular disease.

Why EPA and DHA are so important

A large body of evidence indicates that EPA and DHA are essential to health and that a deficiency of EPA and DHA has played a significant role in the epidemic of modern inflammatory disease. In general, inadequate intakes of EPA and DHA cause systemic inflammation. Systemic inflammation—the body's response, through the production of white blood cells and other substances, to infection or other threats—is associated with nearly every modern chronic disease, from arthritis to Alzheimer's to autoimmune disorders to gastrointestinal diseases. For example:

- Even modest consumption of EPA and DHA (200 to 500 mg/d) reduces deaths from heart disease by 35 percent—an effect much greater than that observed with statin-drug therapy.
- DHA is essential for the proper development of the brain and preservation of brain function as we age. Low levels of DHA in pregnant women are associated with lower scores in learning and memory tasks in their offspring, and low DHA levels in the elderly are associated with multiple markers of impaired brain function.
- Regular consumption of fish or fish oil reduces overall risk of death (that is, total mortality) by 17 percent. Statin drugs reduce total mortality by only 15 percent—and even then, only in populations at very high risk of heart disease.

HOW EATING MORE FISH AND LESS VEGETABLE OIL HELPED MARK TO WALK WITHOUT PAIN

Mark, age sixty-two, had been an avid golfer his entire life. He played eighteen holes at least three times a week for more than twenty years, and he always walked the course. A few years before he came to see me, however, he began experiencing pain in his shoulders and knees. It got so bad that he had to start using the golf cart, and, more recently, he had stopped playing altogether because he couldn't swing a club without pain.

(continued)

I looked at Mark's diet and noticed that he was eating a lot of omega-6 fat. He ate at restaurants every day during the week (he went out to lunch near his office and got takeout for dinner at least twice a week at home) and often on the weekends too, and his main cooking oil was canola (because he was trying to avoid saturated fat). At the same time, Mark wasn't eating much omega-3 at all. The only fish he ate was an occasional can of tuna—which is low in EPA and DHA.

I asked Mark to start bringing a lunch to work and to cut back on takeout at home. Restaurant kitchens use primarily industrial seed oils rich in omega-6 linoleic acid to prepare their food, because these oils are so cheap. I also alleviated his fears about saturated fat and instructed him to cook with ghee, coconut oil, butter, tallow, and lard instead of canola oil. Finally, I told Mark to eat at least four five-ounce servings of cold-water, fatty fish, like salmon, mackerel, herring, or sardines, every week.

After six weeks on this program, Mark came back to the office beaming. He was able to walk without pain for the first time in three years, and he was back out on the golf course—on foot, instead of in the cart. Don't underestimate the power of simple dietary changes!

How to raise your EPA and DHA levels

There are two ways to increase your levels of EPA and DHA:

- Significantly reduce the amount of LA you consume.
- Eat sufficient amounts of preformed EPA and DHA.

Both of these steps are important. As you've read, even when intake of LA is low, the conversion of ALA to EPA and DHA is negligable. And eating too much LA—even with adequate EPA and DHA intake—can be harmful. As I explained in chapter 4, excess LA has been shown to cause vitamin E depletion, intestinal dysbiosis, oxidative damage, and inflammation as well as contribute to weight gain, liver disease, cancer, autoimmune disease, inflammatory bowel disease, and premature aging.

Main dietary sources:

- **Omega-3 ALA:** Found in fruits, vegetables, nuts and seeds, especially walnuts and flax
- **Omega-3 EPA and DHA:** EPA and DHA are found primarily in cold-water, fatty fish, like salmon, mackerel, herring, sardines, anchovies, and bass, as well as in shellfish, like oysters and mussels, and, to a much lesser extent, in meat from grass-fed animals and from wild game. It's important to note that freshwater fish, many species of ocean fish, and farmed fish are generally lower in EPA and DHA and therefore not as beneficial.

FOODS HIGHEST IN EPA AND DHA	
FOOD	**EPA + DHA PER 3 OZ.**
Caviar (fish eggs)	5.5 g
Herring	1.8 g
Salmon, farmed	1.8 g
Anchovy	1.7 g
Mackerel	1.5 g
Salmon, wild	1.5 g
Bluefin tuna	1.3 g
Oyster	1.1 g

Verdict:

- **Omega-3 alpha-linolenic acid (ALA): Consume in moderation** in whole foods like fruits, vegetables, and seeds. Avoid large amounts of flax oil and flax seed, which unnecessarily increase total polyunsaturated fat intake without significantly increasing EPA and DHA.

- **Omega-3 EPA and DHA: Eat liberally.** How much fish should you eat to get the benefits of EPA and DHA? According to some studies, death from heart disease can be reduced by 25 percent or more if you consume about 3.5 grams of EPA plus DHA per week. This is equivalent to about ten ounces a week of wild salmon. However, studies of Western populations without substantial amounts of EPA and DHA in their diets (and with higher amounts of LA in their diet) suggest a continued reduction of cardiovascular disease when an individual consumes up to seven grams of EPA and DHA per week, which is about twenty ounces of wild salmon. With this in mind, I recommend the following:
  - If you're healthy and free of heart disease and your intake of LA is relatively low, aim for the lower-end target of 3.5 grams of EPA/DHA, or ten ounces of fish a week.
  - If you're at risk for heart disease or you're unable to significantly reduce your intake of LA (perhaps you eat out a lot), aim for the upper end of the range at 7 grams of EPA/DHA or twenty ounces per week.

Be aware that, depending on the dose of EPA and DHA, it takes about three to six months to reestablish a healthy balance of long-chain omega-3 polyunsaturated fats in the tissues.

Why not just take twenty grams of fish oil per day to change your tissue levels of EPA and DHA as quickly as possible? The answer is that all polyunsaturated fats are highly vulnerable to oxidative damage—a process associated with cancer, heart disease, and other inflammatory conditions—and EPA and DHA are no exception. In fact, they are the most vulnerable of all fats. A randomized trial showed that six grams per day of fish oil increased oxidative damage in healthy men regardless of whether their diets were supplemented with 900 IU of vitamin E (an antioxidant).

This argues for getting the majority of EPA and DHA from cold-water, fatty fish in the diet rather than from fish oil. Supplementing with fish oil should be reserved for therapeutic purposes and should usually be short-term and limited to two to three grams per day, depending upon background fish intake. The exception would be cod-liver oil, which tends to have relatively low levels of EPA and DHA compared to other fish oils but is rich in important fat-soluble vitamins like A and D. (I'll discuss cod-liver oil and therapeutic supplementation with fish oil in later chapters.)

FATS AT A GLANCE: WHAT TO EAT, WHAT TO AVOID

Saturated fats and monounsaturated fats should form the bulk of your fat intake. The omega-3 fats EPA and DHA and the omega-6 fat arachidonic acid should be consumed regularly, while omega-6 linoleic acid should be consumed only in whole-food form (nuts, seeds, avocados) in moderate amounts. See my website for a printable version of this chart that you can put on your fridge.

EAT LIBERALLY	EAT IN MODERATION	AVOID
Coconut oil	Sesame oil	Soybean oil
Palm oil	Walnut oil	Peanut oil
Olive oil	Pecan oil	Corn oil
Ghee	Almond oil	Safflower oil
Butter	Flaxseed oil	Wheat-germ oil
Lard*	Avocado oil	Canola oil
Tallow (beef and lamb)	Nuts and seeds	Sunflower oil
Duck fat*	Nut butters	Cottonseed oil
Dairy fat		Grape-seed oil
Macadamia oil		Rice bran oil
Eggs, meat, and seafood		

*Choose pasture-raised-animal lard and duck fat. Conventional alternatives are significantly higher in omega-6 linoleic acid, which should be limited.

When choosing fats for cooking, it's important to be aware of their smoke point. The smoke point is the temperature at which the flavor and nutritional integrity of the fat or oil begin to break down. Once an oil exceeds its smoke point, it will usually produce a bluish and pungent smoke that is irritating to the eyes. Oils that have passed their smoke point are likely to contain oxidized fats, which have been shown to damage cells and contribute to numerous diseases.

I've listed the approximate smoke point of various fats and oils below. For high-heat cooking, choose fats with the highest smoke points, such as ghee, extra-light (not extra-virgin) olive oil, palm oil, expeller-pressed (refined) coconut oil, macadamia oil, and beef tallow. Butter, extra-virgin olive oil, and extra-virgin coconut oil have relatively low smoke points and are best for noncooking uses (for example, putting them on previously cooked foods).

FAT	SMOKE POINT (°F)
Ghee	485
Olive oil (extra light)	468
Palm oil	455
Coconut oil (expeller pressed)*	450
Macadamia oil	413
Beef tallow	400
Duck fat	375
Lard	370
Coconut oil (extra virgin)	350
Olive oil (extra virgin)	320
Butter	250–300

*Expeller-pressed coconut oil is nearly odorless and tasteless, which is advantageous for those who do not like the taste of coconut. See my website for specific brand recommendations and information about where to obtain these fats and oils.

FATS: YOUR PERSONAL PALEO CURE

- Saturated and monounsaturated fats from meat, poultry, animal fats, nuts and seeds, avocados, coconut, olives, and dairy products should form the foundation of your fat intake.
- Eat pastured-animal meat and dairy products (if you tolerate them) to obtain conjugated linolenic acid, a healthy form of trans fat.
- Avoid industrial seed oils as much as possible. They are almost completely devoid of nutrients and associated with numerous health problems.
- Eat between ten to twenty ounces of cold-water, fatty fish, like salmon, mackerel, herring, anchovies, or sardines, each week. The higher end of the range is for those who are still eating a significant amount of industrial seed oil and/or who have cardiovascular disease or other inflammatory conditions.
- Avoid high doses (greater than 3 grams a day) of fish oil, which can promote oxidative damage.

CHAPTER 6

Choosing Carbs for Energy: Glucose, Fructose, and Fiber

Carbohydrates are one of the two main energy sources (the other is fat) for humans. They are found in many foods, including refined grains and sugars that have contributed to so much modern disease. But there are many excellent (and often overlooked) dietary sources for healthy carbohydrates that you'll learn about in this chapter as you continue to construct your Personal Paleo Cure.

First, however, let's look at how carbs work. In the body, all carbohydrates in food are ultimately broken down and converted into simple sugars (glucose and fructose) or indigestible fiber. But while glucose, fructose, and fiber are all technically carbohydrates, they each have different effects on the body. Let's look at each of them in more detail.

GLUCOSE

Glucose is a simple sugar (or monosaccharide) found mostly in plant foods like fruits, vegetables, starches, and grains. It can be broken down from sweeteners like table sugar (sucrose) and honey. Glucose has three main uses in the body:

- It forms structural molecules called glycoproteins.

Notes for this chapter may be found at ChrisKresser.com/ppcnotes/#ch6.

- Like fat, it is a source of energy for cells (especially in the brain).
- It's a precursor to compounds that play an important role in the immune system.

Glucose preceded fatty acids as a fuel source for living organisms by a very long time, and it is the building block of foods that have the longest evolutionary history of use by mammals like us. The fact that glucose can be broken down in the body from protein is often used as an argument that we don't need to eat glucose. But rather than viewing this as evidence that glucose isn't important, we might view it as evidence that glucose is so metabolically essential that we evolved a mechanism to produce it even in its absence in the diet.

One of the few differences between the human digestive tract and that of a true carnivore, like a lion, is that humans produce an enzyme called amylase. Amylase allows us to digest starch—a long chain of glucose molecules we can't absorb—into single molecules of glucose that easily pass through the gut wall into the bloodstream.

While glucose from fruits, vegetables, and starches is generally well tolerated, too much of it—in the form of sucrose-sweetened beverages or concentrated sweeteners, for example—can cause weight gain and metabolic problems.

FRUCTOSE

Fructose is another simple sugar found primarily in fruits and vegetables. While it has the same chemical formula and caloric content as glucose, it has a different structure and is processed differently. Rather than being absorbed by the cells, it is shunted directly to the liver for conversion into glucose or fats. About 50 percent of fructose ends up as glucose, 25 percent becomes lactate (a chemical produced during normal metabolism and exercise), and 15 percent or more becomes glycogen, the principal storage form of glucose. The remainder is burned directly for energy, and a small portion—as little as 2 to 3 percent—is converted to fat.

There's little question that excess fructose from high-fructose-corn-syrup-sweetened beverages like sodas contributes to weight gain. One of the main reasons for this is that most people don't cut calories somewhere else to compensate for the additional calories that come from drinking a couple of sodas each day. They simply end up taking in more calories overall. It's also true that excess fructose has distinctly harmful metabolic effects when compared to glucose.

However, despite some claims to the contrary, there's no evidence that we should avoid whole fruit simply because it contains fructose. There's nothing fattening or toxic about fructose when it's consumed in moderate amounts from whole fruits and vegetables. And since whole fruit contains fiber and other nutrients, it's difficult to eat a lot of fruit without also reducing intake of other foods. Fruit has been part of our species' diet for as long as we've been recognizably human. We've adapted to eating it, and we're capable of processing the fructose it contains. Studies overall suggest that eating whole, fresh fruit may actually decrease the risk of obesity and diabetes and that limiting fruit intake has no effect on blood sugar, weight loss, or waist circumference.

While fructose in whole fruits and veggies is unlikely to cause metabolic problems, it can be an issue for some people with digestive disorders. When glucose is present in equal or greater amounts than fructose in a food, as it is in bananas, berries, and cantaloupe, the fructose will be well absorbed (because glucose helps with fructose absorption). However, when there's more fructose than glucose in a food, as is the case for apples, peaches, and papayas, that additional fructose will linger in the gut, where it is rapidly fermented by bacteria. If you have digestive issues, you may wish to limit foods with more fructose than glucose. Please see chapter 20 for more information on this.

FIBER

Fiber is plant matter that is indigestible to humans. There are two types of fiber: **soluble fiber** and **insoluble fiber.** Soluble fiber dissolves in water. It is fermented by bacteria in the colon, and creates a viscous, gel-like substance in the digestive tract. Insoluble fiber does not dissolve in water.

It is not fermented in the colon (with some exceptions), and it adds bulk to the stool. Soluble and insoluble fiber are often lumped together in discussions about the merits of fiber, but their effects on the body are quite different. This has caused confusion and led to dangerous dietary and supplement recommendations.

Many studies suggest that soluble fiber is important for human health. While we can't digest it, some of the one hundred trillion bacteria that live in the human gut can. Intestinal bacteria "eat" soluble fiber by fermenting it. In the process of fermenting the fiber, the bacteria produce short-chain fatty acids like butyrate, propionate, and acetate. These short-chain fats are the primary energy source for intestinal cells in the colon, and butyrate in particular has been associated with several health benefits. It has anti-inflammatory effects, increases insulin sensitivity, delays the development of neurodegenerative diseases, and has shown promise in the treatment of diseases of the colon such as Crohn's, IBS, and ulcerative colitis. Butyrate may play a role in healthy metabolic function, stress resistance, and the immune response. In fact, the benefits observed in epidemiological studies of a diet high in naturally occurring fiber are likely due to the higher butyrate production from these diets.

Soluble fiber may also protect against heart disease. Research shows a strong inverse association between dietary fiber intake and heart disease, heart attack, and peripheral artery disease. In one major study, subjects were followed for more than nineteen years, and those who had the highest dietary soluble fiber intake had a 15 percent lower risk of heart disease and a 10 percent lower risk of cardiovascular events than those who had less soluble fiber in their diets. Soluble fiber binds cholesterol, increases the activity of LDL receptors in the liver (which helps clear LDL from the bloodstream), improves insulin sensitivity, and increases satiety (the feeling of fullness), resulting in lower overall calorie consumption.

By contrast, most insoluble fibers (with the exception of resistant starch, which I'll discuss below) have only partial or low fermentability. Insoluble fibers provide a bulking action and tend to increase regularity, but they do not generate short-chain fatty acids like butyrate and thus don't have the same health benefits as soluble fibers. While soluble fiber has been shown to protect against heart disease, insoluble fiber has not. What's more, excess insoluble fiber can bind to nutrients such as zinc, magnesium, calcium, and iron, preventing their absorption.

The effects of whole-grain fiber (which is mostly insoluble) may be especially harmful. In one study involving men who had previously suffered heart attacks, there were 22 percent more deaths in the high-fiber group (these subjects nearly doubled their grain-fiber intake, going from 9 to 17 grams per day) than in the control group.

Resistant starch is an insoluble fiber with unique properties. Starch exists as large chains of glucose molecules in plants. Since humans produce amylase, an enzyme that breaks down starch, most forms of starch are easily absorbed in the digestive tract. However, resistant starch is unique among starches in that it cannot be broken down in the small intestine and digested by humans. But unlike other types of insoluble fiber, resistant starch can be fermented by gut microbiota in the large intestine to produce helpful short-chain fatty acids like butyrate. Resistant starch has several other benefits, including increasing the uptake of minerals like calcium, boosting levels of *Bifidobacteria* (a beneficial genus of bacteria in the large intestine), reducing harmful pathogens, improving gut motility, and reducing blood-sugar and insulin levels. On a Personal Paleo Cure diet, resistant starch is found in unripe bananas, potatoes that have been cooked and cooled, potato starch, plantain flour, tapioca flour, and some legumes (for those who tolerate them). It can also be used as a supplement for those with digestive and/or blood-sugar problems, which I'll discuss in future chapters.

Fiber is like most nutrients: too little or too much can cause problems. The best approach is to obtain fiber in the context of a whole-foods diet. Though soluble fiber is probably more beneficial than insoluble fiber, many foods in the Paleo diet—such as yams and sweet potatoes, green leafy vegetables, carrots and other root vegetables, fruits with edible peels (like apples and pears), berries, seeds, and nuts—contain both. There's no need to restrict insoluble fiber when it naturally occurs in these foods (unless you have digestive problems, which I'll discuss further in chapter 10). However, grains are high in insoluble fiber and low in bioavailable nutrients and are best avoided.

DOES A HIGH-FIBER DIET PREVENT COLORECTAL CANCER?

The Institute of Medicine recommends a daily fiber intake of thirty-eight grams for adult men and twenty-five grams for adult women obtained from dietary fibers (both soluble and insoluble) and functional fibers (that is, fiber that has been extracted from plant or animal sources and added to other foods). But is there any evidence to support these recommendations?

While initial studies seemed to support the theory that high-fiber diets protect against colorectal disease, later studies have not. Newer, better-designed epidemiological studies involving as many as thirty-eight countries worldwide found that increased dietary fiber was *not* associated with a reduction in colon cancer. Long-term longitudinal studies (a type of observational study that examines a particular variable, like fiber intake, over a long period) that included more than 725,000 participants found no association, and neither did interventional studies (a type of study in which one group receives some sort of intervention — in this case, a higher fiber diet — and the other group receives none). Finally, an analysis of five randomized clinical trials that evaluated almost forty-five hundred subjects found that increased fiber did not reduce the incidence of polyps in the colon. (Colorectal cancer often begins with polyps.)

There is little evidence indicating that very high-fiber diets or fiber supplements prevent colorectal disease. In the vast majority of cases, you can get all of the fiber you need from a whole-foods diet that includes vegetables, fruits, starchy tubers, nuts, and seeds.

WHICH DIETARY SOURCES OF CARBOHYDRATE ARE BEST?

Now that you have a better understanding of the different types of carbohydrate and how they are processed in the body, let's look at the best dietary sources of carbohydrate from a Paleo perspective. These should form the foundation of your carbohydrate intake during the Step 1 Reset. In Step 2, you may choose to reintroduce moderate amounts of other sources of carbohydrate, such as dairy products, certain grains like white rice and buckwheat, and concentrated sweeteners.

In Step 3, you'll explore how much carbohydrate is optimal for you based on your activity level, health status, digestive function, and other factors. During Step 1, the focus is on carbohydrate quality: replacing refined grains and sugars with the more nutrient-dense, whole-food carbohydrates listed below.

During the Step 1 Reset you can aim for approximately **15 percent to 30 percent of calories from carbohydrate.** For a moderately active male eating 2,600 calories a day, that comes out to **100 to 200 grams of carbohydrate** per day. For a moderately active female eating 2,000 calories a day, that comes out to **75 to 150 grams of carbohydrate** per day. Those with blood-sugar issues or who wish to lose significant amounts of weight should aim for 10 percent to 15 percent of calories from carbohydrate, which comes out to 65 to 100 grams on a 2,600-calorie diet, or 50 to 75 grams on a 2,000-calorie diet.

Nonstarchy vegetables

Nonstarchy vegetables include cruciferous vegetables (like broccoli and cauliflower), lettuces, winter greens, summer squashes, onions, tomatoes, asparagus, and more. Nonstarchy vegetables are excellent sources of micronutrients and fiber, but overall they are quite low in carbohydrates. Most have fewer than eighty calories of carbohydrates per pound, and those are typically in the form of glucose and fructose. What's more, some evidence suggests that the human body expends up to forty calories for every pound of nonstarchy vegetables consumed. This suggests a net gain of a mere forty calories per pound of vegetables eaten.

CARBOHYDRATE CONTENT OF SELECTED NONSTARCHY VEGETABLES*		
VEGETABLE	**MEASURE**	**CARBOHYDRATE, G**
Artichokes	1 medium	14
Parsnip	1/2 cup, slices	13
Rutabaga	1 cup, cubes	12
Collard greens	1 cup, chopped	11
Romaine lettuce (raw)	1/2 head	10
Green beans, snap	1 cup	10
Red pepper	1 cup, strips	9
Onion	1 medium	9
Mushrooms, white	1 cup, pieces	8
Turnip	1 cup, cubes	8
Beets	1/2 cup, slices	8
Kale	1 cup, chopped	7
Peas	1/4 cup	7
Broccoli	1 cup, chopped	6
Carrots (raw)	1 medium	6
Zucchini	1 cup, sliced	5
Cauliflower	1 cup (1-inch pieces)	5
Asparagus	4 spears	2

*Cooked, unless otherwise indicated.

Verdict: Eat liberally

I recommend consuming as many nonstarchy vegetables during the day as you like but *not counting them toward your total carbohydrate intake.*

Your optimal intake of nonstarchy vegetables will depend on digestive function (some of them are high in insoluble fiber, which can be hard on an inflamed gut) and personal preference, but approximately one pound per day is a good target for most people.

Fruits

Fruits contain a mixture of glucose and fructose. They also contain a wide range of micronutrients and are a good source of fiber (mostly soluble). Along with starchy plants (see next section), fruits should be a primary source of carbohydrates in your diet.

CARBOHYDRATE CONTENT OF SELECTED FRUITS		
FRUIT	**MEASURE**	**CARBOHYDRATE, G**
Banana	1 medium	27
Pear	1 fruit, medium	27
Pomegranate	1/2 fruit (4-inch piece)	27
Mango	1 cup, pieces	25
Apple	1 fruit (3-inch piece)	25
Pineapple	1 cup, chunks	22
Orange	1 fruit (3-inch piece)	18
Grapes	1 cup	16
Papaya	1 cup, 1-inch pieces	16
Peach	1 medium (2 2/3 inch)	14
Cantaloupe	1 cup, cubes	13
Strawberries	1 cup, halves	12
Watermelon	1 cup, diced	12
Blueberries	1/2 cup	11

FRUIT	MEASURE	CARBOHYDRATE, G
Raspberries	1/2 cup	8
Plum	1 fruit (2 1/8 inch)	8
Tomato	1 cup, chopped	7

Verdict: 3 to 4 servings of fruit a day is fine for most people

Those with insulin resistance, diabetes, or metabolic syndrome may see improvements by restricting fruit intake to one to two servings a day and by choosing fruits that are lower in sugar, like berries and melon. See chapter 18 for more on how to determine your optimal carbohydrate intake.

Starchy plants

Starchy plants include tubers like potatoes and sweet potatoes, roots like taro and yuca, and fruits like plantain and breadfruit. They are primarily broken down into glucose and are thus well absorbed by most people. There are a few caveats to this, however:

- Though all humans produce amylase (the enzyme that breaks down starch), some produce less of it than others and as a result may not tolerate starch as well.
- The intestinal bacteria feed on starch. This is generally a good thing. However, when there's an overgrowth of bacteria in the small intestine (as is often the case with digestive conditions like GERD and irritable bowel syndrome), starch may worsen the problem and cause gas, bloating, and changes in stool frequency.
- Those with diabetes, impaired glucose tolerance, or other problems with blood-sugar regulation may find that starch aggravates the condition.

The key, as always, is to experiment. I have patients with digestive and blood-sugar issues who are able to tolerate moderate amounts of starch without a problem.

HOW STARCHY PLANTS MADE RON REGULAR AGAIN

Ron, forty-six, came to see me complaining of constipation. He averaged only two to three bowel movements per week, and even those were not complete evacuations. His abdomen was bloated and tense most of the time, and his wife constantly complained about his bad breath.

While reviewing Ron's case history, I noticed that he had been on a very low-carb diet for several years. He told me that he wasn't constipated before going low-carb, but he had lost twenty-five pounds on the diet so he had stuck with it over the years. I asked Ron to add some starchy plants, like potatoes, sweet potatoes, taro, plantains, and yuca, back into his diet. I explained that these foods were high in fermentable fibers that feed healthy gut bacteria and that constipation is often caused by an imbalance of good and bad bacteria in the gut.

Ron was concerned about adding these foods back into his diet because of their carbohydrate content. He told me he'd been on a low-fat, high-carb diet prior to switching to low-carb, and he felt the high-carb intake had contributed to his weight gain. However, the carbs Ron was eating prior to going low-carb were almost all processed and refined. I explained to Ron that starchy plants are not only lower in carbohydrates than grain flours and sugar but higher in nutrients and less likely to promote overeating.

Within a few weeks of adding starch back into his diet, Ron began having a complete, daily bowel movement. His energy and sleep also improved, and despite his concern about gaining weight, he actually lost a few pounds.

I've listed several different starchy plants in the table below. If you can't find some of these at your local supermarket, check out ethnic markets in your area. You can often find taro and lotus root at Asian markets, for example, and yuca and plantains at Latin markets. You can make great fries with yuca and great chips with taro, especially if you roast them in duck fat or lard. See chapter 21 for recipes.

CARBOHYDRATE CONTENT OF SELECTED STARCHY PLANTS		
STARCHY PLANT	**MEASURE**	**CARBOHYDRATE, G**
Potato, russet	1 large	64
Tapioca	1/2 cup	63
Plantain	1 cup, slices	48
Taro	1 cup, sliced	46
Yuca* (aka manioc, cassava)	1/2 cup	39
Sweet potato	1 large	37
Yam	1 cup, cubes	37
Breadfruit	1/2 cup	30
Acorn squash	1 cup, cubes	30
Butternut squash	1 cup, cubes	22
Lotus root	10 slices	14

*Yuca should never be consumed raw because it contains toxins. To make it safe, place it in cold water, bring to a boil, and boil it for thirty minutes (make sure you discard the water).

Verdict: Starchy plants, along with fruits, should be the foundation of your carbohydrate intake

Your optimal intake of starchy plants will depend on several factors, which we'll explore in more detail in chapter 18. As a starting place, I'd recommend about one pound per day. That comes out to roughly two to four servings of starchy plants per day.

CARBOHYDRATES:
YOUR PERSONAL PALEO CURE

- Most people should aim to get between 15 and 30 percent of their total daily calories from carbohydrates. If you have blood-sugar issues or are trying to lose significant amounts of weight, aim for between 10 and 15 percent of total calories.
- Eat as many nonstarchy vegetables as you'd like throughout the day. How much you eat depends largely on personal preference and how well you digest them, because they don't make a significant contribution to total carbohydrate intake.
- Eat approximately two to five servings of fruit per day. If you have a blood-sugar issue or are trying to lose weight, aim for the lower end of the range and choose low-sugar fruits, like berries and melon. If you're lean, active, and have no blood-sugar issues, aim for the higher end of the range.
- Eat approximately two to four servings of starchy plants per day. If you're restricting carbs, eat fewer servings and smaller amounts of each serving.
- Avoid grains, concentrated sweeteners, and dairy products as carbohydrate sources during the Step 1 Reset. You'll have a chance to reintroduce some of these if you choose during Step 2.
- Avoid fortified fiber products and most fiber supplements. Soluble fiber or prebiotic supplements may be useful in some situations, which we'll discuss in later chapters.

CHAPTER 7

Proteins for Life:
Optimize Protein Quality

The great thing about protein, an essential nutrient for humans, is that most of us naturally eat the right amount of it without paying much attention. Our brains strongly influence our desire to consume it, based on how much our bodies need. You are probably very familiar with animal sources of protein (like meat and dairy) and plant sources as well (like soybeans). As with fats and carbohydrates, the quality of proteins—and what they do in your body once they are consumed—differs considerably, as you'll soon see.

Protein is vital to life because it is the building block of all body tissues; it can also be converted into glucose for energy. Protein molecules are composed of individual amino acids linked together in a chain. Amino acids can be divided into three categories: essential, nonessential, and conditional. Essential amino acids can't be produced by the body and must be obtained from the diet. Nonessential amino acids can be synthesized from essential amino acids or by breaking down proteins during digestion. Conditional amino acids are usually nonessential but can be essential in certain situations (for example, in times of chronic illness or stress).

There are two things to consider with protein: how much you should eat, and what type. I'll cover *how much* protein each person should eat in

Notes for this chapter may be found at ChrisKresser.com/ppcnotes/#ch7.

chapter 18, where we'll discuss further refining the diet for your particular circumstances. In this chapter we're going to focus more on what *types* of protein are optimal for human nutrition. The factors that determine protein quality include:

- **Amino acid profile.** Complete proteins contain all essential amino acids, whereas incomplete proteins are lacking in one or more essential amino acids.
- **Bioavailability.** No matter how much protein a food has, if you can't digest and absorb it, it won't benefit you.
- **Toxicity.** Some proteins are more likely than others to cause an immune response or allergic reaction.

The best proteins are those that contain all essential amino acids in a bioavailable form and have a low potential for toxicity.

WHICH PROTEINS ARE THE HIGHEST QUALITY?

Over the years, several different methods have been used to measure protein quality. While these methods provide useful information, each of them has significant shortcomings:

- *Protein efficiency ratio (PER).* Protein efficiency ratio determines the effectiveness of a protein by measuring how much weight an animal (usually a rat) gains after being fed a test protein. The problem is that the effects of a given protein on growth in rats doesn't necessarily correlate with its effects on growth in humans.
- *Biological value (BV).* Biological value measures how efficiently the body utilizes a protein consumed in the diet. A food with a high BV indicates a strong profile of essential amino acids. BV is limited in its usefulness, however, because it does not take into account several key factors that influence how protein is digested and absorbed.

- **Net protein utilization (NPU).** Net protein utilization is similar to BV, but it measures the retention of absorbed nitrogen more directly (nitrogen is a by-product of protein metabolism). NPU has the same shortcomings as BV.

To address these shortcomings, the Food and Agriculture Organization of the United Nations World Health Organization created a measure of protein quality called the protein digestibility–corrected amino acid score (PDCAAS). This method combines the amino acid profile of the protein (whether it's complete or incomplete) with the true fecal digestibility of the protein (how much of the protein is actually absorbed). PDCAAS values are expressed on a scale of 0 to 1, with 1 being the highest. This scoring method has been the preferred method for measuring protein value in scientific studies since it was introduced in 1989.

The table below lists the PDCAAS of some common animal and plant proteins.

PROTEIN TYPE	PROTEIN DIGESTIBILITY–CORRECTED AMINO ACID SCORE
Casein	1.00
Egg	1.00
Milk (casein and whey)	1.00
Whey protein	1.00
Chicken (light meat)	1.00
Turkey (ground)	0.97
Fish	0.96
Beef	0.92
Soybeans	0.91
Chickpeas	0.78

(continued)

PROTEIN TYPE	PROTEIN DIGESTIBILITY–CORRECTED AMINO ACID SCORE
Black beans	0.75
Vegetables	0.73
Legumes (average)	0.70
Kidney beans	0.68
Fruits	0.64
Rolled oats	0.57
Lentils	0.52
Peanuts	0.52
Tree nuts	0.42
Whole wheat	0.40
Wheat gluten	0.25

As you can see, without exception, animal proteins are of higher quality than plant proteins like legumes, grains, fruits, and vegetables. It would appear that soybeans are nearly as high quality a protein as beef.

However, although the PDCAAS is the most accepted method of measuring protein quality, one of its shortcomings is that it does not take antinutrients into consideration. Soy contains substances that have been shown to decrease protein absorption in the small intestine. These antinutrients are also present in other legumes (such as lentils and kidney beans) and cereal grains (such as wheat, corn, oats), and they've been shown to decrease assimilation of amino acids in these foods by as much as 50 percent. If the PDCAAS took this data into account, the scores for soy protein, other legumes, and cereal grains would be significantly lower than those listed in the table above.

It's clear that animal protein is superior to plant protein in terms of amino acid composition and bioavailability. But within the animal-protein category, some foods have more proteins than others. For those wishing to boost their protein intake (I'll discuss who might fall into this category in later chapters), it's helpful to know which animal products are the most concentrated protein sources. The table below lists the protein content of various animal foods based on a typical serving size.

PROTEIN CONTENT OF SELECTED FOODS		
FOOD	**MEASURE**	**PROTEIN, G**
Duck	1/2 duck	52
Sockeye salmon	1/2 fillet	43
Halibut	1/2 fillet	36
Rockfish	1 fillet	33
Tuna salad	1 cup	33
Beef, bottom round	3 oz.	30
Chicken, light meat	3 oz.	28
Lamb loin	3 oz.	26
Beef sirloin	3 oz.	25
Ham	3 oz.	25
Swordfish	1 piece	25
Yellowfin tuna	3 oz.	25
Pork spareribs	3 oz.	25
Chicken, dark meat	3 oz.	24
Turkey, light meat	3 oz.	23

(continued)

FOOD	MEASURE	PROTEIN, G
Cottage cheese	1/2 cup	14
Yogurt, whole milk	1 cup	8
Milk, whole	1 cup	8
Swiss cheese	1 oz.	8
Egg, whole	1 extra large	7

As you can see, seafood, poultry, and red meat are the most concentrated sources of protein. While dairy and egg proteins score highest on the PDCAAS, they are generally much lower in protein per serving than fish and meat.

"I ATE ALL THE TIME BUT I WAS STILL STARVING"

Emily, age thirty-two, came to see me complaining of severe fatigue. She could hardly get up in the morning, and she crashed in the afternoons. Up until about six months before our visit, she had been a competitive cyclist, but she had stopped competing because her performance and ability to recover after races and workouts had declined so rapidly. She began to notice extra fat around her waist and in her thighs for the first time in her life. She also had dark circles under her eyes, and her hair was falling out.

"I feel like I've aged about twenty-five years in the past two years," she told me. "I'm scared that I won't be able to ride again, and that this will just get worse." She had become a vegan about two years earlier. (She had been eating a standard American diet prior to going vegan.) At first she felt fantastic, and her performance and energy levels actually improved. But after about nine months she noticed some fatigue and a decline in her performance. She was also hungry all the time, and despite eating every two to three hours, she never felt fully satisfied. As time progressed her symptoms worsened and she decided to get help.

I explained to Emily that vegan diets were low in bioavailable, complete proteins. While on paper, it's possible to get enough protein by eating legumes, grains, and soy products, those proteins are not well absorbed or are lacking in essential amino acids. As she was a competitive athlete, her needs for highly digestible, complete protein were even higher than the average person's, which is why she was feeling so poorly.

After a lot of consideration, Emily decided to begin eating eggs, fish, and chicken again. Almost immediately she noticed an improvement in her energy and sense of well-being. Within a month she was back on her bike and training, and within three months she was ready to start competing again. Her extra body fat melted away, her hair stopped falling out, and the dark circles under her eyes disappeared.

PROTEINS: YOUR PERSONAL PALEO CURE

- Eat the amount of protein you crave. Most people naturally eat the right amount because the brain strongly influences the craving for it depending on how much is needed. In chapter 18 we will discuss optimizing protein intake based on your individual circumstances.
- Meat, poultry, seafood, and eggs should form the bulk of your protein intake during the Step 1 Reset.
- Dairy products are also a source of high-quality protein and may be reintroduced during Step 2 to determine whether you tolerate them.
- Fruits, vegetables, nuts, and seeds are good sources of micronutrients but are low in absorbable protein.
- Grains and legumes are poor sources of protein compared to animal products. They also contain antinutrients that reduce the

absorption of amino acids, as well as proteins that may provoke an immune response. That said, moderate amounts of certain grains and legumes may be tolerated when special steps are taken to reduce their toxicity, and some may wish to reintroduce these during Step 2.

CHAPTER 8

Whole, Organic, and Wild:
Eat Real Food

As we've looked closely at food on a biochemical and molecular level (micronutrients, macronutrients, fatty acids, and toxins), you've learned why certain foods should be a part of your Personal Paleo Cure and why others don't make the cut. Now that you have a good grasp of what should be on your plate, it's time to take a step back and consider food quality. Before you head out to the market to collect ingredients for your next meal, I want to help you understand the importance of eating what I call real food. Real food is:

- Whole, unprocessed, and unrefined
- Local, seasonal, and organic
- Pasture-raised (for animal products) and wild-caught (for fish)

Let's look at each of these in turn.

WHOLE, UNPROCESSED, AND UNREFINED
(OR, IF IT COMES IN A BAG OR
A BOX, DON'T EAT IT!)

Industrial food processing has had more detrimental effects on human health and well-being than any other factor in the past few hundred

---

Notes for this chapter may be found at ChrisKresser.com/ppcnotes/#ch8.

years—and possibly in the entire history of humankind. Food refining has brought us food toxins that destroy health: wheat flour, industrial seed oils, artificial trans fats, and table sugar and high-fructose corn syrup. It has also brought us chemical additives and preservatives, some with known negative effects and others with effects still unknown.

Almost every day, new research is revealing the harm these newfangled processed foods have on us. A study in 2011 found that emulsifiers used in packaged foods ranging from mayonnaise to bread to ice cream increased intestinal permeability (causing a leaky gut, which you'll learn more about in chapter 10) and caused a chain reaction of inflammation and autoimmune disease. Another study showed that diet-soda consumption increases the risk of stroke and causes kidney damage, possibly because of the phosphoric acid used as an acidifying agent to give colas their tangy flavor. High intake of phosphoric acid is associated with premature aging, kidney and vascular disease, and cardiovascular complications in patients with chronic kidney disease. To avoid the harm caused by processed and refined foods, a good general rule is "If it comes in a bag or a box, don't eat it." Of course, not all foods that come in bags or boxes are harmful, so this isn't meant to be taken completely literally. It's just a helpful guideline. Butter is often packaged in a box, and some fruits, vegetables, and salad greens are sold in plastic bags. High-quality frozen organic produce is boxed or bagged. That doesn't mean you shouldn't eat butter, fruits, and vegetables. But in general, if you follow this guideline, you'll avoid most common food toxins. And that's more than half the battle.

ORGANIC, LOCAL, AND SEASONAL

More nutrients

Organic plant foods contain, on average, 25 percent higher concentrations of micronutrients than their conventional counterparts. In particular, they tend to be higher in important polyphenols and antioxidants like vitamin C, vitamin E, and quercetin. Even more relevant in determining your produce's nutrient content is where it comes from, and, more important, how long it's been out of the ground. Most of the produce sold at large supermarket chains is grown hundreds—if not thousands—of miles away, often in areas with longer growing seasons (in warmer states like California, Texas, and Florida, or in countries with year-round tropical climates). This is especially true when you're eating foods that are out of season in your local area, like a South American tomato in midwinter in New York. Possibly weeks have passed since that tomato was picked (hard and unripe, so that it could be shipped without bruising), after which it was packaged and transported thousands of miles through a maze of artificially refrigerated distribution centers before it finally arrived at the store, where it sat on the shelves even longer.

The problem with this (besides producing inferior taste and quality) is that food starts to change as soon as it's harvested, and its nutrient content begins to deteriorate. For example, total vitamin C content of red peppers, tomatoes, apricots, peaches, and papayas has been shown to be higher when these crops are picked *ripe* from the plant. The vitamin C content of supermarket broccoli in May (in season) has been shown to be twice as high as supermarket broccoli in the fall (shipped from another country). Without exposure to light (allowing photosynthesis), many vegetables lose their nutrient value. If you buy vegetables from the supermarket that were picked a week ago, transported to the store in a dark truck, and then stored in the middle of a pile in the produce section, and then you put them in your dark refrigerator for several more days before eating them, chances are they've lost much of their nutrient value. For example, a study at Penn State University found that spinach lost 47 percent of its folate after eight days.

This is why buying your produce at local farmers' markets or, even better, picking it from your backyard garden is preferable to buying conventional produce shipped from hundreds or thousands of miles away. Fruits and vegetables from local farms are usually stored within one or two days of picking, which means their nutrient content will be higher. And as anyone who's eaten a fresh tomato right off the vine will tell you, local produce tastes so unlike (and so much better than) produce shipped in from afar that it could well be considered a completely different food.

Fewer chemicals

A main benefit of organic produce is that it's grown without pesticides, herbicides, or other harmful chemicals that have been shown to cause health problems, especially in vulnerable populations like children. A study published in the journal *Pediatrics* concluded that children exposed to organophosphate pesticides at levels typically found in conventional produce are more likely to develop attention deficit hyperactivity disorder (ADHD) than children who aren't.

In 2010, scientists who had been studying possible links between environmental toxins and cancer concluded that Americans should eat organic produce grown without pesticides, fertilizers, or other chemicals. Their report stated that the U.S. government had grossly underestimated the number of cancers caused by environmental toxins. They also high-lighted the risk to unborn children of the toxins in conventionally grown foods. Fetal exposure to harmful chemicals (through a pregnant woman's consumption of produce grown with toxins) can set a child up for a life-time of endocrine disruption, hormone imbalances, and other problems.

THE DIRTY DOZEN PLUS AND CLEAN FIFTEEN

Each year, the Environmental Working Group publishes a list of the twelve fruits and vegetables highest in pesticide residues (the Dirty Dozen) and the fifteen fruits and vegetables lowest in pesticide resi-dues (the Clean Fifteen). Starting in 2012, the group added two addi-tional crops to the Dirty Dozen (making it the Dirty Dozen Plus) that didn't meet the criteria but were commonly contaminated with pesti-cides that are especially toxic to the nervous system.

If you're on a tight budget and can't afford to buy organic produce exclusively, you'll get the benefits of a diet rich in fruits and vegeta-bles while minimizing the risk of pesticide exposure. Below are the Dirty Dozen Plus and the Clean Fifteen for 2013:

The Dirty Dozen Plus		
Apples	Celery	Cherry tomatoes
Cucumbers	Grapes	Hot peppers
Nectarines (imported)	Peaches	Potatoes
Spinach	Strawberries	Sweet bell peppers
Summer squash	Kale/collard greens	

The Clean Fifteen		
Asparagus	Avocados	Cabbage
Cantaloupe	Corn	Eggplant
Grapefruit	Kiwi	Mangoes
Mushrooms	Onions	Papayas
Pineapples	Sweet peas (frozen)	Sweet potatoes

More and more supermarkets have expanded their organic produce section; it's good business because consumer demand for pesticide-free produce has increased, and it's good for your wallet because as the supply increases, the price drops. Note that this list is also available as a free downloadable app from EWG's website (www.ewg.org/foodnews/). Now you can have this list at your fingertips while you shop.

Supporting local economies and preserving resources

Local produce has more nutrients and fewer chemicals than imported produce, but there are other, non-nutritional reasons to eat it. These were summarized well in Cornell University's Northeast Regional Food Guide:

> Community food systems promote more food-related enterprises in proximity to food production, marketing, and consumption. Such systems enhance agricultural diversity, strengthen local economies (including farm-based businesses), protect farmland, and increase the viability of farming as a livelihood. Local food systems mean less long-distance shipment of the produce we enjoy, which means decreased use of nonrenewable fossil fuels for food distribution, lower emission of resulting pollutants, and less wear on transcontinental highways.

How can you argue with that? I've also found that forming relationships with the people who grow my food leads to a greater sense of community and connection. In an increasingly techno-obsessed, hyperactive world, that is especially welcome.

PASTURE-RAISED AND WILD-CAUGHT: AS NATURE INTENDED

While the reasons to eat pasture-raised-animal products and wild-caught fish span social, political, economic, and health considerations, I'm going to focus on health factors. Several studies have been done comparing the nutrient content of pasture-raised-animal products to that of grain-fed-animal products (that is, animals raised in concentrated animal feeding operations, or CAFOs). Pasture-raised-animal products are superior to CAFO products in two primary respects: (1) they have a better fatty acid profile, and (2) they have higher levels of vitamins and other micronutrients.

Omega-6 and omega-3 content

Studies have shown that grain-fed animals have decreased omega-3 levels, thus raising the omega-6-to-omega-3 ratio. As you'll recall from reading about these fats in chapter 5, too much omega-6 and not enough omega-3 can be problematic. The more grain in a cow's diet, the lower the omega-3 levels in the beef. A 2010 paper published in the *Nutrition Journal* reviewed seven individual studies comparing omega-6 and omega-3 levels in grass- and grain-fed beef. Every study found significantly higher levels of omega-3 in grass-fed beef, and in some cases the difference was almost tenfold. On average, grass-fed beef had an omega-6-to-omega-3 ratio of 1.5:1, compared to 7.7:1 for grain-fed.

Another study compared the omega-6-to-omega-3 ratio of several different types of meat, ranging from pasture-raised bison and beef to wild elk to conventional chicken. They found the following ratios (expressed as parts of omega-6 to one part omega-3):

- Pasture-raised bison: 2.1:1
- CAFO bison: 7.2:1
- Pasture-raised beef: 2.1:1
- CAFO beef: 6.3:1
- Wild elk: 3.1:1
- CAFO chicken breast: 18.5:1

What is apparent from both studies is that pasture-raised beef is much closer to the historical omega-6-to-omega-3 ratio of between 2:1 and 1:1 (what our Paleo ancestors consumed) than beef raised in concentrated animal feeding operations. In fact, the ratio for pasture-raised beef is even better than for wild elk. This means that pasture-raised beef falls within evolutionary norms for the fatty acid content of animals that humans have eaten throughout their history. CAFO beef does not.

You may also have noticed that the ratio of omega-6 to omega-3 of chicken is about nine times higher than that of pasture-raised beef. I don't see this as a reason to avoid chicken, but it does suggest that the fatty acid profile of beef and lamb are superior, and they should be favored in the diet. Studies have shown that meat from pasture-raised animals can actually raise levels of EPA and DHA in the blood, making it the only dietary source of these important long-chain omega-3 fats other than cold-water, fatty fish.

Pastured-chicken eggs

We see a similar difference between eggs from hens raised on pastures and eggs from those raised in confinement. Eggs from pasture-raised hens contain as much as ten times more omega-3 than eggs from factory hens. Pastured-chicken eggs are higher in B$_{12}$ and folate. They also have higher levels of fat-soluble antioxidants, like vitamin E, and a denser concentration of vitamin A.

Wild-caught fish

Farmed fish contain more omega-6 than wild-caught fish. Tests conducted in 2005 show that wild-caught salmon contain ten times more omega-3 than omega-6, whereas farmed salmon have only about four times more omega-3 than omega-6 (despite having more omega-3 fat overall). Another study found that subjects who consumed standard farmed salmon, the kind raised on diets high in omega-6, had higher blood levels of inflammatory chemicals linked to increased risk of cardiovascular disease, diabetes, Alzheimer's, and cancer. Wild salmon also contains four times as much vitamin D than farmed salmon does, which is especially important since up to 50 percent of Americans are deficient in this important vitamin.

Conjugated linoleic acid (CLA) content

Meat, fat, and dairy that comes from pasture-raised animals are the richest source of another type of good fat, called conjugated linoleic acid (CLA). CLA may have anti-cancer properties, even in very small amounts. In animal studies, CLA at less than one-tenth of 1 percent of total calories prevented tumor growth. In a Finnish study on women, those who had the highest levels of CLA in their diet had a 60 percent lower risk of breast cancer than those with the lowest levels. In another study, people with the highest levels of CLA in their tissues had a 50 percent lower risk of heart attack than those with the lowest levels.

Pasture-raised-animal products are the richest known source of CLA in the diet, and they are significantly higher in CLA than grain-fed-animal products. When ruminant animals like cows and sheep are raised on fresh pasture alone, their products contain three to five times more CLA than products from animals fed grain.

Mineral, vitamin, and micronutrient content

Grass-fed beef is also much higher in key micronutrients than grain-fed beef; it has:

- Seven times more beta-carotene
- Three times more vitamin E
- Higher levels of glutathione
- Twice as much riboflavin (vitamin B_2)
- Three times as much thiamine (vitamin B_1)
- 30 percent more calcium
- 5 percent more magnesium

Grass-fed meat also has more selenium than grain-fed products. Selenium plays an important role in thyroid function, has antioxidant effects, and protects the body against mercury toxicity. Grass-fed-bison meat has four times more selenium than grain-fed-bison meat.

SUPERBUGS IN CONVENTIONALLY RAISED MEAT

Here's a good reason to put some thought into how you shop for meat. A 2013 analysis of data by the Environmental Working Group (EWG) found significant levels of antibiotic-resistant bacteria in conventionally raised meat that was being sold in supermarkets across the country. These so-called superbugs can cause serious foodborne illnesses and infections that are becoming increasingly difficult to treat. The EWG reports that antibiotic-resistant bacteria was found in:

- 81 percent of ground turkey
- 69 percent of pork chops
- 55 percent of ground beef
- 39 percent of chicken breasts, wings, and thighs

(continued)

Researchers also found that 87 percent of raw-meat samples were contaminated with both normal and antibiotic-resistant enterococcus bacteria, which indicates that the meat came into contact with fecal matter.

Industrial livestock producers routinely give their animals antibiotics to encourage more rapid growth or prevent infection in overcrowded, stressful, and unsanitary living conditions. Today, 80 percent of the antibiotics manufactured each year are given to food-industry animals.

Superbugs that have evolved because of misuse of antibiotics (in both humans and livestock) have increased the risk that people will succumb to severe infection. An increase in antibiotic-resistant bacteria means that a common problem like strep throat or a scraped knee could be fatal.

- The EWG report recommends the following steps to reduce your exposure to superbugs in meat: Choose meat from organic, pasture-raised animals that have not been given antibiotics. If you're budget-conscious, buy cheaper cuts of meat, like brisket, chuck roast, sirloin, tenderloin, rib roast, shoulder roast, ground meat, bone-in chops, or bone-in thighs and breasts.
- Bag raw meat before it goes in your grocery cart, and be especially careful with ground meats.
- Store meat on the lowest rack in the fridge, away from fresh produce. Thaw it in the fridge, not on the counter.
- Use separate cutting boards for meat and produce. Don't wash meat; splashes spread bacteria.
- Use a food thermometer to ensure that the meat is adequately cooked, which will kill any bacteria. See http://foodsafety.gov for more about how to cook meat safely.

EAT REAL FOOD: YOUR PERSONAL PALEO CURE

- As a general rule, avoid food that comes in a bag or a box. Focus on fresh ingredients.

- Buy organic, locally grown produce as much as possible. Shop farmers' markets or join a community-supported agriculture (CSA) farm. Consider springing for organic varieties of the Dirty Dozen Plus; save money by buying conventional varieties of the Clean Fifteen.
- Buy pasture-raised-animal meat, dairy, and eggs whenever possible. They will have more nutrients and fewer toxins, and they will be less likely to harbor antibiotic-resistant superbugs. Choose tougher, cheaper cuts (which are among the most flavorful, and can be made more tender by slow/wet cooking methods) and buy in bulk or directly from local farmers to save money. If pastured meat isn't available locally, buy it from online vendors. See the Resources section on my website for recommendations.
- Buy wild-caught fish. If fresh wild fish is not available locally, you can buy it canned from online vendors. See my website for recommendations.

CHAPTER 9

Cheaper, More Nutritious, and Better-Tasting: Cooking and Eating from Nose to Tail

One of the most remarkable things about traditional hunter-gatherer diets is that, despite the fact that early humans developed them without the benefits of modern science or even the concept of micronutrients, they often provided all of the nutrients required for optimal health. Our ancestors learned which types, amounts, and combinations of nutrients they needed the old-fashioned way: through experimentation over thousands of generations.

In his book *Nutrition and Physical Degeneration*, Weston Price—the Ohio dentist-turned-documentarian-of-traditional-peoples-and-their-diets (see chapter 1)—recounted the experience of a prospector who went blind while crossing a high plateau in the Rocky Mountains. The prospector was discovered by a Native American, who fed him "the flesh and the head and the tissues of the back of the eyes, including the eyes" of a trout. Within a few hours, the prospector's sight began to return, and a few hours after that, his sight was normal. Today, we know that this type of temporary blindness can be caused by a deficiency of vitamin A. We also know that the eyes and the heads of fish are rich in retinol, preformed vitamin A.

Notes for this chapter may be found at ChrisKresser.com/ppcnotes/#ch9.

Another example is the use of special preconception diets of mothers-to-be (and sometimes fathers-to-be) in traditional cultures like the Masai (see chapter 5), who only allowed marriage and pregnancy after couples spent months drinking nutrient-rich milk from cows who grazed during the lush wet season. Other cultures used special foods like fish eggs, animal glands, spider crabs, or even the ashes of certain plants to supply additional amounts of nutrients that are important for fetal development, such as choline; iodine; vitamins A, D, and K_2; and EPA and DHA. And almost all traditional diets contained liver and other organ meats, bones and skin, fats, seafood, and wild plants, all of which are also high in nutrients crucial for pregnancy and lactation.

Today, unfortunately, much of this ancient and time-tested wisdom has fallen by the wayside. Organ meats, bone broths, skin and cartilage, fish eggs, egg yolks, and many other nutrient-dense parts of animals consumed have all but disappeared from the modern diet. Your grandparents may have eaten these foods, but chances are you don't. This has happened in large part because of the misguided campaigns against saturated fat, cholesterol, and red meat. But it's also a consequence of our love for all things modern and our tendency to discount the knowledge of the past.

The problem is that these now-unpopular foods provide nutrients that work synergistically with those found in more commonly eaten foods and are difficult to obtain elsewhere in the diet. In other words, we may be well fed, but we're undernourished. The solution is to return to the practice of our ancestors and "eat from nose to tail." This means eating not only the lean muscle meat (like steak or chicken breast) of animals but also the organs, skin, cartilage, bones, and fattier cuts.

These parts of the animal contain nutrients that work best when combined with the nutrients found in muscle meats and other lean proteins. For example:

- The amino acid methionine, which is abundant in lean proteins, can't fulfill its important functions without adequate amounts of B vitamins (especially B_6, B_{12}, and folate), choline, and glycine.

- Vitamin A is crucial for a variety of biochemical processes in the body, yet it is found in significant amounts only in the liver of land mammals and the liver oils of fish. Beta-carotene, which is found in vegetables like carrots and red peppers, is often mistakenly referred to as vitamin A. However, while some beta-carotene can be converted into vitamin A in humans, that amount is very small: about 3 percent in the case of raw carrots. Too much vitamin A without enough vitamin D promotes bone loss, whereas too much vitamin D without enough vitamin A leads to kidney and bladder stones and calcification of the arteries. Vitamin K_2 works in concert with vitamins A and D to regulate calcium metabolism.

With this in mind, I suggest balancing your intake of lean meats and fish with liberal amounts of choline, glycine, B vitamins, vitamin A, vitamin D, and vitamin K_2. You can do that by following these guidelines:

- Consume **one-half to one cup of homemade bone broth** daily, in soups, sauces, stews, or as a beverage; eat **tougher cuts of meat, like brisket, chuck roast, oxtail, and shanks;** and don't shy away from **skin and cartilage.** These are all excellent sources of glycine.
- Eat **one to two three-ounce servings of chicken and/or beef liver** per week. See below for tips on how to prepare it. Liver is rich in B vitamins, vitamin A, and several other nutrients.
- Eat at least **four to five egg yolks** per week, preferably from eggs that come from pasture-raised chickens. You're free to eat more if you'd like, since dietary cholesterol does not have a significant impact on blood-cholesterol levels or the risk of heart disease. Egg yolks are the highest source of choline in the diet.
- Take **one-half teaspoon of high-vitamin cod-liver oil** per day. Cod-liver oil is the richest source of vitamin A, but it also contains vitamin D, EPA, DHA, and—in the case of fermented cod-liver oil (see the bonus chapter on supplementation on the website for more info)—vitamin K_2.

- Eat **two servings per day of fermented foods** (for example, sauerkraut, kefir, natto), **cheese and butter** (from pasture-raised cows), and/or **eggs** (from pasture-raised chickens) to obtain adequate amounts of vitamin K_2.

HOW A SIMPLE DIETARY CHANGE CURED AARON'S DEPRESSION

Aaron, thirty-four, came to see me complaining of depression. He had suffered from it on and off for years, but it had gotten worse during the year leading up to our visit. He had tried over-the-counter remedies, like Saint-John's-wort and SAMe, but they didn't help. Aaron wanted to avoid drugs if possible, so he asked me if there was anything else he could do.

I noticed that he had started a strict Paleo diet right around the time his symptoms began to worsen. Aaron was passionate about CrossFit, an intensive strength and conditioning program, so he was eating large amounts of protein to support his workouts. He had been told by the personal trainer who introduced him to Paleo to focus on lean meats and avoid saturated fat. He also consumed whey protein shakes and avoided egg yolks because he had a family history of heart disease and was worried about his cholesterol.

I explained to Aaron that his diet was rich in methionine and low in glycine and that this imbalance could be contributing to his depression. His body wasn't able to produce adequate serotonin on such a diet. I asked him to start eating fattier cuts of meat and egg yolks and reduce his consumption of whey protein. I also prescribed a grass-fed-animal gelatin supplement to provide extra glycine as well as high-vitamin cod-liver oil to provide fat-soluble vitamins (see below). Aaron was skeptical that such simple dietary changes could have any effect, given everything he had already tried. Yet after he spent six weeks on this new regimen, his mood improved significantly. After three months, his depression was completely gone. His sleep had also improved, and he felt calmer and more at ease throughout the day.

ECONOMY, FLAVOR, AND CONVENIENCE

There are three other reasons to eat from nose to tail. The first is economy. Organ meats; more gelatinous cuts, such as brisket, chuck roast, oxtail, chicken breast or legs with bones and skin; and fish heads are typically less expensive than muscle meats, boneless (and skinless) chicken breasts, and fish fillets. Some butchers will even give beef bones away if you ask for them. Grass-fed-animal (or pastured-animal) products are often more expensive than conventional grain-fed alternatives, but choosing the more gelatinous cuts and organ meats of grass-fed animals is one way to make them more affordable. Including these cuts in your diet is less wasteful, as these cuts often go unconsumed, an important consideration in a world with a growing population and dwindling natural resources.

The second reason is flavor. In many cases, to save money you have to sacrifice quality or flavor. Not so with these cuts: they are some of the most flavorful, tender, and delicious parts of the animal if they're prepared properly. This was no secret to our grandparents and our ancestors, who regularly included them in their diet. But today, many people have forgotten how to cook them. Fortunately, there's a nose-to-tail revival happening in culinary circles, and numerous books are available to provide instruction. For some excellent inspiration and recipes, check out two of my favorite books: *The Whole Beast: Nose to Tail Eating,* by Fergus Henderson, and *Odd Bits: How to Cook the Rest of the Animal,* by Jennifer McLagan.

The third reason is convenience. Let's face it: Most of us are busy and don't have time to cook from scratch at every meal. One of the advantages of the fattier cuts of meat is that they tend to be larger and will feed you and your family for more than a single meal. This can save you both time and money.

If you're new to preparing these cuts, here are a few ideas to get you started. Check out my website for recipes.

- *Make a stew.* Chuck roast, chuck shoulder, bottom round roast, round tip roast, and rump roast are good cuts for stew.

- *Make a pot roast.* Pot roast cuts come from the fore- and hindquarters of the cow. You can also use the cuts listed above for pot roast.
- *Make chicken broth.* Roast a chicken and eat the meat for dinner, and then put the carcass in a large pot and make some homemade broth. It's one of the most healing foods you can eat and rich in glycine and minerals. Use it for soups or sauces, or just drink it warm like tea.
- *Make fish-head soup.* Another time-tested remedy, fish-head soup is rich in glycine, iodine, selenium, and other minerals. It can also be used for soup and as a base for sauces, especially in Thai food.
- *Make oxtail soup.* Oxtails are like braised short ribs but with even more flavor. They're incredibly gelatinous and thus high in glycine, and they have all of the other vitamins and minerals beef contains. The segments are vertebrae so they're also rich in nutrient-dense bone marrow.

Organ meats can be prepared in numerous ways. (See the additional meal plans on my website for some ideas.) It's worth pointing out that while some people love the stronger flavor of organ meats, others don't. In that case, here are three ideas for how to include liver (which is one of the most nutrient-dense foods by weight you can eat) in your diet:

- Choose recipes that mask or mellow the strong flavor.
- Mix liver into other meat dishes. See page 43 for instructions.
- Dice fresh liver into pill-size pieces. Arrange them flat on a small baking sheet that will fit in your freezer. Freeze them for at least two weeks to kill any potential pathogens in the raw meat. Then simply swallow several frozen liver pills each day. Aim for about three to six ounces a week, total.

People often object to eating liver because they believe it is toxic, since the liver is the primary organ of detoxification. While it's true that the liver is in charge of detoxification, most of the toxins in the body are stored in fat, not in the liver. (For this reason, it's best to buy pasture-raised and organic items when you're choosing high-fat animal products such as fattier cuts of meat, butter, whole milk, and yogurt.)

WHEN ORGAN MEATS SHOULDN'T BE ON THE MENU

Hemochromatosis is a hereditary condition that causes excess absorption of iron in the body. It's the most common genetic disease in North America, affecting as many as one in two hundred people—a prevalence ten times that of cystic fibrosis. It's associated with a wide variety of disorders, such as diabetes, cardiovascular disease, and Alzheimer's, and if untreated, it can literally rust the organs (especially the liver, pancreas, heart, and brain) and cause early death. Unfortunately, hemochromatosis is often misdiagnosed or simply just missed. A 1996 CDC study found that the average hemochromatosis patient had seen three doctors over a period of nine years before being properly diagnosed. What's more, even mild iron overload that isn't associated with hemochromatosis can cause serious problems, including metabolic disease, male infertility, and severe fatigue.

Iron overload is more common in men and postmenopausal women than in premenopausal women. Why? The only way to get rid of excess iron once it's stored in the body is through bleeding or chelation therapy. Premenopausal women lose a little bit of iron (in the blood) through menstruation each month, whereas men and postmenopausal women simply accumulate iron without losing it.

Ask your doctor about testing your iron levels. If they're high, I'd recommend the following steps:

- Avoid consuming organ meats, clams, and oysters, which are very high in iron.
- Moderate your intake of red meat, such as beef and lamb, and wild game, such as venison, which are also relatively high in iron.
- Donate blood three to four times a year. Men and postmenopausal women can do this as a preventive measure. Studies

have shown that frequent blood donors have better blood-sugar control and lower levels of hypertension.

- Ask your doctor about phlebotomy (the therapeutic removal of blood), the treatment of choice for many cases of iron overload.
- Avoid high doses (over 300 mg/d) of vitamin C or betaine hydrochloride, both of which increase iron absorption.
- Don't consume alcohol with meals containing iron; alcohol also increases iron absorption.

WHAT ABOUT DAIRY?

Dairy often gets a bad rap in the health and nutrition world. It's been maligned by some for its high saturated fat content and condemned by others as unfit for human consumption. Let's take a closer look at each of these criticisms.

Does full-fat dairy contribute to disease?

In the conventional nutrition world, dairy is recognized as an important part of a healthy, well-balanced diet because it's a good source of protein, calcium, and added nutrients like vitamins A and D. However, dairy fat is typically portrayed as being harmful, mostly due to its saturated fat and cholesterol. Mainstream organizations like the American Heart Association and the American Diabetes Association recommend using nonfat, low-fat, or reduced-fat dairy products and have steered consumers away from full-fat or whole dairy for the most part. But does the evidence support this recommendation?

A 2012 paper published in the *European Journal of Clinical Nutrition* reviewed sixteen studies examining the relationship between high-fat dairy intake, obesity, and cardiovascular and metabolic disease. In the majority of studies reviewed, high-fat dairy intake was either inversely associated with obesity and metabolic disease (meaning that those who ate the most high-fat dairy foods had the lowest risk for these conditions) or not associated with them at all.

Some compounds in high-fat dairy products—such as butyrate, phytanic acid, trans palmitoleic acid, and conjugated linoleic acid—have been shown to have beneficial effects. Butyrate provides energy to the cells lining the colon, inhibits inflammation in the gastrointestinal tract, and may prevent colonic bacteria from entering the bloodstream. In fact, butyrate's anti-inflammatory effect is so strong that a dose of four grams per day for eight weeks induced complete remission in a group of Crohn's disease patients. Phytanic acid, one of the fatty acids in dairy fat, has been shown to reduce triglycerides, improve insulin sensitivity, and improve blood-sugar regulation in animal models. In a study of 2,600 U.S. adults, another fatty acid in dairy fat, trans palmitoleic acid, was found to be associated with lower triglycerides, lower fasting insulin, lower blood pressure, and a lower risk of diabetes. Finally, conjugated linolenic acid (CLA), a natural trans fat found in dairy products, may reduce the risk of heart disease, cancer, and diabetes.

Dairy is also a good source of fat-soluble vitamins like retinol (active vitamin A) and vitamin K_2, which are difficult to obtain elsewhere in the diet.

Is dairy unfit for human consumption?

One of the main arguments against dairy, advanced by vegans, raw-foodists, and even advocates of the Paleo diet, is that dairy isn't an appropriate food for humans. They support this argument by pointing out that most humans don't produce lactase after childhood and that no mammals other than humans consume the milk of other animals.

These may seem like compelling arguments on the surface, but they don't hold up under scrutiny. As I mentioned in chapter 1, human evolution didn't stop in the Paleolithic era. While it's true that most of our genes are the same as they were hundreds of thousands of years ago, some of them have adapted in a relatively short time. Lactase persistence is perhaps the best example of this. Our hunter-gatherer ancestors were breast-fed until around age four. Mother's milk was virtually the only food they consumed that contained lactose, or milk sugar, and there was no need for the body to continue producing lactase (the enzyme that digests lactose) after early childhood. But when humans began consuming cow's milk, natural selection went to work, and about eight thousand years ago, a genetic mutation that continued the production of lactase into adulthood began spreading through the population. Now a third of the world's population produces lactase into adulthood (and that figure approaches 100 percent in some parts of Northern Europe).

Humans have also developed technology that addresses some of the potential disadvantages of dairy consumption. For example, fermentation of milk into yogurt and kefir can reduce the lactose content to less than 1 percent—an amount that even someone who doesn't produce lactase should be able to tolerate. Some studies have even shown that consuming fermented dairy products like yogurt may reverse lactose tolerance by increasing levels of lactose-digesting bacteria in the gut.

What about the idea that humans shouldn't drink milk because no other animal drinks the milk of another animal? By this logic, we humans should also avoid cooking our food and drinking coffee and alcohol. I don't know of any other animals doing these things, but that alone is not a sufficient reason for us *not* to do them. We've developed both technological methods and genetic adaptations that enable us to enjoy and benefit from dairy products; other animals don't have these options, so comparing ourselves to them in this case doesn't make sense.

All of this being said, there's no doubt that dairy doesn't work for everyone. Some people are allergic or intolerant to casein, a protein in dairy, or are highly sensitive to lactose. In these cases, dairy must be strictly avoided or additional steps must be taken to make it tolerable. Since there's still no gold-standard test for dairy intolerance, I recommend removing it from your diet during the Step 1 Thirty-Day Reset, and reintroducing it in Step 2. See chapter 11 for guidelines on how to properly reintroduce dairy products.

IS DAIRY RIGHT FOR YOU?

While milk proteins are very well absorbed by most people, they can cause serious issues in a minority of the population. Studies suggest that somewhere between one in two hundred and one in one thousand adults are allergic to milk proteins (which include casein, whey, alpha-lactalbumin, beta-lactoglobulin, and bovine serum albumin, among others). It's also likely that an even larger number of people suffer from intolerance to milk proteins. An intolerance is different than a true allergy in that the body does not produce antibodies to the antigen (milk protein, in this case), but it can still cause serious symptoms.

Unfortunately, there's no accurate and reliable way of testing for milk-protein intolerance, which is why I suggest that everyone remove dairy entirely for at least thirty days during the Step 1 Reset. In chapter 11, I provide instructions for how to add dairy back into your diet if you wish and how to determine if the proteins or the sugar (lactose) is to blame if you have a bad reaction. This is important to know, because if you're reacting to the proteins you won't be able to tolerate most dairy products (with the possible exception of ghee and butter, which are low in protein). However, if you're reacting to lactose, you will likely still be able to enjoy dairy products low in lactose, such as ghee, butter, yogurt, kefir, hard cheeses, and possibly cream.

Parents should be aware that milk protein is one of the most common allergens for babies and young children, with a prevalence ranging from 2 to 3 percent depending on the study. While most children outgrow this (as reflected in the much lower rates of milk-protein allergy in adults), if your baby or child is having symptoms that resemble an allergic response to food (for example, diarrhea, constipation, skin breakouts, abdominal pain, insomnia, or irritability), ask your pediatrician about removing dairy entirely for thirty days to see if that helps.

COOKING AND EATING FROM NOSE TO TAIL: YOUR PERSONAL PALEO CURE

- Eat at least three ounces of organ meats per week. Liver is most nutritious, but heart, kidney, tongue, and even brain are all fair game! Those with iron overload should not consume organ meats.
- Eat one-half to one cup of homemade bone broth (from chicken, turkey, beef, pork trotter, fish, or shellfish) in soups, stews, and sauces.
- Enjoy tougher, more gelatinous cuts of red meat in addition to lean cuts. Brisket, short ribs, chuck roast, rib steak, and 25 percent fat ground meat are good choices. Dark-meat poultry with skin should be consumed in moderation because of its high omega-6 linoleic acid content.
- Eat at least four to six egg yolks (alone or in whole eggs) per week. They are excellent sources of several nutrients, especially choline, which is hard to find elsewhere in the diet. Choose pastured-chicken eggs whenever possible.
- If you eat canned salmon, find a brand that includes the bones. They're soft and safe to eat, and they're a great source of calcium. See my website for recommendations.

CHAPTER 10

Good Gut Feeling: Restore Your Gut Flora and Gut Barrier

Digestive problems have reached epidemic levels in the United States. Consider the following:

- Irritable bowel syndrome (IBS) affects between 10 and 15 percent of the population and accounts for 12 percent of total visits to primary-care doctors.
- IBS is the second leading cause of missed workdays, behind only the common cold.
- On average, 60 percent of adults in the U.S. population experience symptoms of GERD (gastroesophageal reflux disease) in a twelve-month period, and 20 to 30 percent have weekly symptoms.
- Nexium, an acid-suppressing drug prescribed for GERD, generated $6.3 billion in sales in 2010, an amount surpassed only by Lipitor (a statin).

Perhaps by now you've been on the Step 1 Reset Diet long enough to note that your gut is feeling better than it ever has, or maybe you're still tweaking here and there (with further tweaks to come later) and you're getting there. The point is that our Paleo ancestors — with their nourish-

Notes for this chapter may be found at ChrisKresser.com/ppcnotes/#ch10.

ing traditional diets of real foods—probably didn't walk around with heartburn. In our modern world, however, it's a different story. Achieving good gut health is a major part of improving your overall health through your Personal Paleo Cure, because gut problems don't affect only the gut.

We now know that the health of the digestive tract is critical to overall health and that an unhealthy gut may contribute to a wide range of diseases, including diabetes, obesity, rheumatoid arthritis, autism spectrum disorder, depression, and chronic fatigue syndrome. The gut has a distinct nervous system of its own; some researchers even refer to the gut as the second brain, because of its size, complexity, and similarity—in terms of neurotransmitters and signaling molecules—to the brain. And recent studies suggest that approximately 70 to 80 percent of the body's immune cells are in the gut.

Because of this, many researchers and clinicians (myself included) believe that supporting intestinal health will be one of the most important goals of medicine in the twenty-first century. There are two closely related variables that determine gut health: the intestinal microbiota (or gut flora) and the gut barrier. Let's discuss each of them in turn.

THE GUT MICROBIOTA (AKA GUT FLORA)

The gut contains over 100,000,000,000,000 (one hundred trillion!) microorganisms from a thousand different species; there are ten times more microbes in the human body than there are human cells, and together, those microbes have one hundred times more genes than the human genome does. It's not inaccurate, then, to say that at a cellular level, we're more microbe than human. Indeed, according to Stanford microbiologist Justin Sonnenburg, "Humans can be regarded as elaborate vessels evolved to permit the survival and propagation of microorganisms." A hundred trillion microorganisms hitching a ride in your gut may sound like something from a creepy science fiction movie, but it turns out that these passengers are crucial to your health. Among other things, the gut microbiota promotes normal gastrointestinal function, provides protection from infection, regulates metabolism, and is home to the majority of immune cells. And when the gut microbiota is out of balance, you get sick. Changes to the gut microbiota have been linked to diseases ranging from autism and depression to autoimmune conditions like Hashimoto's, inflammatory bowel disease, and type 1 diabetes.

The composition of the gut microbiota

The colonization of the gut by bacteria begins at birth. While the gut of an unborn baby is exposed to some microbes in the womb (via ingestion of amniotic fluid), the vast majority of an infant's gut microbiota is acquired when it passes through the birth canal and swallows the mother's native bacteria. This explains why the method of delivery—vaginal birth or cesarean section—influences how the gut microbiota initially develop. In a vaginal birth, the baby is first exposed to bacteria in the birth canal; in a cesarean, the baby is first exposed to bacteria somewhere in the hospital. Some research suggests that the location of this initial exposure to bacteria affects the composition of the infant's gut microbiota for months or even years. Other studies indicate that children born via cesarean are at greater risk of asthma, obesity, and type 1 diabetes later in life.

The baby's diet (and perhaps, to a lesser degree, the mother's diet) also has a strong influence on the composition of the gut flora. Babies that are exclusively formula-fed have significant differences in gut micro- biota when compared to babies that are exclusively, or even partially, breast-fed. This is important, because pioneer bacteria (the first bacteria to colonize the gut) can alter gene expression to create a more favorable environment for themselves and a less favorable environment for later (and perhaps more beneficial) bacteria.

Diet has a major influence on the composition of the gut microbiota later in childhood and into adulthood as well. The amount, type, and balance of proteins, fats, and carbohydrates, as well as the amount and type of fiber, have a large impact on the gut microbiota. For example, foods that are rich in soluble fiber, such as certain fruits, vegetables, and starchy tubers (like sweet potatoes and potatoes) increase levels of lacto- bacilli, a class of bacteria often used in probiotics because of their beneficial effects on the gut. (Probiotics are good bacteria that help regulate the balance of gut microbiota.)

Other factors that can negatively influence the gut microbiota at all ages include:

- Antibiotics, NSAIDs, and other medications
- Chronic stress
- Chronic infections—especially gut infections

Functions of the gut microbiota

The main functions of the gut microbiota can be broken down into three categories: metabolic, structural, and protective.

(1) Metabolic

The metabolic activity of the gut microbiota is so diverse and important that some researchers refer to it as an organ within an organ. Bacteria in the gut break down dietary compounds that might otherwise cause cancer; they synthesize vitamins like biotin, folate, and vitamin K; they convert nondigestible carbohydrates to short-chain fatty acids, which provide energy and benefit the cells lining the gut; and they help with the absorption of minerals like calcium, magnesium, and iron.

Recent research has revealed a relationship between gut microbes and how we process and store the food we eat. Microbes help us to break down long-chain carbohydrates such as fiber and starch that we can't absorb on our own. During this process, the microbes produce short-chain fatty acids, including acetate, propionate, and butyrate. As I mentioned earlier, butyrate has several beneficial health effects.

(2) Structural

The short-chain fatty acids produced by fermentation (the breaking down of a substance by bacteria or other microorganisms—in this case, by gut microbiota) of carbohydrates have other important effects. For example, they stimulate the growth and differentiation of epithelial cells (the cells that form the inner lining of the colon). Butyrate also inhibits cell proliferation in the colon, which can lead to colon cancer.

(3) Protective

The gut is first and foremost a barrier designed to keep certain things (like pathogens and toxins) out, and let other things (like beneficial nutrients) in. The mucosal lining of the intestine is the primary interface between the external environment and our immune system. Some might assume that the skin plays a more important role in this respect, given its continual exposure to the environment. But the surface area of the gut is approximately one hundred times larger than that of the skin, and the gut contains around 70 to 80 percent of the immune cells in the body. These immune cells form a layer of tissue called the gut-associated lymphoid tissue, or GALT.

Studies have shown that the microbial composition of the gut affects the composition and function of the GALT. It's also true that bacteria in the gut form a crucial line of resistance to invasion by pathogenic microbes. Germ-free mice that have been bred to have sterile guts (with no microbes at all) are highly susceptible to infection, and antibiotics can disrupt the delicate balance of gut microbes and allow overgrowth of pathogenic species like *Clostridium difficile*.

THE GUT BARRIER

Think of the gut as a hollow tube that passes from the mouth to the anus. Anything that goes into the mouth and is not absorbed into the bloodstream will be eliminated as waste and will never enter the body. The gut barrier thus serves as a gatekeeper that decides what gets into our body and what stays out.

Normally, this process works very well. However, when the intestinal barrier becomes permeable (that is, leaky), substances that should not escape the gut—such as large, undigested protein molecules and bacterial toxins—pass into the bloodstream. This triggers an immune reaction, since these particles are viewed as foreign invaders by the body. And we now know that this immune reaction, resulting from intestinal permeability, contributes to everything from autoimmune disease to depression to obesity to skin disease. In fact, some researchers, such as Dr. Alessio Fasano (a pioneer in the study of celiac disease and gluten intolerance), now believe that intestinal permeability is a *precondition* to developing autoimmunity. In other words, it may not even be possible to develop an autoimmune disease unless you have a leaky gut first.

The term *leaky gut* used to be consigned to the outer fringes of medicine, and conventional researchers and doctors originally scoffed at the concept. Yet today it's one of the hottest topics in the scientific literature. Researchers have identified a protein called zonulin that increases intestinal permeability in humans and other animals. Many, if not most, autoimmune diseases—including celiac disease, type 1 diabetes, multiple sclerosis, rheumatoid arthritis, and inflammatory bowel disease—are characterized by abnormally high levels of zonulin and a permeable gut barrier. In fact, researchers have found that they can induce type 1 diabetes almost immediately in an animal by exposing it to zonulin. It develops a leaky gut and begins producing antibodies to islet cells, which are responsible for making insulin.

As you can see, a leaky gut causes an immune reaction that affects not only the gut but also other organs and tissues, including the skeletal system, the pancreas, the kidney, the liver, and the brain. This explains why a person who has a leaky gut doesn't always have gut symptoms, and why the range of symptoms people experience are so diverse. These include (but are not limited to):

- Skin rashes, like eczema or psoriasis
- Anxiety and depression
- Fatigue
- Joint pain
- Acne
- Allergies
- Abdominal pain
- Gas and bloating

- Constipation or diarrhea
- Asthma
- Difficulty concentrating
- Poor memory
- Poor immune function

WHAT CAUSES LEAKY GUT?

Here are several factors that can damage gut-barrier integrity and make it permeable.

Diet

Gliadin is a protein found in wheat that's responsible for the intestinal damage observed in celiac disease. In people with celiac disease (and perhaps in those without it), gliadin activates zonulin signaling, which in turn reduces intestinal barrier integrity and permits the passage of gliadin through the gut barrier. In these cases, wheat and other gluten-containing foods directly contribute to intestinal permeability. This is one reason I recommend that most people do not regularly consume wheat, even if they don't have gluten intolerance or celiac disease.

Diet can also have an indirect effect on gut-barrier integrity via its impact on the gut microbiota. The standard American diet—which is high in refined flours and sugars and industrial seed oils and low in whole fruits, vegetables, and soluble fiber—has been shown to cause undesirable changes in the gut microbiota. These changes to the microbiota make the gut barrier permeable and may increase the risk of autoimmune disease and other problems associated with a leaky gut. By contrast, traditional diets rich in fruits, vegetables, and soluble fibers and with very little processed, modern food cause beneficial changes in the gut microbiota that preserve barrier integrity and improve overall health.

Small intestinal bacterial overgrowth

Small intestinal bacterial overgrowth, or SIBO, is a condition involving inappropriate growth of bacteria in the small intestine. The large majority of the bacteria in the gut should inhabit the colon. However, chronic stress, poor diet, infection, antibiotic use, and other factors can cause bacteria to migrate from the colon into the small intestine. This causes malabsorption of proteins, fats, B vitamins, and other micronutrients. It also causes intestinal permeability.

Chronic stress

Chronic stress has been shown to reduce gut-barrier integrity in both human and animal studies.

Infections

Infection with bacteria (such as *H. pylori,* the bacteria that causes stomach ulcers), viruses (such as HIV), or parasites (such as *Giardia lamblia*) have all been shown to disrupt intestinal-barrier integrity.

Excess alcohol

Excess alcohol can promote the growth of certain types of bacteria in the gut that in turn increase intestinal permeability.

Medications

NSAIDs, aspirin, proton-pump inhibitors (PPIs, prescribed for acid reflux), and several other medications increase gut-barrier permeability. Antibiotics may indirectly disrupt gut-barrier function via their adverse effects on the gut microbiota.

Environmental toxins

Preliminary research suggests that some environmental toxins, such as bisphenol A (BPA), may cause intestinal permeability.

THE GUT-DISEASE CONNECTION

The Greek physician Hippocrates said that all disease begins in the gut. By now, I'm sure you realize how true those words are. Let's look even more closely at the gut-disease connection.

The gut-brain connection

The connection between the gut and the brain is apparent in our language; we all say things like "I have a gut feeling" and "I have butterflies in my stomach." Long before scientists understood how the gut and the brain influence each other, people experienced it firsthand: a nervous stomach before an important speech, or perhaps heartburn during a stressful financial situation.

While most people are aware that stress and emotional states like anxiety affect the gut, fewer people realize that problems in the gut can affect the brain. For example, SIBO (see above) is strongly associated with depression and anxiety in observational studies. Other research indicates that inflammation in the gut can alter mood and cause depression. Inflammatory molecules produced in the gut travel through the bloodstream, cross the blood-brain barrier, and activate specific cells in the brain, known as microglial cells. The microglial cells play an important role in repairing brain cells, but when they are chronically activated, communication among neurons (the functional brain cells) is impaired and depression results. Finally, increased intestinal permeability is much more common in autistic children and may contribute to the development of autism spectrum disorders.

I've found in my work with patients that SIBO, gut dysbiosis (an imbalance between the good and bad bacteria that colonize your gut), and gut inflammation are the most common causes of anxiety, depression, and other psychological and behavioral problems. This is especially true in children.

The gut-metabolism connection

One of the hottest topics in the scientific community over the past few years has been the connection between the gut microbiota and metabolic health. There are several reasons for this link. The gut microbiota is a source of bacterial toxins that provoke inflammation and insulin resistance, both of which contribute to obesity. Changes in the gut microbiota have been shown to increase appetite, increase the rate at which we absorb fats and carbohydrates, and increase the storage of calories as fat. Bad bacteria in the gut can also cause insulin resistance and inflammation of the hypothalamus in the brain, both of which are associated with obesity.

Other gut problems have also been shown to cause obesity and metabolic disease, including bacterial overgrowth in the small intestine, increased intestinal permeability, gallstones, and changes in the enteric (gut) nervous system.

The gut-immune connection

Gut dysfunction is an emerging focus in the study of autoimmune disease. In fact, as I mentioned above, some researchers believe that intestinal permeability is a *precondition* for developing autoimmune disease. In this theory, an environmental antigen (such as a protein from a food) leaks through the permeable gut barrier and initiates an immune response. Though this immune response is designed to protect the body from foreign invaders like bacteria and viruses, when it's continually triggered by food proteins and other environmental antigens penetrating the gut barrier, it can become overzealous and begin attacking human tissue. That's what autoimmune disease is: the body attacking itself.

In addition to contributing to autoimmune disease, disruptions in the gut barrier have also been shown to increase susceptibility to infection and weaken our immune defenses.

The gut-skin axis

There are clear associations between gut disorders and skin conditions in the scientific literature: 14 percent of patients with ulcerative colitis and 24 percent of patients with Crohn's disease have skin rashes, and 25 percent of patients with celiac disease have a skin condition called dermatitis herpetiformis. Celiacs also have a higher frequency of oral mucosal lesions, alopecia, and vitiligo.

One fascinating study found that SIBO is ten times more prevalent in those with acne rosacea than in those without it, and the correction of SIBO in these patients led to either a complete clearing or a significant improvement of lesions in 92 percent of patients. Altered gut microbiota also promotes the release of substance P, a potent neuropeptide that is produced in both the gut and skin and plays a major role in skin disorders. Finally, probiotics have been shown to improve intestinal-barrier function, reduce inflammation, and improve skin conditions. One Italian study involving forty patients with acne found that probiotics plus standard care were more effective than standard care alone.

NOURISHING YOUR GUT

Now that you know how important the gut is to overall health, let's discuss some basic strategies for maintaining your digestive health.

Avoid foods that are harmful to the gut

The basic Paleo approach is an excellent starting place for maintaining gut health. Refined flour, sugar, and industrial seed oils—the staples of the industrialized diet—are harmful because they cause undesirable changes in the gut microbiota and may disrupt the integrity of the intestinal barrier.

Excess alcohol has been shown to cause intestinal permeability, so I recommend limiting alcohol consumption to four to six drinks per week (and eliminating alcohol altogether if you have significant gut issues). Certain foods (such as those in the nightshade family) and nutrients that are well tolerated by most people can be harmful for people with digestive problems. I will discuss these in more detail in the bonus chapter on digestive disorders, available on my website.

Reduce foods that may irritate an already inflamed gut

Vegetables are one of the few foods that every diet philosophy agrees are healthy. That said, vegetables (particularly nonstarchy vegetables) tend to be high in insoluble fiber, which can irritate an inflamed gut. If you have irritable bowel syndrome (IBS), inflammatory bowel disease (IBD), or other digestive disorders, you may benefit from reducing your intake of vegetables that are high in insoluble fiber. These include:

- Greens (spinach, lettuce, kale, mesclun, collards, arugula, watercress, and so on)
- Whole peas, snow peas, snap peas, pea pods
- Green beans
- Kernel corn
- Bell peppers
- Eggplant
- Celery
- Onions, shallots, leeks, scallions, garlic
- Cabbage, bok choy, Brussels sprouts
- Broccoli
- Cauliflower

However, vegetables that are higher in soluble fiber and lower in insoluble fiber tend to have a soothing effect on the gut. These include:

- Carrots
- Winter squash
- Summer squash (especially peeled)
- Starchy tubers (yams, sweet potatoes, potatoes)
- Turnips
- Rutabagas
- Parsnips
- Beets
- Plantains
- Taro
- Yuca

In addition to reducing your overall intake of vegetables high in insoluble fiber, you should also reduce the variety of vegetables you eat at any given meal. Instead of stir-fries with six different vegetables, for example, have a single steamed or roasted vegetable as a side dish.

Note that I'm not suggesting you completely avoid vegetables that are high in insoluble fiber; I'm just suggesting that you limit them. Moreover, there are steps you can take to make these foods more digestible and less likely to irritate your gut:

- Never eat insoluble-fiber foods on an empty stomach. Always eat them with other foods that contain soluble fiber.
- Remove the stems and peels from veggies (such as broccoli, cauliflower, and winter greens) and fruits that are high in insoluble fiber.
- Dice, mash, chop, grate, or blend high-insoluble-fiber foods to make them easier to break down.
- Insoluble-fiber foods are best eaten well cooked: steamed thoroughly, boiled in soup, braised, and so forth. Avoid consuming them in stir-fries, and if you do eat them raw, prepare them as described above.

Finally, fermenting vegetables that are high in insoluble fiber is another option for making them more digestible, since fermentation is essentially a process of predigestion. Many of my patients who can't tolerate unfermented cabbage (raw or cooked) are able to eat fermented cabbage (like sauerkraut) without a problem. See my website for more information about how to make fermented foods. If you choose to buy fermented foods, make sure that they're raw and that they're in the refrigerated section. The sauerkraut you can buy in the condiments section has been pasteurized and won't have the same beneficial effect as raw or unpasteurized sauerkraut. (For more on fermented foods, see below.)

Eat foods that nourish the gut

In addition to avoiding foods that harm the gut, it's important to focus on foods that nourish the gut. These can be broken into three categories: bone broth, fermentable fibers, and fermented foods.

Bone broth

Bone broth is made from water and the meat and bones of animals (it may also contain vegetables and seasonings). It's considered a healing food in many traditional cultures, and it's rich in glycine and gelatin, both of which support digestive health. The nutrients in bone broth are particularly helpful for restoring the integrity of the gut barrier when it's damaged. I recommend consuming one-half to one cup of bone broth per day in the form of soups, stock, stews, or sauces (bone broth makes an excellent base for sauces and stews).

Fermentable fibers

Soluble fibers naturally found in fruits, vegetables, starches, nuts, and seeds provide a food source for the beneficial bacteria in the gut. These bacteria ferment the fiber and produce short-chain fatty acids such as butyrate, which has anti-inflammatory properties, promotes the development of healthy cells in the colon, and may protect against colon cancer. Starches like potatoes, sweet potatoes, plantains, taro root, and yuca are particularly good sources of soluble fibers.

Another option for fermentable fiber is resistant starch. The suggested amount is between twenty and forty grams a day. Unfortunately, it's not easy to come by in whole foods, because cooking tends to destroy it, and foods that contain it in large amounts can't be eaten raw. With this in mind, here are a few ways to add resistant starch to your diet:

- Mix four tablespoons of raw, unmodified, gluten-free potato starch (Bob's Red Mill is a good brand) with water or some other room-temperature food or beverage. Four tablespoons of potato starch provides about thirty-two grams of resistant starch.
- Make plantain chips by cutting a large, green (unripe) plantain into thin slices and placing the slices in a food dehydrator. Eat these as a snack. A single, large, unripe plantain contains about forty grams of resistant starch.
- Eat a green (unripe) banana, which contains about fifteen grams of resistant starch, depending on ripeness.

Note: Some people with gut issues may benefit from reducing intake of fiber for a time.

Fermented foods

These include fermented vegetables, like raw (unpasteurized) sauerkraut, kimchi, and pickles; fermented dairy, like yogurt and kefir; and fermented beverages, like beet kvass, kombucha, and water kefir. Fermented foods contain beneficial microorganisms that have positive effects on several different aspects of gut health. I suggest consuming one to two table-spoons of sauerkraut or other fermented vegetables with each meal and eating additional fermented foods, like yogurt, dairy kefir, water kefir, or beet kvass, throughout the day. (Note that while cheese, sour cream, and alcohol are fermented, they do not have a therapeutic effect like the fermented foods I've listed above do.)

Avoid antibiotics as much as possible

We've known for some time that antibiotics kill beneficial bacteria in the gut. However, more sensitive DNA-sequencing technology developed in the past few years has increased our understanding of just how far-reaching the effects of antibiotic use on the gut microbiota can be. For example, two separate studies published in the past five years have shown that a single course of antibiotics may cause irreversible, permanent changes to the gut microbiota. The clinical significances of these changes are not yet well understood, but given what we know about the importance of the gut microbiota to health, it's likely such changes aren't harmless.

Antibiotics are potentially lifesaving and certainly necessary in some cases, and I'm not suggesting that you avoid them then. But they are often prescribed (or requested by patients) when there's no evidence that they help, such as for colds and flus and other infections that are viral in origin.

Treat gut infections

Gut infections are far more common than most people believe, and you don't have to travel to a foreign country to get one (though that can help!). *Helicobacter pylori*, the bacterium that causes gastritis and ulcers, is thought to infect up to half the global population, with significantly higher rates in developing countries. Parasite infections are more difficult to track because conventional testing does a poor job of identifying them. But using more sensitive lab methods in my practice, I've found them to be quite common. See my website for information on how to find a clinician that can help you test for and treat gut infections.

Manage stress

Chronic stress can cause bacterial overgrowth in the small intestine, inflammation, and intestinal permeability. It also increases disease symptoms in IBS and IBD. However, mindfulness-based stress reduction, hypnotherapy, biofeedback, and other stress-reduction techniques have been shown to improve gut function and reduce gut symptoms. Please see chapter 14 for specific recommendations for stress management.

GUT HEALTH: YOUR PERSONAL PALEO CURE

- Understand the causes of gut dysfunction, which include leaky gut and intestinal dysbiosis.
- Avoid foods that harm the gut, including refined flour, industrial seed oil, and sugar.
- Eat foods that nourish the gut, including bone broths, fermentable fiber, and fermented foods.
- Avoid antibiotics whenever possible.
- Treat gut infections if they are present.
- Practice stress management on a daily basis.

REBUILD YOUR LIFE

CHAPTER 11

Reintroduce Gray-Area Foods

Now that you've finished the Thirty-Day Reset and know how your body feels on a strict Paleo diet, it's time to add some of the gray-area foods back into your diet. These are foods that were not a part of the original human dietary template but that are nevertheless nourishing and health-promoting *when they're well tolerated*. The important thing to understand about these gray-area foods is that different people respond to them in different ways. For example, some people (I happen to be one of them) thrive on dairy products like butter and yogurt. However, those same foods can give other people stomach cramps or make them break out in hives. We don't know why people react so differently to the same food, but genetics, gut microbiota (gut flora), immune health, stress, and emotional and psychological factors each play a role.

Before we get into details about how to safely reintroduce these foods, we should answer the question: *Why reintroduce them at all?* If you're like most of my patients and readers, after the Reset phase, you're probably feeling better than you have in many years — maybe better than you've ever felt in your life. If that's the case, why rock the boat? That's certainly a valid question. If you are feeling better than ever, and you don't miss any of the gray-area foods, then by all means, continue with the Thirty-Day Reset Diet. There's no risk in doing so. That's how our ancestors ate

---

Notes for this chapter may be found at ChrisKresser.com/ppcnotes/#ch11.

for hundreds of thousands of years. The foods permitted in Step 1 are loaded with all of the nutrients necessary for you to be healthy and vital and avoid disease. You could keep eating that way for the rest of your life (likely to be a lot longer than if you stayed on the standard American diet), and many who embrace the Paleo diet do just that.

However, if you're like most of my patients, you might be missing some of the foods that were prohibited during Step 1. I'm sorry to tell you this, but if potato chips and cheese doodles are two of your favorite foods, you won't be reintroducing them in Step 2. The good news is that if you've been missing butter on your sweet potato or that morning bowl of yogurt with berries you love so much or that occasional Thai food meal with white rice, you're in luck. Those are some of the foods you will be reintroducing during Step 2. They're perfectly healthy foods—provided you tolerate them well.

But how do you know if you tolerate them? I've developed a very specific program—tested and refined with thousands of patients and readers—that will help you answer that question. And in my opinion, doing a controlled food reintroduction like I'm about to teach you is the only way you can accurately determine how a particular food affects you. There are many food-sensitivity tests on the market, but all of them have serious limitations or problems that limit their usefulness. It sure would be nice if there was a test that told you which foods you could tolerate and which you couldn't, but so far that test doesn't exist.

While the food reintroduction does require some time and effort, by the end you'll know exactly what does and doesn't work for *you*—which is much better than relying on the experience or advice of others. Just because something works for me, your best friend, or a total stranger on an Internet forum doesn't mean it will work for you.

In the sections that follow, I'll explain some general guidelines about how to successfully reintroduce foods, tell you which foods I think are safe to reintroduce, and provide specific advice about the order in which to reintroduce them.

GENERAL GUIDELINES FOR
FOOD REINTRODUCTION

Food reintroduction requires a methodical approach, and there's both a right and a wrong way to do it. The method I'm going to share below has been tested with hundreds of patients and thousands of readers and listeners around the world, and it is very effective provided you stick with it.

It's important to understand that negative reactions to food can happen in three different ways:

- **Immediate:** You eat a food and almost immediately you notice a reaction. This isn't very common, but it can happen in the case of dairy products when someone is lactose- or casein- (the protein in dairy) intolerant, or when he or she has a true allergy to a food (I'll explain the difference between allergy and intolerance below).
- **Delayed (two to eight hours):** You eat something for breakfast, and by lunchtime you notice you're not feeling so hot. This is probably the most common food-intolerance reaction.
- **Extended (eight to twenty-four hours):** You eat something for lunch, feel fine at dinner, but begin to feel bad the next morning. This tends to be more common in people with slow digestion and constipation, though it can happen in anyone.

The delayed and extended reactions to foods are what make it so challenging to determine how a particular food affects you. For example, let's say you've just finished the Reset phase and are ready to move on to Step 2. You decide you're going to reintroduce butter, since it's the food you've missed the most. So you get up in the morning and cook your eggs in butter instead of coconut oil. You feel fine at lunchtime, so you boldly decide to reintroduce white rice at dinner, which you've also missed. The next morning you wake up with terrible diarrhea. Logic might suggest that it was the white rice, since you ate it at dinner and had problems the next morning. You might even forget that you ate butter at breakfast the day before. It's entirely possible, though, that the butter, and not the rice, is what caused the problem—it simply took a while for the reaction to manifest itself. This illustrates the importance of the first guideline of food reintroduction:

Guideline #1: Reintroduce only one food per three-day period

It's essential that you reintroduce only one food in a three-day period. This gives time for the immediate, delayed, and extended food reactions to happen. If you don't wait this long before introducing the next food, and you have a reaction, you'll never know which food caused it. When I say one food, I'm not referring to an entire category of foods (like dairy products), *but a single food.* For example, you could introduce butter, wait three days, then try cream, wait another three days, then yogurt, and so on. This may seem overly cautious, but it's necessary. I suggest eating one normal-size serving per day of the food you're reintroducing. Make a note in your food diary (see below) of exactly when you eat it, so it's easier for you to track any reaction.

Guideline #2: Keep a food diary

As you've gathered by now, it can be tricky to determine how foods are affecting you as you add them back in. This is where the food diary really shines. Sometimes it's clear how a food affected you only in retrospect, when you look back at your diary to determine a pattern. I've provided a blank diary template as part of the Personal Paleo Cure resources you'll find on my website to make this as easy as possible. You'll be recording what you ate, what time you ate it, how you felt before you ate it, and how you feel at various times throughout the day afterward. If you're a little unclear on how you're doing with a new food you've reintroduced, you can just take out your diary and study the previous two to three days. Has there been any change in your energy level, mood, or digestion compared to the days prior to when you introduced the food? If so, that's probably a sign you're not tolerating the new food very well.

Guideline #3: Low and slow wins the game

If you reintroduce a food and have a reaction to it, it's best to remove that food and wait until your body settles back to where it was before. This usually takes somewhere from one to three days, but if the reaction was severe, it may take longer. If you reintroduce a food and you're not sure how you're reacting to it, remove it, wait three days, and reintroduce it again. Most of my patients need to do this only twice or, at most, three times to determine whether the food is safe for them to eat.

The key is not to rush it. I know it can be frustrating, and you're excited to start eating some of those foods you missed during the Reset phase, but if you move too fast, you risk having to start over again. You've already invested thirty days or more during Step 1, so don't sabotage all that hard work. A little patience here will go a long way.

Guideline #4: Context matters

You might find that you're able to tolerate certain foods well at some times but not others. For example, perhaps when you're feeling well rested and healthy overall, you can eat some yogurt and feel fine afterward. However, if you haven't slept well for a few nights or if you have a cold or the flu or if your typical symptoms are flaring up, even a small amount of yogurt might make you break out or hurt your gut.

This is why context matters. If you're systemically inflamed due to sleep deprivation, an infection, or an autoimmune-disorder flare-up, your body won't respond in the same way to food as it does when you're feeling relatively healthy. Avoid reintroducing new foods if you're sick, stressed, or otherwise unwell, and consider returning to a more basic Thirty-Day Reset Diet during these times in the future, even after you've figured out your own Personal Paleo Cure.

COMMON FOOD REACTIONS

Here's a list of typical symptoms people experience when they are sensitive to a particular food:

- Gas
- Bloating
- Changes in stool frequency (diarrhea or constipation)
- Changes in stool consistency (dry, hard stool, or loose stool)
- Acid reflux
- Skin rashes
- Itchy skin
- Acne
- Difficulty concentrating and memory issues
- Insomnia or excessive sleepiness
- Anxiety
- Depression
- Fatigue
- Malaise
- Muscle or joint aches

This is just a partial list. You also want to look out for an increase of any symptoms that lessened during the Reset phase but were typical for you prior to starting it. If you do experience a reaction, stop eating that particular food and wait a few days for things to settle. This is important. At that point, you can try reintroducing that food again (if you're uncertain whether it was responsible for the reaction), or you can move on to the next food. But do not move on to a new food when you're still in the midst of a negative reaction to something you just reintroduced.

One last thing. It's important to distinguish between food intolerance, which is what we're talking about here, and true allergy. A food allergy involves an immune response to an antigen. An antigen is a substance (in this case, a food) that provokes the production of antibodies by the immune system. The reactions in true food allergies can be very severe and in some cases can even result in anaphylactic shock and death. The most common food allergens are peanuts, tree nuts (for example, walnuts, pecans, almonds), fish, shellfish, milk, eggs, soy products, and gluten-containing products. Fortunately, true food allergies are relatively rare.

Food intolerances are much more common. They involve an adverse reaction that isn't necessarily characterized by an antibody-driven immune response. (One exception to this is gluten intolerance, which does often involve the production of antibodies against gluten.) A food intolerance occurs when something in a food irritates your digestive system or when you're unable to properly digest or break down the food. Intolerance to lactose is the most common food intolerance.

When we talk about reintroducing foods in this section, we're attempting to discover food intolerances rather than food allergies. If you have an allergy to something like peanuts or shellfish, it's likely you already know that. *Do not attempt to reintroduce foods that you have a known allergy to.* Those foods should be avoided for life. However, it's relatively safe to reintroduce foods you suspect, but are not certain, you might be intolerant of, because the intolerance reactions are not life-threatening. They can be very uncomfortable, but they are rarely serious.

FOODS TO CONSIDER REINTRODUCING

I believe the foods below are generally healthy and nourishing when they are well tolerated by the individual. Remember, these aren't mandatory. If you feel great on the Thirty-Day Reset Diet and have no urge to add these foods back in, by all means, continue what you're doing!

Dairy products

While it's true that dairy products have the potential to cause problems, recent genetic adaptations have enabled some people — particularly those of Northern European descent — to digest them without a problem (see pages 33 to 35). In addition, there are several reasons you might wish to bring dairy products back into your diet.

- They're delicious. Most people love the taste of dairy products, like butter, cheese, and yogurt, and they are common ingredients in several different types of cuisine.

- They're nutritious. They contain calcium, high-quality protein, potassium, phosphorus, vitamin B_{12}, vitamin B_6, riboflavin, niacin, and, most important, the fat-soluble vitamin A (and, in the case of raw milk, vitamin K_2).
- They're health-promoting. As you learned in chapter 9, full-fat dairy products have several beneficial impacts on health, including reducing the risks of heart disease, diabetes, and cancer.
- They're a good source of probiotics (when they're raw or fermented). Fermented milk products, like yogurt and kefir, contain probiotic bacteria and yeast that improve digestive function and strengthen the immune system. Raw milk also contains beneficial bacteria, albeit not as much as fermented milk products have.

Of course, if you don't care for dairy or you already know you're intolerant, there's no need to reintroduce it. However, it's worth mentioning that many of my patients who can't digest pasteurized milk are able to tolerate raw dairy products or dairy products that have little or no lactose (like ghee, butter, hard cheeses, and yogurt and kefir). See the next section in this chapter for a specific method of reintroducing dairy that will help you determine which dairy products, if any, you can tolerate.

Grains and pseudocereals

Human beings thrived for thousands of generations without eating substantial amounts of grain. There are no important nutrients in grains that cannot be obtained by eating a diet rich in animal products, fruits, and vegetables. One myth I've seen perpetuated by mainstream nutritionists is that we need to eat grains for fiber. This is not true. We can get all the fiber we need from starchy tubers, fruits, vegetables, nuts, and seeds.

As I explained in chapter 4, grains contain a number of problematic chemical compounds that can damage the human intestinal tract, provoke immune reactions, and interfere with absorption of key nutrients. They are also lower on the nutrient-density scale than meat, fish, vegetables, fruits, nuts, seeds, and dairy products. Keeping this in mind, you might conclude that you should avoid eating grains entirely. I think that's a valid choice, and many people simply feel better when they eliminate grains completely.

That said, there are ways of preparing grains that reduce their toxicity, break down antinutrients like phytic acid, and improve the bioavailability of the nutrients they contain. (The exception to this is gluten-containing grains like wheat, rye, barley, spelt, and kamut. If you have celiac disease or are gluten-intolerant, no amount of preparation will render gluten harmless for you.) Indigenous cultures figured out very early on in the history of agriculture that certain steps taken beforehand made these foods easier to digest. They went to extreme lengths — including soaking, sprouting, fermenting, pounding, mashing, and roasting — to process their grains to make them healthy to eat. Those methods are time-intensive, to say the least.

In the modern world, where most people can barely find the time to cook a quick dinner at home, few are willing to go to these extreme lengths to properly prepare grains. Fermenting grains in your home kitchen is a tremendous amount of work, involving soaking them for up to twenty-four hours at specific temperatures, reserving soaking water, and repeating the process extensively. Even then, you may not be successful in neutralizing phytic acids and other toxins, and the food-processing industry certainly isn't taking these steps. The result is that most Americans end up eating a diet high in unprepared grains, low in nutrients, and high in antinutrients, and their health has suffered as a result.

Because each grain has a different botanical structure and food-toxin profile, each requires a different type of preparation to make it safe to eat. And how safe grains are for you to eat varies significantly based on your genetic heritage, your age, your health (especially your gut health), and what other foods you eat. If you're generally healthy and you soak or ferment grains prior to consuming them to reduce their toxicity and improve their nutrient density, then consuming a modest amount of grain is unlikely to cause harm — provided it doesn't replace more nutrient-dense foods in your diet. However, in my experience, people with digestive problems, autoimmune disorders, or other chronic inflammatory conditions often do poorly with grains, even when they are properly prepared, with the possible exception of white rice and buckwheat. (For links to resources on properly preparing grains through soaking and fermenting, see my website.)

You might be surprised to hear me recommend white rice. It's commonly believed that white rice is less nutritious than brown rice, but scientific research suggests otherwise. Studies that have compared the amount of nutrients absorbed from each type of rice have shown that humans absorb more nutrients from white rice. Why? Because the antinutrients in brown rice, like phytic acid, interfere with the absorption of the nutrients it contains. Brown rice also reduces dietary protein and fat digestibility. White rice doesn't have those problems. Phytic acid and other food toxins are found in the husk or the bran (the outer covering) of the grain. In the case of white rice, the bran has been removed, and what remains is mostly starch. Humans produce an enzyme called amylase that allows us to digest starch efficiently.

This is why I believe white rice is an acceptable food, and my experience with patients suggests that it is generally well tolerated. That doesn't mean everyone does well with it, nor does it mean it should make up a significant portion of your diet or replace more nutrient-dense carbohydrate sources, like sweet potatoes and other starchy vegetables. The point of removing rice (along with all grains) during the Thirty-Day Reset and then reintroducing it is to find out how you tolerate it in moderate amounts. Those with blood-sugar problems, such as hypoglycemia, insulin resistance, or diabetes, may need to minimize or avoid white rice entirely, because of how rapidly it is broken down into glucose. In addition, people who are gluten-tolerant may need to avoid rice. Studies have shown that people who have either celiac disease or non-celiac gluten sensitivity are more likely to react to the proteins in rice.

The other exception is buckwheat. Despite its name, buckwheat isn't even a distant relative of wheat. In fact, buckwheat isn't even a grain; it's a plant in the same family as sorrel and rhubarb. While buckwheat does contain some phytic acid, it also contains significant amounts of phytase, the enzyme that breaks down phytic acid. This means that it's relatively easy to eliminate the phytic acid in buckwheat without extensive preparation. (I do not recommend eating buckwheat without preparing it properly first, however.) On my website, I have a recipe for sourdough buckwheat pancakes in which I explain how to properly prepare buckwheat to make it safe for consumption. If you'd like to eat whole buckwheat (instead of making pancakes with it), simply soak it overnight, rinse, and cook.

What about the pseudocereals quinoa, amaranth, millet, and teff? In general, these pseudograins do contain many of the same plant toxins that other more common grains, like wheat, rye, oats, and brown rice, have. However, we don't have good information about how much preparation is required to neutralize the toxins they contain. For this reason, I generally recommend that people do not eat them regularly.

Legumes

Much of what I said above about grains also applies to legumes. All beans contain phytic acid and thus require a significant amount of preparation. Traditional cultures were aware of this on some level, and reports by anthropologists indicate that they often went to great lengths to prepare the beans before consuming them. In Central America, beans are made into a sour porridge called chugo, which is fermented for several days.

Simply soaking beans at moderate temperatures (78 degrees Fahrenheit) overnight reduces phytic acid by only 8 to 20 percent. Sprouting beans for several days and then cooking them will remove a larger amount. For example, fermenting lentils for three days at 108 degrees Fahrenheit results in about a 70 to 75 percent reduction in phytic acid. Soaking lentils for twelve hours, germinating them for three to four days, and then souring them will likely remove most of their phytic acid. If you're willing to go to these lengths to prepare them, you are healthy, and you don't have digestive issues or any chronic inflammatory conditions, moderate consumption of legumes is unlikely to cause problems. If not, I think they are best avoided.

Nightshades and eggs

If you removed nightshades or eggs due to arthritis or autoimmune problems in Step 1, you may want to reintroduce them in this phase to determine whether they cause problems for you. (Though these two food groups are unrelated, I will be discussing them together because they were removed from Step 1 for the same reasons.)

Eggs are an incredibly healthy food when well tolerated, although they can provoke immune or inflammatory responses in certain individuals. The nightshade family includes peppers, tomatoes, tomatillos, white potatoes, eggplant, and spices like chili, paprika, and cayenne. Nightshades contain toxins called glycoalkaloids, the most prevalent of which are solanine and chaconine. Glycoalkaloids may cause headaches, diarrhea, cramps, joint pain, and body aches in susceptible individuals.

There's nothing wrong with these foods when they're well tolerated. In fact, contrary to popular belief, white potatoes provide substantial amounts of some nutrients, such as potassium, which can be difficult to obtain elsewhere in the diet. But they do sometimes cause inflammation in people with arthritis or immune issues.

Alcohol

Alcohol is another substance that is highly subject to individual tolerance. I advise removing it in the first step not because of its potentially addictive properties but because it can cause leaky gut and other problems in susceptible people.

That said, most research suggests that moderate intake of alcohol is healthy for most people. But not all alcohol is created equal! Beer has gluten, which is probably the biggest offender when it comes to food toxins in grain products. For this reason, I don't recommend reintroducing beer. There are, however, several gluten-free beers on the market made from sorghum, tapioca, or brown rice. Some of them actually taste pretty good, but you'll need to experiment to see if you tolerate them.

Wine and spirits like vodka, tequila, and gin are good choices for those who do wish to drink alcohol. Spirits made from grain (such as bourbon) are fermented, significantly decreasing any antinutrient properties they might have.

Concentrated sweeteners

One of the main things to consider when choosing a concentrated sweetener is its ratio of fructose to glucose. Fructose and glucose are both simple sugars (single-molecule monosaccharides). Glucose is easily absorbed into the bloodstream and taken up as fuel by the cells. Our bodies are designed to run on glucose in moderate amounts. Fructose is a little more complicated. While most people are able to process fructose in moderate amounts (as in whole fruits, for example) without a problem, excess fructose in concentrated sweeteners, juices, and fructose-sweetened beverages can cause metabolic problems and digestive distress.

Fortunately, glucose enhances the absorption and uptake of fructose, so when the two are found together in roughly equal amounts, the body can handle the fructose without much trouble. However, when the amount of fructose in a food or sweetener is significantly higher than the amount of glucose it contains, the excess fructose may be problematic—especially for those with gut issues.

With this in mind, here's a list of sweeteners to favor and avoid:

RECOMMENDED	NOT RECOMMENDED
Coconut sugar	High-fructose corn syrup*
Maple syrup	Table sugar (sucrose)*
Molasses	Agave syrup*
Honey	Brown-rice syrup**
Dextrose	Artificial sweeteners***
Stevia	

*Unfavorable ratio of glucose to fructose, or highly processed
**Recent studies have found high amounts of arsenic, a toxic chemical, in most varieties of brown-rice syrup.
***Some studies suggest a link between artificial sweeteners and cancer, harmful metabolic effects, and digestive problems.

Caffeine

Caffeine is another gray-area food that is highly dependent upon individual tolerance. And individual tolerance is determined by several factors, including adrenal function, mood stability, quality and duration of sleep, and biological factors we don't fully understand.

Caffeine is a compound present in a number of foods and beverages, including coffee, tea, and chocolate. The amount of caffeine varies considerably depending on the type of product. The table below lists the caffeine content of several common beverages:

BEVERAGE	SERVING SIZE	CAFFEINE (MG)
Starbucks grande	16 oz.	330 mg
Brewed coffee	8 oz.	130 mg
Starbucks Tazo Awake Tea	16 oz.	130 mg
Red bull	8.4 oz. (1 can)	80 mg
Black tea	8 oz.	55 mg
Green tea	8 oz.	52 mg
Yerba maté	8 oz.	43 mg
Twig tea	8 oz.	5 mg

Since a lot of people consume their caffeinated beverages at places like Starbucks, I think it's safe to say that they're getting far more caffeine than they think they are. This explains, at least in part, why I see so many patients in my clinic with burned-out adrenals and sleep problems. If you are generally healthy, sleeping well, and have stable energy levels throughout the day, one to two cups of coffee (brewed at home, not a Starbucks grande!) or tea each day is probably not going to harm you. However, if you're dealing with insomnia, anxiety, mood swings, or low energy, I'd recommend eliminating or dramatically reducing caffeine until you overcome these problems.

Chocolate

There's nothing wrong with chocolate itself. In fact, it has a number of health benefits. It's high in magnesium, it's a powerful antioxidant, and it has been shown to have positive effects on the brain and cardiovascular and circulatory systems.

One issue with chocolate is that it is often sold as milk chocolate, which contains a lot of sugar; another problem is that it can have a stimulating effect because of its theobromine content. Theobromine is a bitter compound found in cacao beans that has similar effects as caffeine. Theobromine is generally not as stimulating as caffeine, but some people seem to be more sensitive to its effects than others.

.Chocolate can be safely consumed by eating only dark chocolate (greater than 70 percent cacao content, with greater than 85 percent preferred), limiting your intake to a small serving (about the size of a silver dollar), and not eating it at night if you're sensitive to its stimulating effect.

FOOD REINTRODUCTION SCHEDULE

Now that we've discussed *which* foods you may want to introduce, I'm going to propose a schedule for *when* to reintroduce them based on my experience with how well tolerated they are by the majority of people I work with and on our understanding of their biochemical composition.

If you don't tolerate one food in a particular category, that doesn't necessarily mean you won't tolerate other foods in that category. This is especially true for dairy and nightshades. For example, I have several patients who can't tolerate yogurt, cheese, or kefir but do just fine with butter and cream. Likewise, some of my patients can't eat tomatoes or eggplant but have no problem with white potatoes.

Dairy-products reintroduction

There's a specific order for reintroducing dairy products based on how likely you are to react to them, which is in turn determined by their sugar and protein content. People who are intolerant to dairy are reacting to the sugar (lactose), the proteins (such as casein, butyrophilin, and lacto-globulins), or, in some cases, both. But as I mentioned, some dairy products have negligible amounts of both casein and lactose. These are usually well tolerated, even in cases where people are reacting to lactose or milk protein (provided the reaction is an intolerance, not an allergy).

Since most dairy products contain protein, I'm going to focus on the lactose content of dairy foods. As a general rule, anything below 2 percent lactose can be tolerated by the majority of those who are lactose-intolerant, as long as they don't overdo it. If you find yourself reacting to a dairy food with very low amounts of lactose, it's likely you are intolerant to milk protein and will have to avoid cow's-milk products (with the possible exception of ghee, which contains only trace amounts of protein, and butter, which contains very low amounts). However, goat and sheep dairy products contain a different type of protein than cow dairy products. Because of this, some people who can't consume cow dairy products are able to safely consume goat and sheep dairy. If you determine that you can't tolerate cow-milk products (kefir, yogurt, cheese, milk), then you may want to try goat or sheep dairy during the reintroduction phase.

Dairy products are listed below from lowest to highest lactose content. Ghee was permitted during the Reset, so unless you removed it, you can start with butter and proceed to the next item. If you don't want to reintroduce a particular item on this list, simply move on to the next.

1. Ghee (clarified butter). Ghee is butter with the milk solids removed. You can think of it as butter oil. Butter has almost no lactose to begin with, and the lactose is in the milk solids, so ghee has virtually no detectable lactose. The level of protein is also nearly undetectable in ghee.

2. Butter. Butter is only 0.8 percent to 1 percent of lactose. It is well tolerated by all but the most lactose-sensitive individuals.

3. Kefir. Kefir is milk that has been fermented by strains of beneficial bacteria and yeast. (See my website for instructions on how to make it at home.) Since the yeast and bacteria consume (ferment) the lactose in the milk, the longer the milk is fermented, the less lactose it will have.

I've seen estimates of the lactose content of homemade kefir ranging from 0 percent to 3.5 percent. At twenty-four to thirty-six hours of fermentation, it's likely to contain less than 1 percent lactose. Kefir purchased in the store is often not fermented as long as that and is likely toward the upper end of the range.

4. Yogurt. Yogurt is milk that has been fermented by strains of lactic acid–producing bacteria (again, see my website for instructions on how to make it at home). As is the case with kefir, the longer you ferment yogurt, the less lactose it will have. If you ferment it for twenty-four-plus hours, it's likely to have negligible amounts of lactose and may be well tolerated even by lactose-sensitive individuals. Most varieties of store-bought yogurt, including Greek-style yogurts, are typically fermented for only three to four hours and its lactose content ranges from 4.1 to 4.7 percent. If you react to store-bought yogurt, try making it at home and fermenting it for at least twenty-four hours.

5. Cheese. Hard cheeses like Cheddar, Parmesan, Romano, and so on tend to be very low in lactose, ranging from 0 to 3.5 percent. Soft cheeses often range between 0 and 5 percent lactose. Be aware that cheese does contain a significant amount of casein, so if you're casein-intolerant, you'll need to avoid it.

6. Full-fat (whipping or heavy) cream. Cream is mostly fat and is 2.8 to 3.0 percent lactose. Although it is above the 2 percent safe range, in my experience, moderate amounts of cream are usually well tolerated even by those who are lactose-intolerant.

7. Sour cream. Sour cream ranges from 3.0 to 4.3 percent lactose. If you don't tolerate store-bought sour cream, you can try making it at home. See my website for instructions.

8. Ice cream. Yes, I said it — ice cream! Homemade ice cream is a luxurious occasional treat. It contains 3.1 to 8.4 percent lactose, so it is usually not a good choice for the lactose-intolerant.

9. Buttermilk. Buttermilk is a cultured-milk product that is often added to pancake mixes. It contains roughly 3.6 to 5.0 percent lactose.

10. Milk (whole, 2 percent, 1 percent, nonfat). These are about 3.7 to 5.1 percent lactose. Fluid milk is not well tolerated by most people, so I generally don't recommend it. (The exception would be raw milk, which can be legally obtained in some states. Raw milk is often well tolerated even by those who can't drink pasteurized milk.) Low-fat and nonfat milk have higher lactose content than whole milk. I do not recommend consuming reduced-fat milk products for any reason—this goes for yogurts, cheeses, and other dairy products as well. If you must have milk, go for whole! For at-a-glance information on the foods discussed in this chapter (caffeine content, lactose content, and so forth), see the charts on my website.

WHAT ABOUT FAKE MILKS?

Over the past decade, milk substitutes like soy, rice, and almond milk have grown in popularity. There are two issues with the store-bought versions of these milks that make them a poor choice for regular consumption:

* They are usually quite high in sugar, especially compared to cow's milk or goat's milk.
* They often contain carrageenan, a seaweed extract used to make the milks more viscous. Though there is still controversy about the relevance of this in humans, animal research suggests that carrageenan may cause inflammation and ulceration of the digestive tract, impaired glucose tolerance, insulin resistance, and cancer.

Beyond these two issues, soy milk has additional problems. It may have adverse effects on male fertility. A study at the Harvard School of Public Health found that consuming just one cup per day of soy milk decreased sperm count, especially in men who were overweight or obese. Other studies found that phytoestrogens in soy may adversely affect male reproductive hormones and sperm capacitation (an important process sperm must go through after being ejaculated into the female reproductive tract). Soy phytoestrogens also have potentially harmful effects on women. A large review of forty-seven studies found that soy phytoestrogens reduced levels of LH and FSH, two hormones essential to fertility and reproductive health, and increased menstrual-cycle length.

The research on soy is not black and white. Some studies (like those above) show harm, while others show no harm. I think the precautionary principle applies here: there's nothing essential about soy milk, it's not especially nutrient dense, and it may cause reproductive and endocrine problems (especially in infants fed soy formula), so it's best avoided entirely or consumed only in small quantities.

What about rice milk and almond milk? If you can find varieties without carrageenan and with no added sweeteners, they're fine in moderation. In addition, both rice and almond milks (and other nut and seed milks) can be made simply and quickly at home. Please see my website for instructions on how to make nut milk at home.

Grain, pseudocereal, and legume reintroduction

As I have indicated, extensive preparation is required to make grains and legumes more digestible and improve their nutrient bioavailability. If you really miss grains or legumes in your diet, are healthy and have a strong digestive system, and are willing to take the necessary steps to prepare grains and legumes, then you may reintroduce them in modest amounts (that is, about three to five servings per week) during Step 2.

I suggest starting with white rice and fermented buckwheat, since they are low in phytic acid and other antinutrients and are less likely to irritate the gut. Beyond white rice and buckwheat, I don't think it matters much what order you reintroduce properly prepared grains and legumes in. Just be sure to reintroduce them one at a time, and carefully track your symptoms as you do. And remember, even soaked and fermented grains and legumes should never displace more nutrient-dense foods like meat, fish, vegetables, nuts, seeds, and fruits.

Nightshade and egg reintroduction

If you've been on the autoimmune/arthritis version of the Step 1 Reset, in which you removed eggs and nightshades, you may want to reintroduce these after you've tried dairy and/or buckwheat and white rice.

I suggest reintroducing eggs first, because they're one of the most nutrient-dense superfoods nature has made available to us. They're also tasty, versatile, and easy to prepare. Be aware that some people react negatively to egg whites (one of the most common food allergens). However, it's much less common for people to react to the yolks. This is fortunate, because the yolks contain the majority of the nutrients and are by far the healthiest part of the egg. If you don't tolerate egg whites, you can continue to eat the yolks. Try hard-boiling eggs, then removing and eating the solid yolks if you want a quick source of nutrients without worrying about raw-egg safety or egg-white contamination. You can also make egg-yolk omelets.

There is a lot of variation in how people react to nightshades, but I advise reintroducing them (after eggs) in the following order:

- Ripe, raw tomatoes and tomatillos
- White potatoes
- Eggplant
- Peppers
- Cayenne, paprika

Alcohol reintroduction

Which alcoholic drinks you reintroduce depends primarily on your preference. I haven't noticed one particular class being tolerated better than another. That said, wine does tend to have more sugar than spirits, so if you are sensitive to sugar, it may be wise to start with something like tequila or vodka (if you like them, that is). The reintroduction schedule could look like this:

- Vodka
- Tequila

- Other spirits
- Wine
- Gluten-free beer (rare treat)

In general, I'd recommend limiting alcohol consumption to three to five drinks per week.

Concentrated-sweeteners reintroduction

The particular order of reintroduction of the recommended sweeteners is not important, but this fact is: *sugar is sugar*. Yes, natural sweeteners do have higher nutrient content than the processed sugars, but in general (with the exception of molasses), these nutrients are not enough to make a significant contribution to the diet. Since you will be eating only minimal amounts of these sweeteners, the most important consideration is their glucose-to-fructose ratio—especially if you have digestive problems. Refer to the listing on page 193 for recommended sweeteners; remember to avoid agave syrup, brown-rice syrup, and all artificial sweeteners.

Caffeine reintroduction

I suggest beginning with the lower-caffeine beverages, like green tea and twig tea, first. If you do well with those, you can move on to black tea and coffee. (See the caffeine section on page 194 in this chapter for information on which beverages have the highest and lowest amounts of caffeine, and visit my website for information on the caffeine content of specific coffees, teas, soft drinks, and energy drinks.) Remember that coffee from Starbucks and other vendors can have significantly higher amounts of caffeine than coffee you brew at home! If you notice any worsening of sleep, fluctuations in energy or mood, irritability, anxiety, or agitation when you reintroduce coffee or black tea, remove it again for a few days and then try starting with the lower-caffeine beverages again. Decaf coffee is another possibility, though it is not completely free of caffeine. Most estimates I've seen suggest it has about five milligrams of caffeine.

Chocolate reintroduction

Start with a silver-dollar-size piece of dark chocolate (greater than 70 percent cacao, and preferably greater than 85 percent), and have it earlier in the day—perhaps after lunch. The reason I suggest this is that some people are very stimulated by chocolate, and it can interfere with sleep. If you don't notice that effect, or any other ill effects, you're free to eat one to two silver-dollar-size pieces of dark chocolate per day if you wish. Another great way to enjoy chocolate is to add unsweetened, raw cacao nibs or powder to smoothies. Try combining nut milk, coconut milk, and/or kefir with half a banana and some raw cacao powder for a special treat.

REINTRODUCE GRAY-AREA FOODS: YOUR PERSONAL PALEO CURE

- Reintroducing the foods in this chapter is optional. If you feel great without them and don't miss them, there's no need to add them back into your diet.
- Reintroduce no more than one food every three days.
- Keep a food diary to make it easier to isolate adverse reactions to foods.
- Go slowly! If there's any doubt about how you're reacting to a food, remove it from your diet, wait a few days, and then try again.
- Don't reintroduce new foods if you're experiencing unusual stress, sleep deprivation, a flare-up of a chronic health condition, or inflammation, as these things will affect your response to the new food.

CHAPTER 12

Move Like Your Ancestors

Movement Quiz

Complete the quiz below and use the answer key to determine your movement score.

	POINTS
I sit fewer than five hours per day.	2
I get at least thirty minutes of moderate to vigorous physical activity each day.	2
I walk or bike to work.	2
I do activities to increase muscle strength, such as lifting weights or calisthenics, once a week or more.	1
I do activities to improve flexibility, such as stretching or yoga, once a week or more.	1
I use a standing desk at work or spend several hours standing daily.	2
I typically walk at least eight thousand steps per day (around four miles).	3

(continued)

Notes for this chapter may be found at ChrisKresser.com/ppcnotes/#ch12.

	POINTS
I do not have any injuries or health conditions or symptoms that restrict my ability to exercise (such as asthma, chest pain, or fatigue).	1
I enjoy being physically active.	1
I watch fewer than two hours of television per day.	1
TOTAL	

Answer key

TOTAL POINTS	WHAT YOUR POINTS MEAN	YOUR PERSONAL PALEO CURE
6+	You are likely getting adequate and healthy levels of physical activity.	Complete the *Paleo Cure* 3-Step program. No additional personalization is required.
3–5	You may benefit from incorporating additional movement into your day.	Complete the *Paleo Cure* 3-Step program and add the recommendations in this chapter.
0–2	You are likely getting an inadequate amount of physical activity.	Complete both steps above. This should be a major focus for you, and ignoring this area may stand in the way of improvement elsewhere.

Our Paleolithic ancestors didn't worry about the benefits of cardio versus weight training, and they weren't concerned about whether they should do Pilates to strengthen their cores or squats to sculpt their glutes. They didn't exercise or work out; they just lived. For the vast majority of evolutionary history, humans had to exert themselves—often quite strenuously—to survive. They naturally spent a lot of time outdoors in the sun walking, hunting, and gathering.

Anthropological research suggests that our ancestors sprinted, jogged, climbed, carried, and jumped intermittently throughout the day. They walked an average of six miles and ran an average of one-half to one mile per day. Women were as active as men; although they rarely took part in large-game hunting, they spent hours walking to and from sources of food, water, and wood, and they carried their children (whom they breast-fed for up to four years!) for extended distances. Our ancestors also alternated strenuous and demanding days with days of rest. This instinctual response protected them from injury and fatigue, which in turn improved their chances of survival.

Contemporary hunter-gatherers are also active. Studies show that they walk an average of ten thousand steps (about five miles) per day, with frequent bouts of more intense activity. Anthropologist Kim Hill spent thirty years living with and studying the Ache hunter-gatherers of Paraguay. His GPS data indicated that they covered more than six miles a day on average while they hunted, running in hot pursuit of their quarry for half a mile to a mile, all while "ducking under low branches and vines about once every 20 seconds all day long, and climbing over fallen trees, moving through tangled thorns, etc." Closer to home, contemporary Amish people who have retained their traditional ways take between fourteen thousand and eighteen thousand steps per day. One way of measuring an individual's fitness is the VO_2 max, the volume of oxygen that can be consumed while exercising at maximum capacity (VO_2 max is measured in milliliters of oxygen per kilogram of body weight per minute). Today, the average sedentary person has a VO_2 max of 35 ml/kg/min, and the average elite endurance athlete has one around 70 ml/kg/min. The estimated VO_2 max in modern hunter-gatherers is 52, which places them in the excellent-to-superior fitness category; it's likely our ancestors were equally fit. In other words, if we want to get and stay highly physically fit, we can move more like our ancestors.

Many concepts in this chapter were inspired by the Enduring Mover framework created by Dan Pardi, a researcher on human behavior and the CEO of Dan's Plan. As Enduring Movers, we maintain optimal health and fitness by incorporating both low- and high-intensity activity into our daily lives, just as our ancestors did. I'll have more to say about the Enduring Mover framework and Dan's Plan later in the chapter.

AN EPIDEMIC OF INACTIVITY

In most Western societies, people were highly physically active until—you probably guessed it—the Industrial Revolution. In the 1800s, approximately 90 percent of jobs in America required manual labor; today, only 2 percent do. Now, thanks to dramatic changes in the way we live, communicate, travel, use technology, and get and consume our food, the typical American adult walks only about 5,900 to 6,900 steps per day.

Simply put, we've become a nation of sitters, whether we're working at our computers, watching TV, playing video games, or commuting. The typical U.S. adult is now sedentary for 60 percent of his or her waking hours and sits for an average of six hours (and often much more, in the case of those who work primarily on computers). A sedentary office worker expends only ten calories per pound each day, down from the hunter-gatherer's average of forty-three to fifty-five calories per pound per day.

Why sitting is dangerous to your health

We weren't born to sit all day. We're genetically designed to be physically active. All this increased sitting and decreased physical activity has a profound, negative effect on almost every aspect of human health, from the cardiovascular and pulmonary systems to the immune system. In fact, a whole new subfield, called sedentary physiology, has evolved to address the health risks of being too sedentary. Here are a few specific ways being sedentary harms us:

- Sitting wrecks our metabolic functions.
- Sitting decreases the activity of the enzyme lipoprotein lipase (LPL), which is associated with higher triglyceride levels, lower HDL levels (the good cholesterol), and an increased risk of cardiovascular disease.
- Even a single day of prolonged sitting has been shown to reduce insulin action.
- Sitting weakens the bones.

Up to two-thirds of professional cyclists, who spend long hours in a seated position, have lower levels of bone mass, studies have shown. Both humans and animals experience dramatic reductions in bone mass following spinal-cord injuries, long-term bed rest, or time in zero gravity. After just twelve weeks of bed rest, healthy men and women experienced reductions in bone-mineral density of 1 to 4 percent. What's more, studies suggest that vigorous exercise alone isn't enough to prevent the changes in bone metabolism caused by too much sedentary behavior.

Sitting harms the blood vessels

Although the data in this area isn't as robust as it is with metabolic and bone health, initial findings suggest that sedentary behavior has harmful effects on the vascular system. Just five days of bed rest can increase blood pressure and decrease arterial diameter. Other studies have found that after two months of bed rest, subjects had decreased blood flow and increased damage to the cells in the fragile lining of the blood vessels.

Sitting increases the risk of death

In an Australian study that followed participants over a six-and-a-half-year period, researchers found that high levels of TV time were significantly associated with increased risk of death from heart disease as well as all other causes. Each hour of TV daily was associated with an 11 percent and 18 percent increase in all-cause and cardiovascular mortality, respectively. By contrast, those who watched less than two hours of TV a day had an 80 percent lower risk of death from cardiovascular disease and a 46 percent lower risk of death from all causes when compared to those who watched more than four hours. These associations were independent of exercise and traditional risk factors such as smoking, blood pressure, cholesterol levels, waist circumference, and diet.

A U.S. study based on twenty-one years of follow-up of 7,700 men found that those who reported spending more than ten hours a week sitting in automobiles or more than twenty-three hours a week of combined TV and automobile time had an 82 percent and 64 percent greater risk of death from cardiovascular disease compared to those who spent less than four hours a week in cars or less than eleven hours a week of combined sedentary time, respectively. Regular physical activity is one of the best predictors of long-term health and survival in large, observational studies. In fact, your fitness level (as measured by performance on a treadmill exercise test) has been shown to be a better predictor of how and when you'll die than age, body mass index, or even cardiovascular risk factors.

In other words, if you want to live longer, you have to be physically active on a regular basis.

And if you want a better quality of life, physical activity's the answer too. Adults who exercise report higher quality of life, and studies have shown that physical activity improves cognitive function in the elderly. These benefits are evident from the earliest years; physically active children report greater body satisfaction and self-esteem than their sedentary peers. Finally, getting adequate exercise during the day promotes deeper and more restful sleep at night and reduces pre-sleep anxiety and insomnia.

Working Out Isn't the Answer
(Or, the Active-Couch-Potato Problem)

Maybe you're thinking, *Okay, I sit a lot—but I also work out a lot, so I'm good.* Here's the shocker: too much sitting and sedentary time is harmful *even if you're getting enough exercise.* This means you could be meeting the recommended government guidelines for exercise (that is, thirty minutes of moderate to vigorous activity five days a week) but still be at high risk of heart disease if you sit for long periods each day. In fact, a large study involving over one hundred thousand U.S. adults found that those who sat for more than six hours a day had up to a 40 percent greater risk of death over the next fifteen years than those who sat for less than three hours a day *regardless of whether the participants exercised.* Canadians who reported spending the majority of the day sitting had an increased risk of death compared to those who reported less time sitting. As with the American study, this association was apparent even among those who exercised regularly. Perhaps you're one of these active couch potatoes. If you work in an office, commute by car, and watch a few hours of TV each night, it's not difficult to see how you could spend the vast majority of your waking hours sitting on your butt. Imagine the following hypothetical day:

- 7:00 a.m.: wake up
- 7:15–7:45 a.m.: go for a jog (exercise)
- 8:00–9:00 a.m.: breakfast and drive to work (sitting)
- 9:00–12:30 p.m.: work on computer (sitting)
- 12:30–1:00 p.m.: lunch (sitting)
- 1:00–5:00 p.m.: work on computer (sitting)
- 5:00–6:30 p.m.: drive home and eat dinner (sitting)
- 6:30–9:30 p.m.: watch TV, read, check e-mail (sitting)
- 10:00 p.m.: go to bed

If you did this routine five days a week, you'd meet the typical guidelines for exercise (at least one hundred and fifty minutes of moderate exercise a week), but you'd also be sitting for at least twelve hours a day.

Other problems with exercise as an intervention

The evidence clearly indicates that sitting too much is harmful in itself and that exercise alone isn't enough to reverse the harmful effects. But there are other problems with looking at exercise as solely an intervention.

In an effort to overcome inactivity when they're not exercising, some people are overtraining. Exercise is a stressor. Not all stress is harmful; in the right dose, it can cause a positive adaptation and better equip you to face that stressor in the future. This is referred to as hormesis. Weightlifting is a great example of the hormetic effects of stress. When you lift weights, you stress the muscles, and this causes them to get stronger.

However, when stress exceeds your capacity to adapt, it stops having a beneficial, hormetic effect and begins to cause damage. (See the section "Are You Overtraining?") Just as we didn't evolve to sit so much, we're not adapted to perform excessive amounts of exercise. A large and growing body of evidence has demonstrated that excessive exercise, such as marathons, ultra-marathons, full-distance triathlons, and very long-distance bicycle rides, is associated with damage to the heart, muscles, and joints. Overtraining has been associated with increased injury, oxidative damage, inflammation, and cognitive decline, as well as with decreased immune function, fat metabolism, and cardiovascular health. Consider the following:

- A study of one hundred middle-aged marathon runners found higher levels of coronary calcium (a marker of heart-disease risk) as compared with non-runners, and the marathoners' risk of cardiovascular events during the follow-up period was similar to that of people with preexisting heart disease.
- A study of elite runners found that those who participated in a large number of long-distance races had increased scarring (fibrosis) of the heart tissue, and the degree of scarring was directly correlated with the number of marathons or ultra-marathons completed and the number of years spent training.
- Finally, a study of marathoners between fifty and seventy-two years of age who ran an average of thirty-five miles a week found that they were more than three times more likely to have heart damage than non-runners.

Too much exercise may harm people in less obvious ways as well. If you get up a half-hour early to exercise to offset all that sitting, that's better than doing nothing, of course, but you're also cutting into valuable sleep time. You may simply trade one problem (too much sitting) for another (chronic sleep deprivation). As you'll see in the next chapter on sleep, that's not a good trade! Some research suggests that people who exercise intensely (like marathon runners) are actually more likely to be sedentary when they're not exercising. They may assume—incorrectly—that their exercise regimen protects them from the harmful effects of too much sitting.

THE SOLUTION: SWAP YOUR WAY TO HEALTH

So how do we find the sweet spot and ensure that we get enough—but not too much—physical activity? Once again, we can look to our ancestors for clues on how to be naturally active throughout the day: sitting less, incorporating more movement into our daily routines, and engaging in moderate-to-vigorous exercise periodically.

The best way to accomplish this is by becoming what Dan Pardi of Dan's Plan calls an Enduring Mover. The Enduring Mover framework involves three elements that can be expressed in the acronym SWAP: Stand, Walk, and Push. (Please see my website for a great infographic that Dan created to inspire the Enduring Mover in you and a link to Dan's Plan, where you can find additional information about this approach.)

Stand

To undo the harmful effects of sitting, stand up! Standing engages postural muscles that increase helpful LPL activity, among other benefits. Standing and walking slowly increases energy expenditure by two and a half times; employees who stand while they work burn up to 75 percent more calories per day than people in sedentary jobs. An analysis by Dan Pardi showed that simply standing and engaging in light activity throughout the day burns as many calories over the course of a week as one to three intense spinning classes!

Studies show that the more breaks you take from sitting, the lower your waist circumference, body mass index, and triglycerides and the more stable your blood sugar. In fact, some research suggests that regular light physical activity throughout the day—including standing and walking—is more effective than short periods of vigorous exercise in reversing the harm caused by too much sitting.

If your day typically involves sitting for long periods, here are a few ways to reduce your sitting time:

- Follow the guidelines in "How to Make Your Workspace Paleo-Friendly" on page 214.
- Take standing breaks. Stand up for at least two minutes every thirty to forty-five minutes. Take a brief walk or do some light stretching. Even short breaks like this can make a big difference. (They're great for relieving eyestrain too.) Try setting an alarm on

your phone each time you come back from a break and sit down again, and do this until the break becomes second nature.

- Stand up at long meetings. If you're worried about what your colleagues might think, just tell them you have a bad back!

Goals:

- Stand for about half of the day.
- Take a standing break every thirty to forty-five minutes.

Walk

Again, let's keep it simple: Walk more, sit less. Of course, light physical activity, such as gardening or performing household chores, is also beneficial. In fact, all that fidgeting your parents and teachers told you to knock off—pacing around, being restless, doing a whole lot of nothing—is actually good for you. Studies show that fidgeting alone can increase energy expenditure by 50 percent when compared to sitting motionless; that translates to burning off an extra 350 calories a day—that's thirty-five to forty pounds a year! Besides, it's easier (and cheaper) to integrate a low-intensity activity into your daily life than an intensive, formal workout (like that pricey class at a gym you have to drive to).

You don't have to do intensive exercise to improve fitness. Even a relatively low to moderate level of physical activity will lower your postmeal blood sugar, insulin levels, and triglycerides, as well as reduce your waist circumference. People who are lean tend to be physically active for more than 50 percent of the day, whereas people who are obese tend to be active for less than 40 percent of their day. The benefits of incorporating more activity and walking don't stop with fitness. For years, I suffered from back pain and persistent muscle aches. I tried numerous treatments, from acupuncture to anti-inflammatory nutrients like curcumin to yoga. Nothing worked. When I started writing this book, the pain got even worse, since I was now spending two or three additional hours a day sitting at my computer—and I was only on the first chapter! I also had a fifteen-month-old daughter, a busy private practice, and several other obligations encroaching on my exercise-and-physical-activity time. I had to do something.

My first step was to install a standing desk in my office, and I began alternating between standing and sitting as I wrote. (I'll talk more about the benefits of this routine later in this chapter.) It took me only about half a day to get used to writing while standing. My back pain improved slightly, but my muscles still ached. So I installed a treadmill under my standing desk. In the beginning, I averaged about eight thousand to ten thousand steps a day as I wrote. I felt a little sore at first, simply because I wasn't accustomed to walking this much. But I also noticed a decrease in muscle pain at other times of day, and my back pain was significantly reduced. Encouraged, I slowly increased the amount of time I spent working at my treadmill desk. After a couple of weeks, I settled into an average of between fifteen thousand and eighteen thousand steps per day.

The improvements were nothing short of miraculous. Back pain? Gone. Muscle pain? Gone. I noticed other benefits as well, from an increase in mental clarity and sharpness to an improvement in the quality of my sleep.

You don't need to match my steps to see a major improvement — just aim for ten thousand steps a day for optimal health. Walking that distance — about five miles a day — might seem impossible if you commute by car to work and spend most of the day at a computer, but here are a few tips for increasing your steps:

- **Take walking meetings.** If you have a meeting scheduled with someone in your office, why not suggest taking a walk while you do it?
- **Use the stairs whenever possible.** You might want to take the elevator if you work on the fiftieth floor of a building (at least some of the time), but do you really need to take it if you work on the third floor?
- **Walk or bicycle to work.** Get creative. If you live too far away to walk or ride exclusively, consider driving part of the way and walking or cycling for the remainder.
- **Do your own chores.** Rather than outsourcing cleaning, laundry, gardening, washing the car, and other household chores, do them yourself.

- **Get a dog.** Dogs need to be exercised regularly for optimal health, just like people. You might not be motivated to take a walk yourself, but if you have a dog, you're more likely to do it.
- **Choose a hobby that requires physical activity.** Ballroom dancing, bowling, and cooking are fun choices, but it's especially great to pick a hobby that gets you outdoors, like bird-watching, gardening, snorkeling, camping, or hunting.
- **Extra credit: work at a treadmill desk!** See the sidebar "How to Make Your Workspace Paleo-Friendly."

Goals:

- Aim for ten thousand steps each day.
- Integrate light activity throughout your daily routine.

HOW TO MAKE YOUR WORKSPACE PALEO-FRIENDLY

The most important changes you can make in your workspace is decreasing the amount of time you spend sitting and sitting more actively when you do sit. Here are four of the best ways I've found to accomplish this goal:

- **Use a standing desk.** There are several types of standing desks, ranging from stationary models to adjustable desks that move from seated to standing work positions. Many employers permit standing desks now, and more will follow once they understand the benefits in terms of reduced absenteeism, lower health-care costs, and higher productivity in their employees. Ask your boss for one; if you get any resistance, educate him or her on the benefits to the bottom line—healthy workers are better workers. See my website for more information on where to find standing desks (including how to make one yourself).

- **Use a treadmill desk.** Treadmill desks are similar to standing desks, except they have a treadmill underneath them. I use one daily and it allows me to walk while I'm working. As with standing desks, there are several options for configuration. You can buy a treadmill for your existing standing desk, as I did, or buy a desk that fits above your existing treadmill. However, if you're just starting out, the best option might be to buy a preconfigured treadmill desk. I use a brand called TrekDesk but there are other options (see ChrisKresser.com for an article I wrote on treadmill-desk options).
- **Sit on a balance disk.** Balance disks are squishy cylinders about four inches thick. When you slip one onto your chair and sit on it, you'll find it's almost impossible to slouch. The disk forces you (in a good way) to engage your sitting muscles and continually readjust your position. There are several different brands of balance disks on the market. I use one made by Fitter First.
- **Sit on a yoga ball.** Try using a yoga ball in place of your chair for certain periods throughout the day. Like balance disks, they require small postural adjustments while you're sitting. I like my Natural Fitness Professional yoga ball because it's so sturdy, but there are several other good brands.
- **Take frequent breaks.** I recommend taking a micro-break every ten to fifteen minutes, during which you look away from the computer screen and shift your position, and macro-breaks every thirty to forty-five minutes, during which you stand up, walk, or do some strength-training or conditioning exercises or perhaps some stress reduction. If you have trouble remembering to take breaks, you can use an app like Time Out (Mac) or Workrave (Windows) to remind you.

The ideal approach would be to switch between standing, walking, sitting in your chair, sitting on a balance disk in your chair, and sitting on a yoga ball throughout the day. If you do that, even if you have to work for ten hours straight, you'll be sure to get plenty of physical activity and continue to burn calories.

Push

Push here is short for push yourself. The goal is for you to include intense physical activity in addition to standing and walking throughout the week.

Modern research has confirmed that intense, intermittent exercise results in reductions in weight and improvements in blood-sugar regulation similar to equivalent amounts of lower-intensity continuous activity. In fact, some studies suggest that high-intensity, intermittent strength training is even more effective at improving resting metabolic rate (which helps burn fat) than lower-intensity, traditional strength training.

However, our ancestors didn't overdo it. They instinctively conserved their energy, strength, and stamina for the daily tasks they needed to perform to survive. As one researcher put it, "Retirement was not an option for hunter-gatherers." Studies of contemporary hunter-gatherers indicate that they likewise alternate difficult or strenuous days with easier rest days whenever possible. Modern research suggests that following a strenuous-workout day with a less demanding workout the next day leads to superior fitness and lowers risk of injury.

With this in mind, I recommend following Dan Pardi's guidelines for moderate-to-vigorous activity:

- 150 minutes of moderate-intensity activity per week (like jogging, yoga, or dancing); or,
- 75 minutes of vigorous intensity activity per week (like running, Zumba, or playing sports); or,
- 30 sets of highest-intensity exercise per week (like sprinting, jumping rope, or resistance training—see "How to Strength Train in Your Home or Office," page 217); or,
- some combination of the above.

Moderate exercise, vigorous exercise, and highest-intensity exercise are defined as follows:

- Moderate: 50 to 70 percent of maximum effort

- Vigorous: 70 to 90 percent of maximum effort
- Highest-intensity: greater than 90 percent of maximum effort

I use these percentages because one person's moderate activity might be someone else's all-out highest effort. If someone has been completely sedentary, he might consider even a leisurely jog or a yoga class high intensity, whereas a fit person would likely classify the same activity as moderate intensity. A set of squats or bench-presses performed to failure—that is, until you can't do one more repetition—would always be considered highest intensity, since by definition you've exerted maximum effort.

You can do your Push activity in designated workouts or simply integrate it into your daily routine (see "How to Strength Train in Your Home or Office," below). I incorporate SWAP into my day through working at my treadmill desk and taking regular micro- and macro-breaks. I use micro-breaks to look away from the computer monitor and give my eyes a rest and to do some light stretching; during longer macro-breaks, I do some sets of pull-ups or other exercises, or I go outside and jump rope. By the time my workday is done, there's no need for me to go to a gym!

Most of my patients and readers report huge improvements in energy levels and cognitive function and reductions in muscle and joint pain and soreness when they sneak in moderate to vigorous activity throughout the day. Of course, if you can't do this at work or you simply prefer a predictable workout schedule, that's fine too. The important thing is to Push!

Goal:

- Push it for 150 minutes of moderate-intensity activity, 75 minutes of vigorous activity, 30 minutes maximal or near-maximal activity each week, or some combination of these.

HOW TO STRENGTH TRAIN IN YOUR HOME OR OFFICE

Resistance training, or strength training, is a proven way to build up and maintain muscle, which helps keep your metabolism revved, helps keeps you mobile, and helps prevent injuries. Stressing your body with a load makes it stronger, whether that load is a dumbbell or your own body. Lifting weights at the gym a few times a week is a great option, but for those of you with less time or without gym access or who wish to pursue a more natural pattern of movement, try incorporating your strength training throughout the day using relatively affordable tools you can keep in your home or office. This is the strategy advocated by Dan's Plan with their inTUNE daily movement practice. The acronym inTUNE stands for "integrative and opportunistic training." The idea is for you to integrate short bursts of physical activity throughout your day. You might, for example, do three sets of push-ups, three sets of pull-ups, and three sets of lunges interspersed with periods of sitting or standing at your desk (or walking at it, if you have a treadmill desk).

With this approach, you'll reap great health benefits in very little time and without leaving your home or office. You're far more likely to find multiple two-minute opportunities for exercise across your day than you are to find one larger chunk of time. Also, it's no-cost (if you use your body, as when you do push-ups or lunges) or low-cost; no need for an expensive gym membership. And the more time-efficient and convenient your exercise routine is, the more likely you are to stick with it. Here are some tools that make incorporating exercise throughout the day easier than ever:

- **Push-up handles.** Around twenty dollars, these amp up the intensity of push-ups.
- **Pull-up bar.** Around twenty-five dollars, this can be attached to a door frame so you can do pull-ups and chin-ups.
- **PowerBlocks.** These dumbbells are pricier — around three hundred dollars — but they can adjust from fifteen to ninety pounds, so you don't need a whole set of weights taking up room.
- **Abdominal wheel.** Around twenty dollars, this gives your abs a super-intense workout.
- **Weight bench.** You can find this at any price point to add more range to your strength-training workouts.

- **Weight vest.** For about thirty-five dollars, this makes pull-ups, push-ups, and dips more intense.
- **Suspension trainers.** These straps are pricey — one hundred to three hundred dollars — but they turn a doorway into an instant gym — and they're portable. I take mine along when I travel.

TRACKING YOUR PROGRESS

If you want to make a change stick, then track your progress. Getting visual confirmation that you're meeting or even exceeding your goals is one of the best ways to stay motivated and inspired. Tracking your SWAP program is easy if you've got the right hardware and software.

There are lots of hardware gadgets to choose from: FitBit, Nike + Fuel Band, Jawbone's Up, BodyMedia FIT, Striiv, or a simple pedometer can each do the job. I use a FitBit every day and I get a lot of value from it. The FitBit includes a pedometer that measures the number of steps you take each day. (It can also track sleep and calories.) It then syncs up wirelessly to the FitBit dashboard, which e-mails you progress reports.

There are a zillion apps to help you monitor your progress. My favorite tracking software by far is a free Web-based application called Dan's Plan (DansPlan.com). The goal of Dan's Plan is to bring more attention to lifestyle habits and encourage daily actions that support health. It combines several variables (for example, sleep, physical activity, weight) into a Health Zone Score, which gives you a quick visual indicator of whether you're reaching your daily health goals. Dan's Plan integrates with several popular hardware tracking tools, such as the FitBit (for sleep, step, and weight data). But Dan's Plan also helps you track the kind of daily movement practice we've been discussing in this chapter. Exercise is measured in a simple, flexible way so you get credit for any type that you do. Your total physical activity is also tracked and reported, so you can be sure you're getting enough overall activity to promote health. Dan's Plan is simple to use and takes only a few minutes each day, but it provides powerful feedback that quickly tells you whether you're living in your

Health Zone. I use Dan's Plan myself and I recommend it to all of my patients.

ARE YOU OVERTRAINING?

Most of my patients know when they're not getting enough exercise; they're less likely to know when they're overtraining.

Competitive athletes who specialize in endurance sports as well as any people who perform intense, strenuous exercise several times a week are at the highest risk for overtraining. You may be at risk too, even if you don't put yourself into those categories, because if you're chronically ill, injured, sleep deprived, or restricting calories, it's possible to be overtrained at much lower levels of physical activity. This is why it's so important to customize your exercise and other activities to your unique circumstances and needs—which often change over time. (I also recommend you work with a qualified trainer who can monitor you and tell you if you're overdoing it.)

How do you know if you're overtrained? Typically you'll experience one or more of the following signs and symptoms:

- Decreased performance
- Increased recovery time
- Fatigue or lethargy
- Insomnia
- Difficulty concentrating and memory issues
- Muscle and joint pain
- Low libido
- Amenorrhea in women
- Anxiety or depression

The longer you overtrain, the more severe these symptoms become, and the more difficult it is to recover. Remember, sometimes less is more. You don't have to train like an Olympic athlete to stay fit. In fact, unless you actually are an Olympic athlete, training like one is likely to cause more harm than good.

If you think you're overtrained, here are some suggestions for recovery:

- **Reduce or even stop anything more than moderate physical activity for a while.** How long depends on how severe your symptoms are and how long you've been overtraining. Most people benefit from at least a month of reduced activity, but some will need three months or even longer.
- **Focus on gentle, nourishing activities like walking, gardening, leisurely hiking, and so on.** Low-level physical activity is unlikely to exacerbate the problem and will protect against too much sedentary time.
- **Spend time outdoors.** Spending time in nature and getting exposure to sunlight seem to be particularly helpful for recovery.
- **Get plenty of sleep and rest.** At least eight hours a night but preferably ten or even more if you're significantly overtrained. If you're tired during the day, take a nap.
- **Eat!** Do not diet or restrict calories when you're overtrained. Your body needs an adequate supply of macronutrients (especially protein) and micronutrients to repair itself.
- **Read the bonus chapter on adrenal fatigue syndrome** (available on my website) and follow the suggestions on treatment. The brain-adrenal axis is typically most affected by overtraining.

I know scaling back might be difficult for you. But consider this: the more you rest and take care of yourself, the faster you'll recover and be able to resume a more normal level of activity. I've seen people string their recovery out for years by not taking the necessary time to rest or by going back to their high-intensity routine too quickly. That just deepens the hole they're already in and makes it harder to ever get out.

GO BARE: WHY BAREFOOT IS BEST

Our ancestors walked, ran, and performed other physical activities barefoot or in simple leather shoes. I recommend you do the same.

Today's running and fitness shoes are often highly cushioned with elevated heels and other features that impair range of motion and create an unnatural gait. Studies have shown that most athletic shoes increase the risk of overuse walking and running problems like plantar fasciitis, ankle sprains, Achilles tendinitis, hamstring tears, and lower back pain. Other studies have shown that simpler shoes that don't restrict range of motion or change natural foot-strike dynamics are less likely to cause injury and are better for long-term orthopedic health than typical fitness or running shoes. For these reasons, walking, running, and exercising barefoot or with minimalist footwear have become increasingly popular. Some of the more popular minimalist footwear brands include Vibram, VivoBarefoot, and Inov-8. Brands like New Balance, Merrell, and Patagonia also offer minimalist options. (Some of these companies also make shoes with flat, thin soles for work and casual wear.) I go barefoot or wear minimalist shoes almost exclusively at this point (including while I'm walking at my treadmill desk).

Barefoot running is not without controversy, however. Some recent studies suggest that runners who go barefoot or wear minimalist shoes are still prone to injuries—they're just prone to different injuries than runners who wear traditional running shoes. That said, most experts in barefoot or minimalist running believe that the injuries associated with it are due primarily to poor technique and making the transition from traditional to minimalist footwear too quickly.

So if you decide to give this a try, it's crucial to focus on proper biomechanics and make the transition slowly—especially if you're a runner. Here are a few tips for making the switch:

- **Go slowly.** Don't expect to be able to run your typical mileage when you first move to barefoot or minimalist shoes.
- **Run on a hard surface to begin with.** This allows you to determine if you're heel-striking, and it provides more immediate feedback on your form. We evolved to run lightly on the balls of the feet, not to hit the ground hard with the heels, as people do when they wear typical running shoes.

- **Try alternating running and walking at two-hundred-meter intervals.** This can help you make the transition to barefoot/ minimalist training.
- **Do most of your barefoot/minimalist running on level ground to start with**—for at least the first month, if not longer. Running uphill or downhill puts additional stress on your body.
- **Pay extra attention to good biomechanics.** Christopher McDougall, author of *Born to Run: A Hidden Tribe, Superathletes, and the Greatest Race the World Has Never Seen,* has some instructional videos on his site. See my website for links.

Once you're accustomed to going barefoot or wearing minimalist footwear, consider doing your walking or running on soft, natural surfaces such as grass and dirt and over uneven terrain. This was the norm for humans until very recently. It's difficult to imagine a situation in the past when humans would have walked for miles on solid, flat, hard surfaces—yet this is exactly what most modern runners do. No wonder we get so many injuries! A preliminary study reported that some runners who transitioned from typical running shoes to minimalist footwear developed a stress injury called bone-marrow edema. It's unclear whether this injury developed because the runners were putting in miles on unforgiving pavement, because they transitioned too quickly from highly cushioned footwear to uncushioned footwear, or for some other reason. The authors of the original study suggested that runners transition "very slowly and gradually in order to avoid potential stress injury," which makes good sense to me.

Go barefoot and you'll never go back.

MOVE: IT WILL CHANGE YOUR LIFE

I've told you about how my back pain and fatigue dissipated once I began to SWAP. Given my profession, I was naturally open to the benefits of exercising this way, but even I was amazed at my improved physical and mental state—and I'll never work the old way again. For my patient Terry, the benefits of SWAP improved his quality of life tremendously.

When thirty-five-year-old Terry came to see me, he had a laundry list of complaints: metabolic syndrome/pre-diabetes, very high cholesterol, and obesity, as a start. "I'm tired all the time," he told me. "My back's so bad I've got to take painkillers just to get to sleep."

A computer programmer, Terry sat for eight to twelve hours a day, five or six days a week. He was on Metformin for his blood sugar and statins for his cholesterol. "Time to get moving, Terry," I told him. Since he worked from home, I had him get a treadmill desk for his office along with TRX straps, PowerBlocks, kettle bells, an abdominal wheel, and push-up bars. I set Terry a goal of walking at least ten thousand steps a day (which he built up to slowly). I also had him sprinkle higher-intensity strength-training exercises throughout his workday.

Terry lost twenty pounds in the first thirty days, and sixty pounds over the first six months. "I can't believe it!" he told me. "My back pain disappeared! My blood sugar and cholesterol are back to normal! I haven't had this much energy in years!" His doctor even stopped his medications.

Like me, like Terry, and like our Paleo ancestors who walked, ran, and simply moved throughout their day for basic survival, you can easily incorporate movement into your daily routine. It will make your life better—and probably longer.

MOVE LIKE YOUR ANCESTORS: YOUR PERSONAL PALEO CURE

- Stand for half of your day.
- Take a standing break every thirty to forty-five minutes.
- Aim for walking ten thousand steps a day.
- Integrate as much light activity into your day as possible.
- Aim for 150 minutes of moderate-intensity activity per week, or 75 minutes of vigorous activity per week, or 30 sets of highest-intensity activity per week, or some combination of the above.

CHAPTER 13

Sleep More Deeply

Sleep Quiz

Complete the quiz below and use the answer key to determine your sleep score.

	POINTS
I have not been diagnosed with a sleep disorder, such as sleep apnea	1
I regularly sleep more than eight hours per night.	2
I rarely feel sleepy or struggle to remain alert during the day.	1
I rarely have difficulty falling asleep.	2
I rarely wake up earlier in the morning than I would like to.	1
I never have thoughts racing through my mind, preventing me from getting to sleep.	1
I rarely have trouble concentrating at work or school.	1
I have never fallen asleep while driving.	1
I almost never doze off while watching TV, reading, or sitting in a car.	1

(continued)

Notes for this chapter may be found at ChrisKresser.com/ppcnotes/#ch13.

	POINTS
I have never been told that I snore.	1
I do not expect a problem with sleep during the week.	1
I feel full of energy.	1
It is easy for me to get up in the morning.	2
I do not experience vivid dreams or hallucinations upon falling asleep or awakening.	1
After taking a nap, I feel refreshed.	1
I have never worked in a job that involves shift work or night work.	1
I rarely travel across times zones (east-to-west travel).	1
I rarely use an electronic device with a screen (TV, laptop, cellphone, iPad) within one hour of going to sleep.	1
My sleep environment is quite (or completely) dark.	1
I feel that the quality of my sleep is satisfactory.	1
TOTAL	

Answer key

Give yourself the correct number of points to all of the questions you answered yes to. Then use the chart below to determine your sleep score.

TOTAL POINTS	WHAT YOUR POINTS MEAN	YOUR PERSONAL PALEO CURE
7+	You are likely getting an adequate amount of sleep during the week.	Complete the *Paleo Cure* 3-Step program. No additional personalization is required.
4–6	You're probably not getting enough sleep, or the quality of your sleep is poor.	Complete the *Paleo Cure* 3-Step program and add the recommendations in this chapter.

TOTAL POINTS	WHAT YOUR POINTS MEAN	YOUR PERSONAL PALEO CURE
0–3	You may be experiencing a sleep disorder or very low-quality sleep.	Complete both steps above and see a health-care provider for additional assistance. This should be a major focus for you, and ignoring this area may stand in the way of improvement elsewhere.

There are few things more important to health than a good night's sleep. A large body of evidence suggests that most people require seven to nine hours of sleep each night for optimal function and prevention of disease. But an increasing number of people in industrialized countries are falling far short of this ideal. According to data from the National Health Interview Survey, approximately one-third (35 percent) of U.S. adults sleep fewer than six hours a night. This may not seem unusual today, but it's a relatively recent phenomenon: just fifty years ago, only 2 percent of Americans averaged fewer than six hours of sleep a night. During that period, American adults and adolescents lost between one and a half to two hours of sleep a night, and chronic sleep loss and sleep disorders are now estimated to affect seventy million Americans. The consequences of chronic sleep deprivation are nothing short of catastrophic. The sleep-wake cycle—an important part of the twenty-four-hour biological clock known as the circadian rhythm—affects nearly every aspect of human physiology, including brain-wave patterns, hormone production, cell regulation, immune function, and metabolism. In fact, studies suggest that the circadian cycle controls from 10 to 15 percent of our species' genes. This may explain why disruption of the sleep-wake cycle is associated with numerous health issues, such as depression, obesity, memory loss, type 2 diabetes, and cardiovascular disease, as well as an increased risk of death.

Perhaps not surprisingly, understanding of the negative impacts of sleep deprivation has increased during the very period that sleep duration has decreased so precipitously. We're effectively engaged in a giant, society-wide experiment using ourselves and our children as test subjects, and so far the results are not encouraging. Despite current attitudes ("I'll sleep when I'm dead"), sleep is not optional. It's crucial to the proper function of every system of the body, and we can't escape the consequences of getting too little of it. Improving the quality, duration, and timing of your sleep is one of the single most powerful interventions you can make to improve your health.

MODERN THREATS TO SLEEP

The prevailing theme of this book is that human beings are biologically adapted and genetically designed for a particular diet and lifestyle and that we are currently mismatched with our current environment. This is as true for sleep behavior as it is for diet and physical activity. For the vast majority of humans' evolutionary history, our species lived in harmony with natural rhythms of day and night, without exposure to artificial light. They were active during the day and rested at night; they did not have ready access to stimulants like caffeine and tobacco; and they didn't have cell phones, computers, tablets, video games, and other electronic devices. Today, these influences are ubiquitous—and their effects are profound. They include:

- **Light pollution (excess artificial light):** Artificial light has many benefits—such as increasing productivity and making recreational activities possible at night—but it hasn't come without a cost. Exposure to artificial light at night affects circadian rhythms (along with nearly every other aspect of human physiology) and shifts the natural biological clock. It does this primarily by suppressing the production of melatonin, an important hormone that helps regulate the sleep-wake cycle and plays a role in numerous other biological functions.
- **Electronic media use:** Electronic media—including television, computers, tablets, mobile phones, and video games—is another

relatively new phenomenon that has become ubiquitous in modern society. Too much electronic media use at night has been shown to interfere with getting a good night's sleep.

- **Changes in work habits:** Work is the primary activity exchanged for sleep, and work hours in the United States have been steadily increasing over the past several decades. But it's not just how much we work that is eating into our sleep time; it's the way we work. Twenty percent of the population in industrialized countries now work beyond the normal hours in various types of shift work or flexible work schedules, and thanks to cell phones, laptops, and the Internet, the barriers that previously separated work and leisure time have dissolved.

- **Jet lag:** Jet lag is another modern phenomenon that affects the natural rhythms of the circadian clock. Chronic jet lag—which is associated with regular travel across time zones—has been shown to decrease sleep quality, reduce cognitive function, raise cortisol levels (a sign of stress), and even increase the risk of cancer (due to disturbances of melatonin levels).

- **Other aspects of the modern lifestyle:** Physical inactivity, excess alcohol consumption, illicit-drug use, cigarette smoking, and caffeine are all associated with decreased sleep duration and quality.

Now you know how much less people are sleeping and why, but what, exactly, does chronic sleep deprivation do?

HOW SLEEP LOSS DESTROYS YOUR HEALTH

Changes in sleep duration and quality increase the risk of everything from heart disease to diabetes to overall mortality; there's little doubt that sleep loss is directly contributing to the modern epidemic of chronic inflammatory disease.

Let's examine the effects of poor sleep on three particular areas in more detail.

Cardiometabolic disease

Cardiometabolic disease refers collectively to diabetes, cardiovascular disease, and obesity. It is by far the most common cause of death and disability worldwide in industrialized countries. While most people are aware of the connection between lifestyle factors like diet and physical activity and cardiometabolic disease, the contribution of chronic sleep deprivation is less well known.

This is already changing, though, since numerous scientific studies have shown that sleep loss directly affects cardiovascular and metabolic function in several ways:

- A single night of partial sleep deprivation causes insulin resistance even in healthy subjects with no preexisting metabolic disease. Exposure to even low levels of artificial light at night may contribute to weight gain by promoting late-night snacking and disrupting metabolic signals.
- A randomized controlled trial with 225 participants found that restricting sleep over five consecutive nights led to increased calorie intake (especially late at night) and weight gain.

The effects of sleep deprivation on food intake alone could almost single-handedly explain the connection observed between obesity and impaired sleep. One study showed that restricting sleep for eight consecutive days increased subjects' calorie intake by 566 calories per day, with no changes in energy expenditure. Imagine this pattern over the long term: Eating an extra five hundred calories a day with no changes in how many calories you burn is equivalent to gaining a pound a week, or fifty-two pounds in one year! But the connection between sleep and obesity goes both ways: obesity has been shown to worsen sleep quality, usually due to a higher prevalence of sleep disorders such as sleep apnea.

HOW BETTER SLEEP HELPED JEN SHED THE FINAL FIVE POUNDS

Jen, twenty-eight, came to see me complaining of difficulty reaching her target weight. She had started a Paleo diet nine months prior to our visit, and she lost twenty-five pounds—almost all of the thirty pounds she wanted to lose—over the first five months. But no matter what dietary modifications she made, Jen couldn't lose those final five pounds. "It's so frustrating," Jen told me. "I'm eating perfectly and exercising every day, but nothing changes. I'm completely stuck."

I reviewed Jen's case history, and I noticed she had a habit of staying up until midnight or later. She often used her laptop or iPad at night to check e-mail or chat with her friends on Facebook. She woke up frequently through the night and sometimes had trouble falling back asleep. And though she was often in bed for eight hours, she woke up feeling unrefreshed. I suggested to Jen that inadequate sleep and too much exposure to artificial light at night might be disrupting her metabolism and preventing her from losing those last five pounds. I suggested she try:

- Getting to bed by ten or ten thirty each night
- Stopping electronic media use at least two (and preferably three) hours before bedtime
- Wearing orange glasses that filter out melatonin-suppressing blue light after dark (see below for more on this)
- Making her sleep environment pitch-dark, cool, quiet, and free of electronic devices (Jen had a habit of leaving her phone on the nightstand)
- Getting exposure to natural light first thing in the morning by taking a fifteen- to twenty-minute walk outside

After making these simple changes, Jen the found the quality of her sleep improved dramatically, and she was finally able to lose those last five pounds. "I have so much more energy when I wake up," she reported, "and I feel much calmer throughout the day. But the best part is that I don't feel hungry all the time anymore, and I've lost the extra weight without even trying."

Immune dysfunction

Disrupted circadian rhythms and chronic sleep loss alter immune responses, leading to an increased risk of cancer, greater susceptibility to infection, and more inflammation. Melatonin plays a key role in the inhibition of cancer development and growth and the enhancement of immune function. In a remarkable study at Johns Hopkins University, researchers injected two groups of mice with a known cancer-causing agent. Then they exposed one group to sixteen hours of daylight and the other to sixteen hours of darkness. The rats in the group that experienced darkness had melatonin levels significantly higher than the other group's, and not a single animal developed cancer. However, in the group that was exposed to light, 90 percent of the animals developed cancerous tumors. The authors of the study speculated that adequate periods of darkness each day and seasonally throughout the year were necessary for proper immune function. Human studies have found similar results. People who are exposed to light at night on a regular basis (such as shift workers or those who stay up late using the computer or playing games) experience melatonin suppression and are at higher risk of developing several different types of cancer, including breast, colon, prostate, and endometrial cancer, as well as influenza and chronic infections.

Stress tolerance, cognitive function, and mood

Perhaps the most immediately noticeable effects of sleep loss are the changes that occur in stress tolerance, cognitive function, and mood. If you have children, you might recall how you felt during those early months when the baby wasn't sleeping through the night. You may have been more emotionally reactive, less tolerant of stress, and less able to focus and think clearly than normal. Numerous studies support this connection between sleep loss and emotional, cognitive, and neurological functions:

- Sleep-deprived people report significantly greater subjective stress, anger, and anxiety in response to low-grade stress than normally sleeping people. Sleep loss increases cortisol levels. High cortisol levels are a sign of stress and are associated with several diseases.

Poor sleep has multiple effects on cognitive functions: decreased short-term memory, reduced learning capacity, a decline in mental stamina, an inability to sustain attention, and a decrease in performance in tasks requiring complex thinking.

Perhaps the best way to think about sleep loss in this context is as a chronic stressor. The body is constantly working to maintain a state of internal balance, or homeostasis, in which it functions optimally. Sleep deprivation overloads the body's capacity to maintain homeostasis, which results in the numerous changes and increased risk of disease and death we've reviewed in this section. This is why getting a good night's sleep is so crucial to maintaining health.

HOW TO SLEEP LIKE A PRO

Now that we understand why sleep is so important, let's take a look at what to do if you're not getting enough.

Make sleep a priority

If you don't allow adequate time for sleep, the rest of the suggestions I'm going to make below won't help much. The amount of sleep that's required for optimal function varies from person to person and throughout a given individual's life, but research suggests that most adults need between seven and nine hours each night.

As a starting place, I recommend allowing eight hours for sleep. For many of you, this will mean going to bed earlier, as you may have less control over when you wake up due to your work schedule. Patients often tell me they're naturally night owls, and they've always preferred to stay up late and sleep in. But in truth, there's nothing natural about this. For millions of years of human history, sleep patterns likely were synced with the daily variation in exposure to daylight and darkness. This is what our bodies are adapted for. Having a lot of energy late at night and being excessively tired in the morning is often a sign that your circadian rhythm is out of whack. In most cases, if you follow the suggestions here, you'll start to get tired earlier and wake up with more energy.

Control your exposure to light

Light is the primary determinant of our circadian rhythm and sleep/wake cycles. Exposure to light at night suppresses melatonin production (which impairs sleep), and exposure to light in the morning resets the internal biological clock and improves sleep at night. It follows, then, that controlling exposure to light is a powerful tool for regulating sleep. The first step would be to reduce your exposure to artificial light at night. This can be done by:

* Avoiding or minimizing the use of computers and tablets within three hours of your bedtime
* Dimming, covering, or removing anything that emits light in your bedroom, such as an alarm clock
* Using blackout shades to make your bedroom as dark as possible
* Wearing a face mask when you sleep to further block light

Of course, unless you want to go back to living by candlelight, you will inevitably be exposed to some artificial light at night. One way to mitigate the impact of that is to wear specialized orange-tinted glasses that block out the spectrum of light that suppresses melatonin. These glasses are remarkably effective in reversing artificial light's melatonin-suppressing effects in clinical studies, and they've been shown to improve sleep quality as well as mood. My patients with sleep difficulties have had great improvements in sleep from wearing them after dark. Simply put them on after the sun goes down and wear them until you go to bed. They're especially important to wear if you're using electronic media (such as computers, tablets, smartphones, or the TV) after dark. See my website to learn the brands that I recommend and where to buy them.

The next step would be to increase your exposure to light in the morning and during the day. Again, this mimics humans' natural evolutionary pattern and has been shown in studies to regulate the circadian rhythm and sleep/wake cycle. The circadian system evolved in order to synchronize human physiology and behavior to the natural periods of day and night imposed by the earth's rotation. Because the cycle length of the earth's rotation is close to—but not exactly—twenty-four hours, the circadian rhythm must be retrained to the twenty-four-hour day on a regular basis. This would have happened without conscious effort in our ancestors who lived outdoors and in harmony with the natural cycles of light and darkness. However, in modern society, exposure to light and darkness can be much less regular.

In these circumstances, purposely exposing yourself to bright light first thing in the morning can help reset your circadian rhythm and thus improve your sleep at night. If it's bright outside in the morning when you wake up, going outside (without sunglasses) and perhaps taking a walk for fifteen to thirty minutes is the best choice. If you have to rise before it gets light, another option is to buy a light machine that emits ten thousand lux of light and sit in front of it for fifteen to twenty minutes after rising. These machines have been studied extensively for seasonal affective disorder (SAD) and depression, but research suggests they can also be effective in resetting the circadian rhythm. Please see my website for a specific recommendation.

Move your body

Physical activity is positively associated with sufficient sleep, as extensive research shows. In one study of roughly fifteen thousand ninth- to twelfth-graders, students who engaged in more than sixty minutes of daily physical activity had significantly higher odds of getting adequate sleep than students who got less than sixty minutes of daily activity. Studies also suggest that too much sedentary time (that is, sitting) may decrease the quality and duration of sleep. For optimal sleep, follow the recommendations I made in chapter 12 for movement. This means not only getting enough exercise but also, and even more important, reducing sedentary time and increasing non-exercise physical activity.

Optimize your sleep nutrition

Some people sleep better after eating only a light dinner. This is especially true for those with digestive issues. Others—such as people with a tendency toward hypoglycemia—do better with a snack before bed (and possibly even during the night). In general, it's best to be neither overly full nor hungry when you go to bed.

I haven't seen any research on this, but in my experience working with patients, I've found that both low-fat and low-carbohydrate diets can cause insomnia. Long-chain saturated and monounsaturated fats such as butter, lard, tallow, olive oil, and palm oil contribute to satiety and help prevent hunger throughout the night. Carbohydrates increase the ability of the amino acid tryptophan to enter the pineal gland; tryptophan is the precursor to serotonin and melatonin, both of which are crucial for sleep. If you're on a low-carb diet and you're experiencing insomnia, try adding a little carbohydrate back in—especially at night.

Certain amino acids that are found in muscle meats and eggs compete with tryptophan for transport across the blood-brain barrier and entry into the pineal gland. However, gelatinous animal products like skin, cartilage, and bones don't have this effect because they aren't rich in the amino acids that compete with tryptophan. Balancing your intake of muscle meats and eggs with fattier cuts of meat and bone broth can promote the uptake of tryptophan and production of serotonin and melatonin in your brain.

Ditch the stimulants

Many people can drink a cup of coffee or two a day without any adverse effects on their sleep. But if you're having trouble sleeping, one of the first things you should do is stop all caffeine intake for at least thirty days. In some cases this single change alone can completely cure insomnia. However, if your sleep doesn't improve while you're off it and doesn't worsen when you start again, it's probably safe to assume that caffeine isn't an issue for you.

Remember, caffeine is a drug, and like all drugs, stopping cold turkey is not easy. If you've been consuming large amounts of caffeine for many years, you may need to cut back slowly instead of stopping all at once to reduce the potential for withdrawal symptoms. For example, you might reduce your intake by 25 percent each week over four weeks, meaning that it will take you a month to stop entirely.

Regulate your nervous system throughout the day

Many people run around all day like chickens with their heads cut off and then wonder why they can't fall right to sleep as soon as their heads hit the pillows. If your nervous system has been in overdrive for sixteen hours, it's unrealistic to assume that it can switch into low gear in a matter of minutes simply because you want it to. This is why sleeping pills are growing in popularity each year.

One of the keys to getting a good night's sleep is managing your stress levels throughout the day. See chapter 14 for specific tips on how to do that.

Create an environment that is conducive to sleep

In addition to taking the steps above aimed at optimizing your physiology for sleep, you also need to optimize your environment for sleep. This includes:

- Using your bed (and preferably bedroom) for only sleep and sex. Avoid working and using electronic media in the bedroom, especially near bedtime. Do not bring your phone into the bedroom. (Be aware that if you read in bed, sometimes a good book with a gripping plotline can hook you—and prevent you from sleeping—as easily as more high-tech forms of entertainment!)
- Creating a pleasant and relaxing environment. Make your bed as comfortable as possible; control the temperature (most people sleep better in a slightly cool room); and create an ambiance that is conducive to sleep and rest.
- Avoiding emotionally upsetting conversations or activities. Just before bed is not the time to get into a heated discussion with your partner or a family member, and it's not a good idea to review your stock portfolio after a bad day in the markets. Create an emotional buffer between the rest of your day and the thirty to forty-five minutes prior to bedtime.
- Using blackout shades and a face mask if necessary to darken the room and decrease your exposure to light.

- Reducing the noise level. If there's a lot of noise outside your bedroom, use earplugs and/or a white-noise machine to block it out.

WHEN SLEEP HYGIENE ISN'T ENOUGH

Let's say you've incorporated all of the sleep-hygiene tips in the last section, but you're still having trouble sleeping. Perhaps you toss and turn for hours before you fall asleep, or maybe you have no trouble falling asleep but you wake frequently through the night or don't feel refreshed when you get up in the morning. In these cases, you may need some additional support. See chapter 14 for tips on managing stress (a key step to improving sleep), and visit my website for a list of natural supplements and stress-management techniques that are especially helpful for sleep.

SLEEP MORE DEEPLY: YOUR PERSONAL PALEO CURE

- Make sleep a priority. Individual sleep needs vary, but as a starting place, aim for spending at least eight hours in bed per night.
- Control your exposure to artificial light at night by minimizing the use of electronic devices before bed, dimming or covering anything that emits light in your bedroom, using blackout shades to darken your bedroom, and wearing orange-tinted glasses that filter out blue light.
- Get plenty of exercise and physical activity during the day.
- Optimize your sleep nutrition: find your optimal ratio of carbohydrates and fats, and make sure to consume bone broth and gelatinous cuts of meat in addition to lean meats.
- Create an environment that is conducive to sleep: use your bedroom only for sleep and sex, keep it slightly cool, and use white-noise machines or earplugs to reduce outside noise.
- If you're having sleep difficulties, avoid caffeine, chocolate, tobacco, and other stimulants.

CHAPTER 14

Manage Your Stress

Stress Quiz

Complete the quiz below and use the answer key to determine your stress score.

	POINTS
I actively pursue a hobby.	1
I belong to a social or activity group that meets at least twice a month.	1
I practice some form of relaxation exercise at least five times a week	1
I have a place in my home to which I can go to relax or be by myself.	1
I practice time-management techniques daily.	1
I do not bring work home with me.	1
I know exactly which situations make me feel stressed.	1
My average day always includes time for exercise and fun.	1
I rarely have a hard time coping with stress.	1

(continued)

Notes for this chapter may be found at ChrisKresser.com/ppcnotes/#ch14.

	POINTS
I feel that I'm able to control my anger.	1
I can forgive people after they've hurt or angered me.	1
I have an activity, a hobby, or a routine I use to release my feelings of stress.	2
I avoid unnecessary conflict and stress (such as Internet debating with strangers)	1
I get seven to eight hours of sleep every night.	1
I have an income adequate to meet basic expenses.	2
TOTAL	

Answer key

TOTAL POINTS	WHAT YOUR POINTS MEAN	YOUR PERSONAL PALEO CURE
10+	You are likely controlling your stress well.	Complete the *Paleo Cure* 3-Step program. No additional personalization is required.
4–9	You may benefit from additional stress-relieving efforts/activities.	Complete the *Paleo Cure* 3-Step program, and add the recommendations in this chapter.
0–3	You may be dealing with serious or uncontrolled stress.	Complete both steps above and see a health-care provider for additional assistance. This should be a major focus for you, and ignoring this area may stand in the way of improvement elsewhere.

I believe stress management is one of the most important—and also most neglected—steps you can take to improve your health. Why?

Because no matter what diet you follow, how much you exercise, and what supplements you take, if you're not managing your stress, you will still be at risk for modern conditions like heart disease, diabetes, hypothyroidism, and autoimmunity.

I see this every day in my practice. I have a lot of patients that are following a "perfect" diet, and yet they are still sick. Stress is often the cause. (I'll define stress more clearly in a moment.) Yet as pervasive as stress is, many people don't do anything to mitigate its harmful effects. The truth is, it's a lot easier to make dietary changes and pop some pills — whether drugs or supplements — than it is to manage stress. Stress management bumps you up against core patterns of belief and behaviors that are difficult to change. It also forces you to slow down, to step back, to disengage — if only for a brief time — from the electric current of modern life and to prioritize self-care in a culture that does not value it.

Not surprisingly, those who are the most stressed out and in the greatest need of stress management are also the least likely to carve out the time for it. While I empathize with the difficulty of managing stress in such a hectic and crazy world and still struggle to find the time for it myself on occasion, I won't sugarcoat this: *If you're not doing some form of regular stress management, you will sabotage all of your best efforts with diet, exercise, and supplements.*

In this chapter I'm going to teach you how to effectively manage stress and reduce its harmful effects. Before I do that, though, I'm going to define stress more clearly, discuss its evolutionary purpose, and describe how too much of the wrong type of stress causes disease.

WHAT IS STRESS?

Stress isn't all bad. In fact, we couldn't survive without it. Stress helps us adapt to our environment and meet and overcome challenges. When the body experiences acute stress, a range of physiological responses occur to prepare us for fight or flight: heart rate and respiration increase, nutrients are mobilized, the immune system is activated, and awareness heightens. At the same time, resources are diverted from processes that aren't needed for immediate survival, such as digestion and reproduction. This exquisitely regulated response to stress provided our ancestors with the energy and wherewithal they needed to survive in a dangerous natural environment.

Exercise is another example of the adaptive effects of stress. During exercise you stress your muscles and cardiovascular system. In response, your body will build larger muscles and increase the capacity of your heart and lungs so you can meet the same challenge (the same distance on a run or the same amount of weight lifted) more effectively in the future.

This beneficial type of stress is referred to as eustress, or positive stress, by some researchers. It motivates, focuses energy, improves performance, and enhances your ability to thrive in whatever environment you live in. It is typically short-term, and it is perceived to be within an individual's coping abilities. But what happens when stress exceeds your capacity to adapt? It becomes *distress*, or negative stress. In contrast to eustress, distress feels unpleasant, decreases performance, and can lead to mental, emotional, and physical problems. It can be both short- and long-term, but it is more commonly chronic stress that causes distress.

Why does distress cause disease? The human body is constantly working to keep critical physiological variables, like blood pressure, glucose, pH, and hormones, within the narrow range required for optimal health. This delicate and dynamic state of internal balance is called homeostasis. Under conditions of eustress, the body is able to maintain homeostasis, or return to homeostasis fairly quickly if it's disturbed. For example, if you go to the gym and lift weights, you're placing stress on your muscles and cardiovascular system, but your body will recover fairly quickly after you finish your workout (assuming you're not overtraining; see pages 220–221 in chapter 12). However, with distress, your body cannot maintain homeostasis because the intensity or frequency of the stressor exceeds its capacity to cope. This might occur with the death of a loved one, a divorce, legal or financial problems, or chronic injury or illness. In these cases stress is no longer adaptive — it's destructive.

But what determines whether you experience something as distress?

What makes stress stressful? When a person is faced with a potential stressor, he (consciously or unconsciously) asks himself the following questions:

- Does this matter to me?
- Do I have the resources to cope with this?

A stressor caused by something that is important and that exceeds the capacity to cope will be perceived as negative, while a stressor that is relatively trivial and is well within one's capacity to cope may be experienced as positive or may not be experienced as stress at all. This suggests that the same stressor could be perceived differently depending on the circumstance or the meaning assigned to stressor. For example, a flood would be a direct threat (and therefore a stressor) for a human being, but not necessarily for a bird. The loss of a job for a single, young professional who was ready to quit is much less of a stressor than the loss of a job for a salaried employee whose family depends on his or her income. A pregnancy for a woman in her midthirties with a strong social and financial support system would be far less stressful than it would be for a teenager with limited resources and no desire to have a child. In other words, how one experiences stress is subjective and depends a lot on internal resources and perspective. This is important to understand, because it suggests that strengthening those resources and changing your perspective can buffer you against the effects of stressors that can't be avoided. (I'll discuss this in more detail shortly.)

HOW STRESS WREAKS HAVOC ON YOUR HEALTH

When the body perceives a stressor, the hypothalamic-pituitary-adrenal (HPA) axis is activated. This axis consists of the hypothalamus and pituitary gland, located in the brain, and the adrenal glands, located on top of the kidneys. This axis causes the release of several different hormones, such as cortisol and epinephrine (aka adrenaline), that orchestrate and govern the stress response.

The first stage of the stress response is called the alarm reaction. It includes the following changes:

- Heart rate, respiration, and blood pressure increase to supply more oxygen to the muscles and brain.
- Blood flow is shunted to the brain and skeletal muscles and diverted from the gut, kidneys, liver, and skin.
- Reproductive and immune functions are suppressed.
- Natural painkillers are released into the bloodstream.
- Stored fats and sugars — the body's primary fuel sources — are mobilized to provide energy.
- The senses of vision and hearing become sharper, and awareness heightens.

Cortisol is the hormone responsible for many of these changes. It's a diurnal hormone, which means it is not secreted uniformly throughout the day. Cortisol levels are highest at about 8:00 a.m. and then decline throughout the rest of the day and into the evening. When cortisol is produced in appropriate amounts at the right times, it protects the body from excessive stress. However, when cortisol production is too high for too long or when it is secreted at the wrong time (like at night), numerous problems ensue. These include:

- High blood sugar
- Depressed immunity
- Intestinal permeability (aka leaky gut)
- Increased craving for comfort and junk foods
- Poor cognitive function and memory
- Poor thyroid function
- Increased fat storage in the liver and abdominal area
- Anxiety and depression

As you can see, the negative effects of stress affect nearly every system of the body. This explains why chronic stress is associated with a wide range of diseases and health conditions. Chronic stress has been shown to:

- Contribute to both type 1 and type 2 diabetes by reducing blood-sugar control
- Play a role in weight gain by promoting overeating, snacking, and consumption of junk food (By contrast, studies have shown that managing stress facilitates weight loss.)
- Increase circulating inflammatory markers, such as C-reactive protein, which are associated with many chronic diseases
- Play an important role in both the onset and exacerbation of asthma and allergies
- Impair cognitive function and mental health via cortisol's direct effects on the brain
- Trigger or worsen numerous autoimmune disorders, including multiple sclerosis, Crohn's disease, psoriasis, and rheumatoid arthritis

This is by no means a complete list. In fact, there are few chronic inflammatory diseases that stress is *not* associated with.

"MANAGING MY STRESS FINALLY CLEARED UP MY SKIN"

Celeste, age forty-three, came to see me complaining about persistent acne. "It's so embarrassing," she said. "I'm forty-three years old, but I look like a teenager." Celeste was under a lot of stress. She worked long hours as a VP of a Fortune 500 company; she had two young children; she was concerned about her mother, who was beginning to show signs of dementia; and she was struggling in her relationship with her husband.

I told Celeste about the relationship between stress and the skin and suggested that she incorporate some stress-management practices into her routine. Initially she was resistant. "I don't have time for stress management!" she told me. "I can barely fit everything in as it is." Of course, people in such situations are the ones who need stress

(continued)

management most, and Celeste was no exception. After trying a few other treatments with limited success, Celeste agreed to commit to a short daily meditation practice and a weekly yoga class. She also started getting acupuncture once a week.

After Celeste had been on this regimen for about six weeks, her skin had improved significantly. After three months, her skin was almost entirely clear. She also noticed other benefits, such as improved sleep, better digestion, and more stable moods. "At first I couldn't imagine how I'd find the time for stress management," she told me. "Now I can't imagine my life without it."

MINIMIZING THE IMPACT OF STRESS

There are two different approaches to minimizing the impact of stress, and both are important.

1. Reducing the amount of stress you experience

Reducing stress means just what it sounds like: reducing your total exposure to all forms of stress, whether psychological or physiological. Of course, it's never possible (or even desirable) to *completely* remove stress from your life, but even in the most pressure-packed circumstances, it's still possible to reduce it.

The first step is to avoid unnecessary stress. Obvious — but it's a challenge for most of us because it's easy to overlook habitual patterns of thought and behavior that cause unnecessary stress. Here are a few guidelines for how to avoid this kind of stress:

- **Learn to say no.** Know your limits, and don't take on projects or commitments you can't handle.
- **Avoid people who stress you out.** You know the kind of person I'm talking about. Drama kings and queens. People who are constantly taking and never giving. Limit your time with these people or avoid them entirely.

- **Turn off the news (or at least limit your exposure to it).** If watching the world go up in flames stresses you out, limit your exposure to the news, especially given the sensationalistic nature of so much of today's news coverage. You'll still know what's going on in the world, but you'll be in control of what you're exposed to.
- **Give up pointless arguments.** There is obviously a place for discussion and debate and working toward change. But have you noticed that heated, highly emotional arguments don't lead to real change? In fact, they tend to have the opposite effect—each side becomes more defensive and entrenched in his worldview. Find other ways to get your point across, learn to listen with empathy, and know when it's time to walk away.
- **Escape the tyranny of your to-do list.** Spend some time in every morning really considering what needs to be done that day. Drop unimportant tasks to the bottom of the list. Better yet, cross them off entirely. The world will go on.
- **Reduce your exposure to online stress.** Social media can be a fun way to connect, but it's truly a mixed bag, peppered as it is with strangers primed for endless arguments (not to mention those Facebook "friends" from college who want to debate you about your political views). Pay attention to how much energy you expend Tweeting, texting, e-mailing, and commenting—do you really need to respond to everything? Trying to do so is quite stressful—and you can never really have the last word when it comes to online exchanges.

The second step in reducing the amount of stress you experience is to address any physiological problems that are taxing your adrenal glands. These include anemia, thyroid issues, blood-sugar swings, gut inflammation, food intolerances (especially gluten), essential fatty acid deficiencies, and environmental toxins. The basic three-step Reset, Rebuild, and Revive approach will help with many of these conditions, and I discuss more specific strategies for addressing some of them throughout the book and in the bonus chapters on my website.

2. Mitigating the harmful effects of stress you can't avoid

Obviously, there are times when stress just can't be avoided. Maybe you have a high-stress job, or you're caring for an ailing parent, or you're having difficulty with your partner or spouse. In these situations it's not about reducing stress itself but about reducing its harmful effects.

How do you do that? There are several different strategies:

- **Reframe the situation.** We experience stress because of the meaning we assign to certain events or situations. Sometimes changing your perspective is enough to relieve the stress. For example, being stuck in traffic can be a disaster or it can be an opportunity for contemplation and solitude.
- **Lower your standards.** This is especially important for you perfectionists out there. Don't let the perfect be the enemy of the good. Let good enough be good enough.
- **Practice acceptance.** One of my meditation teachers used to say, "All suffering is caused by wishing the moment to be other than it is." Many things in life are beyond our control. Learn to accept the things you can't change.
- **Be grateful.** Simply shifting your focus from what is not okay or not enough to what you're grateful for or appreciative of can completely change your perspective — and relieve stress.
- **Cultivate empathy.** When you're in a conflict with another person, make an effort to connect with his or her feelings and needs. If you understand where he or she is coming from, you'll be less likely to react and take it personally.
- **Manage your time.** Poor time management is a major cause of stress. When you're overwhelmed with commitments and stretched too thin, it's difficult to stay present and relaxed. Careful planning and establishing boundaries with your time can help.

In addition to everything I've listed above, other important ways to mitigate the harmful effects of stress include cultivating more pleasure and play in your life and spending more time outdoors. I will cover these in more detail in chapters 15 and 16, respectively.

In the next section, we'll discuss specific strategies for managing stress that I've found to be helpful in my own life and in my work with my patients.

STRATEGIES FOR STRESS MANAGEMENT

There are many different clinically proven ways to manage stress, from yoga to deep breathing to biofeedback to acupuncture. Now I'm going to share the practices I've found to be most helpful for myself and my patients over the years. This isn't meant to be an exhaustive list, and if you're drawn to something that I don't mention here, by all means, go check it out! The important thing is not the type of stress-management practice you choose but that you do it on a regular basis. By *regular*, I mean every day, or as close to it as possible.

Here are a few general tips for incorporating a stress-management practice into your life:

- **Start small.** Instead of committing to one hour of meditation each day, which will be hard to follow through on if you're new to it, start with just five minutes. Then gradually increase the time as you become accustomed to the practice.
- **Make it a priority.** I ask my patients to put stress management on their calendars in the same way they schedule important appointments.
- **Choose a mix of practices.** Some days you might be so wound up that doing a movement-based stress-management technique such as yoga or tai chi is preferable to simple meditation. On other days, you might be so exhausted that a more sedentary technique, like mindfulness-based stress reduction or deep breathing, might be better.
- **Be gentle with yourself.** Don't beat yourself up if you miss a session, and don't treat this as another thing you have to be good at. Stress management should feel like a peaceful and restorative break from your normal routine.

- **Find a teacher.** Many of these practices can be learned at home with books or recordings, but there's something to be said for finding an experienced instructor to work with.

Finally, a note about exercise. While it's true that exercise relieves stress, I'm purposely not including it here. The techniques I mention below induce a particular pattern of brain-wave activity that exercise does not. I view exercise and stress management as complementary, not as interchangeable.

Meditation

In spite of the fact that I'm listing it in this section, I don't consider meditation a form of stress management, although it can certainly have that effect. Meditation is an awareness practice. Through meditation, you learn to witness your thoughts, feelings, and sensations and dis-identify with the stories you tell yourself about them. You learn to stay present in your life, even in the face of great difficulty or pain.

Contrary to popular belief, you don't have to be able to relax in order to meditate. Sometimes people are relaxed during meditation; sometimes they are quite agitated. We don't meditate to manipulate our feelings but to learn to observe them without reacting to or becoming them.

One of the books I often recommend to people who'd like to learn more about meditation practice is *Opening the Hand of Thought*, by Kosho Uchiyama. Another excellent resource is *Meditation for Beginners*, by Jack Kornfield. If you do pursue meditation, I recommend working with an experienced teacher. You might consider doing a beginners' meditation retreat at a retreat center, finding a local teacher in your area, or doing an online class. See my website for links to specific resources.

FINDING JOY IN THE HEART OF PAIN

In her book *Finding Joy in the Heart of Pain*, my late Zen teacher Darlene Cohen posed these questions:

How do we live through unbearable situations like catastrophic diseases without being destroyed? How do we deal with the mundane anguish of our everyday lives? How do we continue to live under crushing stress? And, even further, how do we not just get through these things but have rich, full, and worthwhile lives that we actually want to live—under any circumstances?

For me, and for many others who have had experiences similar to mine, meditation is the answer. As I explained at the start of this book, I was seriously ill for several years. I was scared, exhausted, and in great pain during this period. I had tried so many things and seen so many doctors that it was hard not to lose hope. Yet my meditation practice taught me how to find joy in the heart of pain, how to stay present in circumstances that felt unbearable, and how to love and forgive myself through it all—whether I felt sick or well, sad or happy, frustrated or at peace.

Have you ever taken a walk in the woods or on the beach only to realize after ten minutes that you've been completely lost in your thoughts and have hardly experienced your surroundings? Compare that with a time that you were completely present to what was happening around you: the feeling of the breeze against your skin and the sand between your toes, the sound of the waves crashing against the shore, and the taste of salt in the air. When you are fully present and aware, your experience of life becomes far more rich and full. Your senses are heightened, your heart is opened, and your connection to the world around you deepens.

Meditation practice is what taught me how to slow down, remain present, and experience these moments of joy, peace, and connection even in the midst of severe illness and unrelenting pain. Those moments are what made my life worth living and prevented me from succumbing to darkness and despair.

Mindfulness-Based Stress Reduction

Mindfulness-based stress reduction (MBSR) combines mindfulness meditation and yoga to help cultivate greater awareness of the unity of mind and body and of the unconscious thoughts, feelings, and behaviors that can undermine emotional, physical, and spiritual health. Dr. Jon Kabat-Zinn developed the mindfulness-based stress reduction program at the University of Massachusetts Medical Center in 1979, and clinical research at the University of Massachusetts and elsewhere has demonstrated that MBSR positively affects a range of autonomic physiological processes; for example, it has been shown to lower blood pressure, reduce overall arousal and emotional reactivity, and improve sleep—particularly slow-wave sleep. MBSR is offered as an eight-week intensive training course in hospitals and medical centers around the world. It is also offered as an online course, and it can be done via home study with books and audio recordings. MBSR is particularly effective for anyone struggling with chronic illness or pain. I've found it to be particularly helpful in my own life and in my work with patients.

Yoga

The word *yoga* comes from the Sanskrit *yuj*, which means "to unite." Today *yoga* is used as a general term to refer to physical, mental, and spiritual disciplines that originated in ancient India. Yoga has been shown to reduce stress as well as improve cardiovascular and respiratory health, flexibility, cognitive performance, and overall well-being. It is particularly effective in relieving stress-induced or stress-related disorders such as insomnia, anxiety, depression, hypertension, and asthma.

Yoga is a great choice for stress management for several reasons. First, it's a movement-based practice, which is often suitable for people who are new to stress management or who have very busy minds and find it difficult to sit still. Second, yoga is often practiced in a group or class setting, which has additional benefits. Third, because of its popularity, it's now easy to find a class in most places.

Massage

Touch is vital to human health. In fact, touch is so important that infants deprived of it are unlikely to survive. Human beings are highly social creatures, and touch is part of the way we relate to and communicate with others. This is one reason that massage can be such an effective stress-management strategy.

Massage has been shown to cause beneficial hormonal shifts, such as an increase in oxytocin and a decrease in the hormone ACTH, that help regulate the HPA axis and decrease stress. I will discuss the benefits of touch and massage in more detail, along with specific recommendations for how to incorporate it into your life, in chapter 15.

Feldenkrais (Awareness through Movement)

Feldenkrais (awareness through movement) classes are, as the name implies, movement lessons that bring awareness to our everyday actions. They help people become aware of tension patterns that are unconscious and cause stress, fatigue, and pain. Through this awareness and through learning new patterns of movement, people report feeling more relaxed and at ease moving through their day, which often leads to better sleep at night. People also notice an improvement in how they do everyday activities, from sweeping the floor to working out. Though Feldenkrais isn't as well known as yoga, acupuncture, massage, or other stress-management modalities, I've found it has more profound and longer-lasting results in many cases. See my website for information on how to find a class in your area.

Biofeedback

Biofeedback is a process of becoming aware of the body's physiological functions. Specialized sensors deliver information about blood pressure, heart rate, skin temperature, and muscle tension, which the participant uses to learn to modify his or her physiological response to stress.

Biofeedback has been shown to significantly reduce stress and anxiety in groups of people who are highly stressed, such as nursing students and physicians. It has also been shown to reduce chronic pain associated with stress, to improve sleep in soldiers in combat zones, and to lessen preoperative anxiety in children with cancer. In the past few years, low-cost, portable biofeedback devices have been developed that work with smartphones and tablets. (Emwave2, BioZen, and Quantum Life are examples.) This is perhaps the easiest and most accessible way to learn biofeedback.

SUPPLEMENTS FOR STRESS MANAGEMENT

There are a number of supplements that support the HPA axis and help with stress management. However, don't be tempted to think you can simply take the supplements and ignore all of the behavioral and lifestyle changes I've discussed in this chapter. That won't work. Supplements can be an important part of a stress-management program, but they should never be seen as a substitute for making the necessary changes to reduce the amount of stress you experience.

Please see my website for additional stress-management techniques, including links to free instructional audio recordings that you can download.

MANAGE YOUR STRESS: YOUR PERSONAL PALEO CURE

- Reduce the amount of stress you experience by learning to say no, avoiding people who stress you out (when possible), turning off the news, giving up pointless arguments, escaping the tyranny of your to-do list, and addressing physiological problems (such as blood-sugar swings, gut infections, chronic inflammation, and so on) that are taxing your adrenals.
- Reduce the impact of stress you can't avoid by reframing the situation, lowering your standards, practicing acceptance, cultivating gratitude and empathy, and managing your time.
- Make stress management a priority. Give it as much attention as you give other aspects of staying healthy, such as diet, exercise, and sleep.

- Commit to a regular stress-management practice. Choose a mix of techniques that suit your temperament and lifestyle, such as meditation, yoga, massage, Feldenkrais, mindfulness-based stress reduction, acupuncture, and biofeedback.
- If you're new to stress-management practices, start small and be gentle with yourself. Consider finding a skilled teacher who can help you get started and deepen your practice.

CHAPTER 15

Cultivate Pleasure and Connection

Pleasure and Connection Quiz

Complete the quiz below and use the answer key to determine your pleasure and connection score.

	POINTS
I have a close friend or confidant that I regularly confide in.	1
I am in a committed, loving relationship.	2
I have a strong social-support network.	2
I enjoy regular touch and physical contact (for example, massage, sex, or partner dancing).	1
I listen to music that inspires or relaxes me on a daily basis.	1
I have supportive family around me.	1
I play an instrument and practice or make music at least twice a week.	1
I engage in activities that make me laugh out loud at least three times a week.	1

Notes for this chapter may be found at ChrisKresser.com/ppcnotes/#ch15.

	POINTS
I have a good sense of humor and tend not to take life too seriously.	1
I volunteer for an organization or cause I believe in.	1
I have a dog, cat, or other pet.	1
I have one or more friends to confide in about personal matters.	1
I set aside time to play, exercise, or interact with my pet at least three times a week.	1
TOTAL	

Answer key

TOTAL POINTS	WHAT YOUR POINTS MEAN	YOUR PERSONAL PALEO CURE
6+	You're likely doing well with pleasure and connection.	Complete the *Paleo Cure* 3-Step program. No additional personalization is required.
3–5	You may benefit from more focus on pleasure and connection.	Complete the *Paleo Cure* 3-Step program, and add the recommendations in this chapter.
0–2	You are likely suffering from a lack of pleasure and connection.	Complete the *Paleo Cure* 3-Step program, and add the recommendations in this chapter. This should be a major focus for you, and ignoring this area may stand in the way of improvement elsewhere.

For the vast majority of our species' history, humans lived in tight-knit, extended family or kin groups with regular social contact. Like all other primate species, we're inherently social animals: we thrive when we feel a sense of connection and belonging, and we suffer when we feel isolated and alone.

Socially isolated people have a higher risk of disease and death even after controlling for traditional risk factors like physical health, smoking, and alcohol consumption. By contrast, having a positive social-support system has been shown to extend life span and improve cardiovascular, endocrine, immune, and mental health. Unfortunately, both the quality and quantity of social relationships in the industrialized world is decreasing. Humans have gone from living primarily in extended-family or tribal units to living in single-family or even individual units; they are more mobile and thus less likely to put down roots; they get married later; and they have more dual-career families. Perhaps most disturbing, over the past two decades, the number of Americans who report having no close confidants has increased threefold and is now the rule rather than the exception.

This is ironic in a world characterized by electronic hyperconnectivity. Never before have people been able to communicate with such speed and ease. A written message that used to take weeks if not months to travel from one end of the world to the other can now be sent in less than a second, and social media allows everyone to interface with more people in a month than he or she would have met in an entire lifetime just a few hundred years ago. Yet the findings given above suggest that, despite these increases in technology and global connectivity, people are becoming more — rather than less — socially isolated.

Like social connection, pleasure is not only part of our species' cultural heritage but also essential to our health. The experience of pleasure releases powerful chemicals that promote health and prevent disease. Pleasure protects against the harmful effects of stress; it strengthens and regulates the immune system and improves mood. In many ways, pleasure is the *antithesis* of stress.

Yet in our increasingly busy and hectic world, many people have difficulty finding time for pleasure. Though leisure time has actually increased over the past forty years, much of those hours are devoted to distraction, not pleasure. Distraction and pleasure might seem similar on the surface, but they're fundamentally different. Distraction is something that prevents you from giving full attention to yourself and your life. Pleasure is almost exactly the opposite. When you experience pleasure, you are more fully present to life, more grounded in your body, more alive and aware. While there's a time and place for distraction, it shouldn't be substituted for pleasure. Unfortunately, statistics suggests that this substitution is what's happening today. The average American now devotes half of his or her leisure time each day to watching television, and computer activities like checking e-mail and using social media are also on the rise.

Social connection and pleasure are vital to everyone's health and well-being, and we'll all benefit from bringing more of each into our lives.

WHY WE NEED PLEASURE AND CONNECTION

In chapter 14 we talked about how chronic stress contributes to everything from insomnia and anxiety to obesity and heart disease. Scientists have devoted vast amounts of attention to understanding the mechanisms of the fight-or-flight response. They've found that when a person is faced with stress, the sympathetic nervous system triggers a cascade of physiological changes that result in increased blood flow and spikes in adrenaline levels.

But there's another nervous system response that's just as important as fight-or-flight to human survival and yet is often ignored in the scientific literature and in mainstream articles about stress. Humans are designed not only to deal with stress and challenges but also to enjoy life, to relax, to bond, and to heal. This is the parasympathetic state, often referred to as the rest-and-digest or calm-and-connect response. It produces the opposite biochemical effects on the body as the fight-or-flight response does: heart rate and respiration slow down; blood pressure drops; blood flow to the digestive tract, skin, and reproductive organs increases; and stress hormones decrease.

Both fight-or-flight and calm-and-connect are essential to life. We need the ability to meet challenges and mobilize our physical and mental resources to take action. But we also need to digest food, replenish our energy stores, and heal ourselves. It's likely that these different systems were in a state of relative balance in our Paleo ancestors. Imagine a day of mostly relaxing, interacting with others, and gathering food or building shelters. This might be punctuated by an acutely stressful event, such as a hunt or an encounter with a predator. But it would likely be followed again by more rest-and-digest or calm-and-connect time, such as gathering around a fire and feasting on the day's hunt. Human beings adapted to this balance of pressure and calm, stress and relaxation, sympathetic and parasympathetic stimulation.

Unfortunately, most of us today do not have this balance. In modern times, fight-or-flight is rarely a temporary state that quickly passes. Instead, it's an almost continuous reaction to the excessive demands placed on us by modern life. Worrying about money, watching upsetting news, being skipped over for a promotion, and driving in traffic may not literally threaten your survival, but your body reacts as if they do. All of these elicit the exact same physiological fight-or-flight response, only to a lesser degree.

PLEASURE: THE ANTIDOTE TO CHRONIC STRESS

Stress is the antithesis of pleasure: it feels unpleasant, raises heart rate and blood pressure, weakens the immune system, and makes people sick. And if stress is the antithesis of pleasure, it follows that one of the best ways to fight stress is with pleasure.

The reactions of the human nervous system are relatively black-and-white. Either you're experiencing stress, and the sympathetic nervous system (fight-or-flight) is activated, or you're in a state of relative ease, and the parasympathetic nervous system (rest-and-digest) is activated. This suggests that if you're experiencing pleasure, you're not experiencing stress, and it explains why pleasure is such a powerful antidote to stress.

Endorphins are the body's feel-good chemicals. They have similar structures and effects as opium, the poppy-derived narcotic that has been used for thousands of years to induce euphoria and reduce pain. Endorphins are responsible for intensely pleasurable experiences like orgasm and the runner's high some people experience with exercise. In fact, animal research has shown that endorphin levels can be up to eighty-six times higher after animals experience multiple orgasms. But endorphins are released, albeit at lower levels, in more mundane daily activities as well, such as when you're playing with a pet, watching a funny movie, listening to your favorite music, visiting a favorite place, or connecting with loved ones. In addition to counteracting stress hormones and improving mood, endorphins also:

- Improve immune function by producing antibacterial substances
- Enhance the killer instincts of various infection-fighting white blood cells, such as B cells, T cells, and natural killer (NK) cells
- Enable certain immune cells to secrete their own endorphins as a way of improving their disease-fighting capacity

In other words, endorphins don't just make us feel good; they improve our health and protect us from disease. This explains why experiences that bring pleasure—such as warm, caring touch, listening to music, and interacting with pets—are associated with a greater sense of well-being as well as longer life spans.

SOCIAL CONNECTION: NO MAN (OR WOMAN) IS AN ISLAND

For almost two million years, humans lived in tight-knit extended-family or tribal groups. They had regular daily contact with family members and others they were close to, and they had an inherent sense of community and belonging. Yet today, most people in the industrialized world live either alone or with only the immediate family.

Throughout this book we've discussed the idea that there's a mismatch between our current diet and lifestyle and the one humans adapted to. The decline in the quality and quantity of close relationships and social connection is yet another way that this mismatch manifests in the modern, industrialized world. And while you might suspect that diet and other lifestyle factors, like sleep and exercise, would have a far greater impact on health than social support, research suggests otherwise. A landmark study published in 2010 involving over three hundred thousand participants found that social support was a stronger predictor of survival than physical activity, body mass index, hypertension, air pollution, alcohol consumption, and even smoking fifteen cigarettes a day! The researchers found that people with adequate social relationships had up to a 90 percent greater likelihood of survival than those with poor or insufficient relationships. This is likely a conservative estimate, because this study didn't take the *quality* of relationships into account, and previous studies have shown that negative relationships actually *increase* the risk of death. Had the researchers examined the effects of positive relationships separately, the percentage almost certainly would have been higher.

There are several theories to explain why social support is so important to health. One theory is that social relationships help buffer the effects of chronic stress by providing emotional and other forms of support. Another theory holds that social relationships directly influence health through their effect on physiology, behavior, and mood. Whatever the case, it's likely that a hormone called oxytocin is involved.

Oxytocin plays a critical role in both the causes and the effects of positive social interaction, and it is associated with a general feeling of mental and physical well-being. Oxytocin stimulates a sense of calm, improves trust, reduces fear, and enhances the desire to connect with others. (Some even refer to it as the tend-and-befriend hormone.) It is secreted during sex, caring touch, nonverbal expressions of love, eye contact, and mother-infant bonding, including during breast-feeding. Studies have shown that men and women who report great support from their partners have higher oxytocin levels than those who don't; other studies indicate that administering oxytocin encourages close and intimate contact. By contrast, low levels of oxytocin are associated with social isolation, cardiovascular disease, psychiatric problems, and decreased quality of life.

A lack of social support also causes harm in ways that don't directly involve oxytocin. For example, lonely people have higher blood pressure and heart rates and greater amounts of atherosclerosis than people with adequate social support. They also suffer from more inflammation, insomnia, infectious disease, cancer, depression, and stress. People who are more socially integrated have lower serum levels of proteins associated with inflammation, like C-reactive protein (CRP) and interleukin-6 (IL-6); are less likely to experience cardiovascular disease and infection; and have longer life spans.

Most people recognize the inherent value of pleasure and social connection, but my guess is that few realize how important these things are to physical health and longevity. Yet the studies we've covered in this chapter suggest that, together, pleasure and social connection may have as much of an influence on well-being as the food people eat, how much exercise they get, and how well they sleep. With this in mind, let's explore some ideas for how to bring more pleasure and connection into your life.

SIX WAYS TO BRING MORE PLEASURE AND CONNECTION INTO YOUR LIFE

1. Touch

Touch is the first sense to develop in the womb, and it's the most fundamental means of relating to the world. It plays an important role in social interactions, governs emotional well-being, stimulates the release of potent chemicals that influence all aspects of health, and serves as a clear — but often overlooked — form of communication.

Unfortunately, touch is often actively discouraged in the United

States and some other industrialized societies, like the United Kingdom, because of concerns about litigation and changes in public attitudes. This has led Dr. Tiffany Field (who has published over one hundred research articles documenting the beneficial effects of touch) to speculate that many people living in modern societies are suffering from what she calls "touch hunger." Although long-distance forms of communication, like phone calls, text messaging, e-mail, and social media, are widely available, these cannot compensate for a lack of flesh-to-flesh contact; electronic communication simply does not have the same impact on the body and the mind that physical touch has.

Numerous studies have documented the beneficial health effects of touch. For example:

- A study of fifty-nine women found that more frequent hugs with their partners increased oxytocin levels and decreased blood pressure.
- A study of ninety-five students at UCLA found that massage was associated with an increase in oxytocin and reductions in hormones associated with stress.
- A study of 183 men and women found that, compared to a control group, subjects who had brief episodes of warm, physical contact prior to a stressful event had significantly reduced blood pressure and lower heart rates upon exposure to that event.

If you're suffering from touch hunger, here are some suggestions for bringing more nurturing physical contact into your life:

- **Be a hugger.** Hug your spouse, your kids, your friends, and those you love and see the most. You might even consider hugging people you don't know quite as well. (In European cultures, the default greeting for strangers of both genders is often a kiss to each cheek.)
- **Receive or give bodywork or massage.** If you can get a professional massage or another form of bodywork on a regular basis, that's fantastic. But another option is to take a massage class with

your partner, spouse, or a close friend and then trade off giving
and receiving massages. This is a great way to cultivate intimacy
as well as experience more touch.

- **Have sex.** Sex releases more oxytocin than any other form of
  physical activity.
- **Take a partner yoga class.** Partner yoga is a nonsexual form of
  yoga in which two people rely on each other's support to keep correct body alignment, balance, and focus in a posture. This is a
  great activity to do with a spouse or romantic partner, but you can
  also do it with a friend or even a stranger you meet in the class.
- **Take a dance class.** Ballroom dancing, tango, contact improvisation, and other dance forms that involve partner-to-partner contact are also great nonsexual ways to experience more touch.

2. Intimate relationships

Researchers have known for decades that in general, married people have
lower rates of disease and greater life satisfaction, happiness, mental
health, and life expectancy than single people. (This is also true for people who are living together in committed relationships but who aren't
married.) Additionally, single adults without close confidants have three
times the risk of premature death than singles with confidants or married
people. Recent research has provided deeper insight into exactly which
relationships are most beneficial and what it is about relationships in general that promotes health and protects against disease. For example, we
know that poor-quality marriages don't carry the same benefit as higher-
quality marriages. Chronic relationship stress—characterized by mis-
trust, conflict, and instability—has been tied to greater levels of
inflammatory chemicals over time. Hostile married couples have higher
levels of these chemicals when compared to couples with supportive relationships, and married women with rheumatoid arthritis who experienced criticism from their spouses had higher markers of disease activity
than those who didn't.

Of all the types of social support, *emotional* support is the most consistent predictor of better health. More specifically, social support that

engenders feelings of intimacy and belonging have the greatest health benefits. One study examining the effect of social support on blood pressure found that support in general did not change blood pressure one way or the other; however, emotional support was significantly associated with lower blood pressure. Other studies have shown that trusting and satisfying relationships are associated with lower levels of inflammatory cytokines, such as interleukin-6 and C-reactive protein, and lower levels of stress hormones, like cortisol. The beneficial effects of emotional support are especially pronounced in women, perhaps because oxytocin has a stronger impact on the female nervous system.

Here are some suggestions for cultivating intimacy in your current relationships and creating new supportive connections with others.

- **Be honest, open, and vulnerable.** Intimacy is based on mutual trust, and mutual trust is based on honesty, full disclosure, and a willingness to let your guard down. Sharing heartfelt feelings can be difficult and scary, especially for men, but true intimacy isn't possible without such open communication.
- **Schedule regular time for intimacy.** In today's busy and hectic world, many couples have trouble finding time for intimate contact. Try scheduling regular dates and times to be alone with each other, and stick to them just like you would any other appointment. You could do a monthly romantic dinner, a weekly massage, a short walk in the morning before work, or perhaps a shared activity that you both enjoy.
- **Get professional help.** If you're struggling in your relationship, seek out professional help. Plodding along in a toxic, hurtful relationship is not only alienating and painful but harmful to your health. If you can't afford therapy, consider going to a student clinic where therapists are being trained (they're often quite good) or to a low-income therapy clinic in your neighborhood. You might also consider peer-to-peer counseling methods such as cocounseling. See my website for recommendations.

- **Don't be a martyr.** If your relationship is not meeting your needs, and you've done everything you can to make it work (including getting help), consider a separation or divorce. This can be terrifying for many people, but ultimately it may save not only your sanity but also your life.

- **Join a friendship network.** As social media has become more prominent, the quantity of our connections to other people has increased dramatically. But a growing body of research suggests that we're more isolated and alienated than ever before. Recently, new organizations have sprung up dedicated to helping people form friendships (real, not virtual!) with others in their local community. See my website for recommendations.

- **Put yourself out there.** If you're looking for a partner, online dating is a great option. But another way to increase the chances of meeting that special someone is to surround yourself with people who share your interests and values. Volunteer for a cause you support, join a book club or some other activity group, play coed softball or soccer, learn ballroom dancing, go to parties, and get out and about!

3. Pets

Pets—especially dogs—have been part of human culture for a long time. Most scientists believe that dogs were first domesticated about ten thousand years ago, right when humans shifted from nomadic, hunter-gatherer lifestyles to agricultural lifestyles. However, some recent archaeological findings suggest that dogs may have been human companions as far back as thirty-three thousand years ago. Why such a strong mutual attraction? While there are probably many answers to this question, one of the most significant reasons is the human need to give and receive affection. Pets aren't just pets; they're our friends and family members. We love them, play with them, touch them, care for them, and grow old with them. In return, they love us unconditionally, make us laugh, and are always there when we need them.

On top of all that, pets make us healthier:

- Pets improve physical fitness by encouraging exercise.
- Pets decrease anxiety and the fight-or-flight response.
- Pets decrease loneliness and depression by providing companionship.

A study of roughly 480 subjects found that people who had pets were more likely to be alive one year after a heart attack than people who did not have pets. Other studies have shown that pet owners have lower blood pressure and triglycerides, greater stress tolerance, improved immune health, and fewer minor health problems than nonpet owners. These beneficial effects aren't limited to dog owners; caring for a cat or a bird or even watching fish in an aquarium all appear to promote relaxation.

Here are some tips for how to benefit from pet ownership:

- **Choose the right pet.** Most of the research on the benefits of pet ownership has involved dogs. But if you're not a dog person, don't feel you have to get a dog! Get a pet that you and your family members can all agree on and that will be a good fit for your temperament and lifestyle.
- **Choose the right breed.** If you're a runner, don't get a bulldog. If your mobility is limited and you can't take your dog for long walks (or runs) every day, you should probably think twice about a vizsla or border collie.
- **Train your dog.** A trained dog means a happier dog — and a happier guardian. An untrained dog can be a source of stress and frustration, and that's the opposite of what you want! I think positive training methods (like clicker training) are more likely to increase pleasure and connection than negative ones, and they're very effective.
- **Make time to play.** Once you have your pet, be sure to carve out time in your schedule to play with it. That's one of the best ways

to connect with your pet, and play has its own benefits, as I'll explain in the next chapter.

- **Volunteer at a local shelter.** If pet ownership isn't for you right now, volunteering at a shelter will give you the opportunity to connect and interact with many different animals while supporting a good cause. And as you'll see, volunteering is one of the six ways to bring more pleasure and connection into your life.

4. Music

Music has been part of human experience for thousands of years—and perhaps much longer. In traditional hunter-gatherer groups, such as the Aboriginal Australians, music was an important part of ceremonial and cultural life. In the sixth century, the Greek philosopher Pythagoras wrote about music's contribution to health. He prescribed music and a specific diet to restore the harmony of the body and soul. In the mid-1800s, the now-renowned nurse Florence Nightingale used music in hospital wards to accelerate the healing process for soldiers injured in the Crimean War.

Today, we know that music affects us by engaging specific brain functions involved in memory, learning, and multiple motivational and emotional states. Music can enhance positive and calming emotions and is used therapeutically in everything from surgery to intensive care to pain relief.

It's important to note that not all music has a relaxing effect. Some types of music are calming and reduce blood pressure and other biological markers of stress, while other types may actually increase blood pressure, heart rate, and other indicators of stress. It appears that the tempo of music is the most important factor, with slow and flowing music with sixty to eighty beats per minute showing the most positive outcomes on relaxation and pain relief. Research also suggests that music intended for relaxation should be nonlyrical (without words), have predominantly low tones, be made up mostly of strings with minimal brass and percussion, and reach a maximum volume of sixty decibels.

Of course, this doesn't mean you shouldn't listen to faster tempo, more upbeat music; it just means that that kind of music will have a different physiological effect. Faster, more rhythmic music — especially when you dance to it — is more likely to release endorphins and other feel-good chemicals associated with pleasure, play, and celebration. This is great, and it also has a healing effect; it's just not calming and relaxing. The important thing is for you to know what you need in a given moment and be able to choose the right music for the job.

Here are some tips for using music to bring more pleasure and connection into your life:

- **Build playlists for specific purposes.** Make a playlist with slow, flowing, melodic, and meditative music for listening to while working or at other times when you need to take the edge off. Make a playlist with faster, more upbeat music for when you need to get the endorphins and feel-good chemicals flowing.
- **Be selective.** Why listen to the radio with a bunch of intrusive advertisements and a lot of music you don't like when you can use services like Pandora to build your own smart radio station that learns your preferences? Music that appeals to you is more likely to boost chemicals associated with pleasure and stress reduction, so don't settle for music you don't like.
- **Expand your horizons.** We have more access to music, and a wider variety to choose from, than ever before. Maybe you'd like to try Afro-Cuban music, or Gregorian chanting, or Tibetan throat singing, or classical. Whatever your taste, there's something out there for you, and thanks to the Internet, you can add it to your playlist. Ask friends for recommendations and search out new music that makes you happy.
- **Start or join a music exchange.** Consider starting or joining a group of friends who share music with one another. This is a great way to get exposed to new music.
- **Learn how to play and sing.** Maybe you didn't receive music instruction as a child, but it's never too late to learn. Making

music has additional benefits above and beyond listening to it. We all have music in us, and there's an instrument out there for everyone. Playing music in groups—like in a drum circle or band—is especially beneficial.

5. Humor

The idea that humor can heal can be traced back to biblical times; in Proverbs 17:22, you'll find the maxim "A merry heart doeth good like a medicine." More recently, physicians like Norman Cousins and Patch Adams have advocated the use of humor in medicine, and some researchers have argued that humor may have evolved specifically as a strategy for coping with stress. The American psychologist Rollo May believed that humor allowed people to distance themselves from their problems, view them from a different perspective, and thus reduce the feelings of anxiety and helplessness they experienced. And the British philosopher Bertrand Russell once said, "Laughter is the most inexpensive and most effective wonder drug. Laughter is a universal medicine."

Humor has been shown to reduce stress, relieve pain, and improve the overall quality of life. Laughter can lead to changes in heart rate, skin temperature, blood pressure, pulmonary ventilation, skeletal muscle activity, and brain activity. It may also improve immune function by blocking the production of stress hormones (like cortisol, ACTH, and adrenaline) and stimulating the production of feel-good chemicals (like endorphins). Laughter may increase the activity of natural killer cells, which help fight infection and keep cancer at bay.

Here are some tips for benefiting from humor and laughter:

- **Lighten up.** Learn not to take yourself and your life so seriously. Take a step back, get some perspective, and remember that this too shall pass.
- **Watch a funny movie (or TV show).** If you watch TV, you might as well watch shows that are funny and improve your health. Just don't watch too much, or the benefits of laughter might be outweighed by the harm of sitting on your butt for too long.

- **Go to a live comedy show.** Watching a live stand-up comic or improvisation performance has the added benefit of laughing with a group of people. Watch for listings in your area and make this a regular event.
- **Go on a news diet.** Let's face it: the news is often depressing. While I believe it's important to stay informed and not avoid or deny tragedy when it occurs, your life will not be enriched by hearing about every murder, car crash, and catastrophic event that happens in the world. Consider limiting your news consumption to fifteen minutes per day on most days, with perhaps a longer read of the Sunday paper.
- **Avoid people who bring you down.** This isn't always possible, and there's a certain amount of interpersonal struggle we all have to face in life. But there's no reason to go looking for it or to invest your limited time and energy in relationships that are a constant drain on you.
- **Play with your kids and pets.** Kids and animals are experts in humor, play, and fun. Learn from them.

6. Volunteering

Whether as a parent, spouse, partner, parishioner, or friend, each of us has experienced the joy of giving. Giving and receiving are essential to who we are and how we relate to others, as necessary to our survival in the modern world as breathing, eating, and sleeping. Perhaps it won't surprise you, then, to learn that research has shown that people who help others experience satisfaction, happiness, and self-esteem from giving. People who volunteer have longer life spans than people who do not, and they're less likely to suffer from disease.

There are a number of reasons why volunteering might yield both mental and physical health benefits, but one of the strongest is that it increases meaningful social connection. People who give social support have lower blood pressure, and they're more likely to report having greater social support (what goes around comes around!) and a greater sense of self-efficacy, as well as less depression and less stress, than people with a lower tendency to give support to others. As I'm sure many of you have experienced, giving increases one's sense of value and purpose and makes life more meaningful.

Here are some tips for volunteering and giving:

- **Find a cause you believe in.** Volunteering for a cause you believe in will make your volunteer work even more beneficial, since you'll be working toward developing a world more in line with your values and ideals. It's also a great way to meet like-minded people and expand your social network. Consider a service like Volunteer Match to help you find the right fit.
- **Volunteer at your church, temple, mosque, or religious organization.** Some of the research on volunteering suggests that those with the strongest faith receive the greatest benefits.
- **Volunteer in person.** Volunteering remotely (for example, doing computer work for an organization across the country) is still worth doing, but research suggests that volunteer work that involves live contact with other people is likely to be more beneficial.
- **Don't overextend yourself.** Informal giving and volunteer work have been shown to benefit health, but extreme giving (such as caring for a disabled or very sick person) is detrimental to health. Of course, there are times when that is necessary and unavoidable, but don't overextend yourself if you don't have a compelling reason to do so.

THE HEALING POWER OF PLEASURE AND CONNECTION

I'd like to finish this discussion by sharing a personal story. At one point in my long struggle with illness, I felt I had reached the end of my rope. I was demoralized, discouraged, and exhausted. I had tried at least six special diets; I had a cupboard full of supplements that had done nothing for me (or made me even worse); and I'd seen at least fifteen specialists in all different fields without much of anything to show for it. I came to a place where I simply didn't know what to do, and I didn't have the energy or will to focus on yet another diet or supplement program.

So I did something radical—or at least, it seemed radical to me at the time. I decided to focus almost exclusively on cultivating more pleasure and connection in my life and not to worry much about diet or supplements. I was feeling isolated and somewhat disconnected from my life after being sick for so long, and intuitively, I knew that I had to nourish myself on a deeper level than food or supplements could offer in order to regain my strength. I created a weekly pleasure-and-connection program that involved a massage trade, acting/improvisation classes, regular social visits with friends, dancing at least once a week, and volunteering as a meditation teacher at the San Francisco county jail. During this time, I continued to eat a healthy diet, but I resolved not to be overly restrictive or think too much about what I was eating. In fact, I made sure to eat plenty of things that brought me pleasure—even if they didn't fit my concept of healthy foods.

After about three months on this program, I felt like a different person. I was more calm, relaxed, and happy. I didn't feel so alienated and alone. But the benefits weren't just psychological and emotional; I felt more energetic, my digestion improved, I gained about ten pounds that I had lost during my illness, and my sleep became more restorative. In fact, nearly everyone who knew me remarked on how much more vital and healthy I looked.

There's no question that diet and exercise are crucial to health. But experiencing pleasure and feeling connected to others are also important and, in certain circumstances, maybe even more so than diet. You may not need to go to the lengths I did to reap the benefits of pleasure and connection, but I hope this story inspires an appreciation of just how powerful they can be.

PLEASURE AND CONNECTION: YOUR PERSONAL PALEO CURE

- Make pleasure and connection as much a priority as eating well, managing stress, and getting enough sleep and exercise.
- Get plenty of physical contact and touch from hugs, massage, sex, partner dance, and partner yoga.
- Cultivate intimate relationships and expand your social-support network by being open and honest, scheduling time with loved ones, joining a friendship group, and putting yourself in situations where you're likely to meet people you'll connect with.
- Get a dog, cat, or other pet; if you already have one, set aside time to play and interact with your pet.
- Listen to music that makes you feel alive, happy, relaxed, and at peace. Use software or music-exchange groups to discover new music and expand your horizons.
- Volunteer for a cause you believe in, and focus on giving more to the people in your life.

CHAPTER 16

Go Outside

Nature and Sunlight Quiz

Complete the quiz below and use the answer key to determine your nature and sleep score.

	POINTS
I often spend a large portion of my day outside.	2
I am outside for more than thirty minutes daily.	2
I frequently walk or bike to work or to do errands.	2
I don't always cover my skin with sunblock or clothing when I go outside.	1
I live in an environment with a lot of green space, parks, and/or natural attractions.	1
My office or place of work has many windows.	1
I spend less than eight hours a day looking at a screen (computer, television, and so on).	1
Most of my physical activity takes place outdoors.	1
I have frequent interaction with nature (trees, water, plants, and animals).	1
TOTAL	

Notes for this chapter may be found at ChrisKresser.com/ppcnotes/#ch16.

Answer key

TOTAL POINTS	WHAT YOUR POINTS MEAN	YOUR PERSONAL PALEO CURE
6+	You are likely spending adequate time outside.	Complete the *Paleo Cure* 3-Step program. No additional personalization is required.
3–5	You may benefit from more focus on time outside.	Complete the *Paleo Cure* 3-Step program, and read this chapter for additional tips on how to bring more outside time into your life.
0–2	You are likely not spending enough time outside.	Complete both steps above. This should be a major focus for you, and ignoring this area may stand in the way of improvement elsewhere.

Most people intuitively know that spending time outdoors is good for them. But researchers are now beginning to understand that nature may be as essential to health as sleeping, exercise, and eating a healthy diet.

Humans evolved over hundreds of thousands of generations in a natural, outdoor environment rich in sunlight (in what is now modern-day Africa), and our species has inhabited urban environments for only a few hundred years. Human beings have never in history spent as little time in contact with plants and animals as they do today. And though the consequences of this profound separation are not yet entirely clear, recent evidence suggests that too much artificial stimulation and time spent in purely human-made environments may cause everything from fatigue and a loss of vitality to a decline in health. Just as we didn't evolve to eat an industrialized diet full of processed and refined foods, we also didn't evolve to live lives with little or no contact with nature. This disconnection from the natural world is yet another way that humans are mismatched with the current environment, and it is likely contributing to the epidemic of modern disease.

There are three features unique to spending time outdoors that are essential to health: exposure to sunlight, making contact with nature, and getting outdoor exercise. Let's look at them in more detail.

SUNLIGHT IS NOT OPTIONAL

Our Paleo ancestors spent about half of their days in the light of the sun. But today, frequent sun exposure is actively discouraged because of fears that it will encourage skin cancer, and modern lifestyles often involve long hours spent indoors under artificial light. While there's no doubt that too much ultraviolet radiation in the form of sunlight can increase the risk of skin cancer in fair-skinned people, not enough sunlight can also cause problems.

One of the primary benefits of sunlight is that it stimulates vitamin D production. Vitamin D is formed when a particular type of ultraviolet light (ultraviolet-B) interacts with 7-dehydrocholesterol, a molecule in the skin. Fair skin produces about 10,000 to 25,000 IU of vitamin D in response to twenty to thirty minutes of summer skin exposure, while those with darker skin may need to spend up to two hours in the sun to obtain the same amount.

We now know that vitamin D deficiency is a major predisposing factor in at least seventeen varieties of cancer, as well as heart disease, stroke, hypertension, autoimmune disease, type 2 diabetes, depression, birth defects, infectious diseases, and more.

Yet as important as vitamin D is, exposure to sunlight isn't absolutely necessary to obtain it, and it's possible to use supplements to ensure an optimal vitamin D level, checking lab tests to avoid toxicity. Does that mean we don't really need sun exposure for optimal health? No. A growing body of evidence suggests that sunlight has additional benefits above and beyond its capacity to stimulate vitamin D production, including reducing the risk of cardiovascular disease and regulating the immune system.

Scientists observed a connection between sunlight and cardiovascular disease as far back as the 1970s, when clinical studies of hypertension showed that blood pressure was consistently lower in summer than winter. Later studies showed that both the prevalence of hypertension and average blood pressure is directly correlated with latitude; in other words, those living in higher northern or southern latitudes (with less sunlight) had more hypertension and higher average blood pressure than those living closer to the equator. While some have argued that this variation may be due to genetic differences, it has been found that when people migrate from one place to another, their risk of death changes to match that of their new place of residence — which of course suggests that latitude and sun exposure, not genetics, are the responsible factors. In the United Kingdom, the risk of death from heart disease is directly correlated with latitude; there are more deaths at higher latitudes, even when researchers take into account all other known risk factors (like obesity and family history) and possible protective factors (like fruit and vegetable consumption and physical activity). Finally, clinical experiments have provided direct evidence that ultraviolet light reduces blood pressure. In one study, researchers exposed one group of people to lamps that gave off ultraviolet light as well as heat and another group to lamps that gave off only heat. In the group that received both heat and ultraviolet light, blood pressure dropped significantly after just one hour of exposure, whereas those that received heat alone experienced no change in blood pressure.

How does sunlight lower blood pressure and reduce the risk of cardiovascular disease? Sunlight stimulates the production of a chemical called nitric oxide in the skin. Nitric oxide helps blood vessels to relax and expand, which in turn reduces blood pressure. This is important because high blood pressure is one of the strongest risk factors for cardiovascular disease, and even relatively small reductions in blood pressure can dramatically reduce the deaths from both heart attack and stroke. For example, a drop of 20 mmHg in systolic blood pressure (blood pressure is expressed in terms of variations in pressure — for example, 120/80 — and *systolic* refers to the number on the top) leads to a twofold reduction in the overall risk of death in both men and women between the ages of forty and sixty-nine. Sunlight may also reduce the risk of cardiovascular disease by putting the brakes on inflammation. These beneficial effects of sunlight are likely to extend to other organs and tissues as well, since both blood pressure and inflammation have widespread effects in the body.

Another effect of sunlight that isn't mediated by vitamin D is its ability to regulate immune function. Studies have shown that the more hours of sun there are where you were born, the lower the risk you'll develop multiple sclerosis. Along the same lines, the more exposure to sun people have where they work and live as adults, the lower their rates of MS, and relapse rates for MS are higher in winter than in summer. Evidence for benefit from sunlight is strong for other autoimmune diseases as well, such as type 1 diabetes. Finally, exposure to sunlight may improve endocrine function, elevate mood (via its effects on certain brain chemicals, like serotonin), increase DNA repair capacity, and reduce skin lesions in psoriasis, eczema, and vitiligo. Researchers aren't entirely clear on how sunlight protects against autoimmune disease, but one possibility is that ultraviolet radiation suppresses the immune system. This explains why too much sun exposure can cause skin cancer: the excessive ultraviolet radiation breaks down natural defense mechanisms in the body that keep the growth of cancer cells in check. But it also suggests that not enough sunlight could lead to an *overactive* immune system that starts attacking its own organs and tissues. Importantly, these immune-suppressing effects of sunlight appear to be completely independent of vitamin D. With all of this in mind, how much sun exposure is just right? How can you minimize your risk of skin cancer while optimizing vitamin D levels and getting the additional cardiovascular and immune benefits of sunlight? Just follow these guidelines for you and your family members:

- If you have fair skin, aim for spending about half the amount of time in the sun that it takes for your skin to turn pink (without sunscreen) two to three days a week. This could be as little as ten minutes for those with very fair skin. If you have dark skin, you may need up to two hours per day to generate the same amount of vitamin D (which is why supplementation may be necessary for those with darker skin).

- Never burn yourself in the sun. Cover yourself with light clothing; wear a hat; shade yourself with an umbrella, a tree, or a canopy; wear sunglasses; and use a safe sunscreen (see sidebar below) to prevent sunburn if you're going to be exposed to sunlight for a prolonged period.
- Pay attention to the time of day, latitude, and season. This probably goes without saying, but you need less sun exposure at midday during the summer on the equator to generate a given amount of vitamin D than in the late afternoon during the winter in New York City. Vary your exposure accordingly.
- Infants under six months old don't have much of the protective pigment melanin in their skin. It's best to avoid direct sun exposure at midday, use protective clothing and a hat, and limit exposure to the morning or late-afternoon hours. Infants may be particularly susceptible to the toxic effects of some sunscreen ingredients, so use clothing or shade when possible and closely follow the recommendations in the sidebar on sunscreen.

NOT ALL SUNSCREENS ARE CREATED EQUAL

According to a report from the Environmental Working Group, only 25 percent of eight hundred sunscreens that were tested were effective at protecting the skin and didn't use potentially harmful ingredients. The report made the following recommendations for choosing a safe and effective sunscreen:

- Look for zinc oxide, titanium oxide, Mexoryl SX, or avobenzone (3 percent) as an active ingredient.

(continued)

- Use lotions, not sprays or powders. Many sunscreens contain tiny nanoparticles of zinc oxide and titanium dioxide. While these don't generally penetrate the skin, they can be inhaled from sprays or powders — with unknown health consequences.
- Don't be fooled by high SPF ratings. If you buy higher than SPF 50, you may think you have a free pass to stay in the sun for as long as you'd like without skin damage. But research suggests that SPF ratings higher than 50 are a hoax. Stick with SPF 15 to 50, depending on your skin tone and sun intensity.
- Avoid sunscreens with vitamin A (retinyl palmitate). While vitamin A is beneficial when consumed in the diet, some studies suggest that rubbing it on the skin may increase the risk of skin cancer.
- Avoid oxybenzone, a synthetic estrogen that can penetrate the skin and disrupt hormone regulation.

See my website for a link to the Environmental Working Group's sunscreen guide, which has a list of recommended products that meet these criteria.

HOW NATURE SOOTHES YOUR BODY AND MIND

For as long as cities have existed, humans have sought out nature as a refuge from the business, noise, and pollution of urban environments. More than two thousand years ago, Taoists in China created gardens and greenhouses that they believed promoted health. At the end of the seventeenth century, the book *English Gardener* suggested that readers "spare time in the garden, either digging, setting out, or weeding; there is no better way to preserve your health." By the 1890s, landscape architects and park planners were developing large urban parks for health purposes. Parks were considered the "lungs of the city," and the health benefits of exposure to nature were an unquestioned article of faith. Without nature, there would be no life. Humans are entirely dependent upon the natural environment for food, water, and shelter. But nature is more than just a source of raw materials; it's necessary to our psychological, emotional, and spiritual well-being. Frederick Law Olmsted, the famous nineteenth-century American landscape architect, believed that nature "operates by unconscious process to relax and relieve tensions created by the artificial surroundings of urban life." Yet over the last few hundred years, people have become profoundly disconnected from the natural world. As they moved from rural areas to cities and transitioned from working primarily outdoors (on farms) to working primarily indoors (in offices), they lost their vital contact with nature, and their health suffered as a result. A recent review of studies found that people living in the United States, Japan, and Spain are spending on average between 18 and 25 percent less time in wilderness or natural environments today than they did in 1981.

In his book *Last Child in the Woods*, Richard Louv refers to this disconnection from nature and its effects as nature-deficit disorder. It affects children and adults of all economic, social, and cultural backgrounds and leads to "diminished use of the senses, attention difficulties, and higher rates of physical and emotional illnesses." According to Louv, the disorder can affect individuals, families and communities, perhaps even changing human behavior in cities, since the absence of parks and open space has long been associated with high crime rates, depression, and other urban maladies. Louv and other commentators point to a growing body of evidence suggesting that regular contact with nature is important to health, and a lack of such contact contributes to both physical and mental problems. For example:

- Natural environments have restorative and rejuvenating effects, reduce stress and blood pressure, and improve one's outlook on life.
- Patients in hospital rooms recover faster when they're exposed to plants or nature; prison inmates whose cell windows face nature have fewer illnesses than those whose cell windows face the prison courtyard; and office workers with views of trees and flowers feel that their jobs are less stressful and more satisfying than those with windowless offices.

- Spending even a little time outdoors can reduce the symptoms of ADHD—even among kids who failed to respond to medication.
- Nature can improve the capacity to tolerate stress and can reverse mental and physical fatigue.

What's happening here? Why is contact with nature so essential to health? The simplest answer is that nature is in our DNA. For hundreds of thousands of generations, humans lived, worked, ate, played, and slept outside in undeveloped, natural environments. Living indoors with artificial light, air-conditioning, and central heating has been common for only a few generations, and we're still biologically adapted to life on the savanna. This concept—that humans have an innate affinity for the natural world—was labeled the biophilia hypothesis by Harvard University scientist and Pulitzer Prize–winning author E. O. Wilson. It's supported by more than a decade of research demonstrating how strongly people respond to open, grassy landscapes, scattered stands of trees, meadows, water, winding trails, and elevated views—exactly the environment that humans evolved in. But there are other reasons contact with nature improves our health. Studies using geographic information databases have found a strong correlation between greater amounts of parks and open, green spaces in an area and increasing levels of cycling, walking, and other forms of physical activity. In preschool children, time spent outdoors is the single most predictive factor of how physically active they will be. In addition to encouraging activity, nature protects against the harmful effects of air pollution. According to the California Air Resources Board, indoor air-pollutant levels are 25 to 62 percent greater than outside levels, and this difference poses a serious risk to health. And while crowding, high temperatures, and noise have all been linked to increases in aggression and violence, natural settings appear to have the opposite effect.

Here are a few tips to increase your exposure to nature:

- **Put plants in your home and office.** Studies have shown that caring for and seeing plants in your home and workspace has beneficial effects on health.

- **Get to know your local parks.** Many urban environments have great parks and open green spaces you can take advantage of without leaving town. Studies have found associations between use of urban green spaces and stress reduction, regardless of an individual's age, sex, or socioeconomic status.

- **Limit your screen time (and your children's):** Studies consistently show that increased screen time leads to less time spent outdoors.

- **Exercise outdoors.** Outdoor exercise has some unique benefits, which I'll cover in the next section.

- **Go camping.** Camping is a great way of getting out of the city and interacting with nature.

- **Get a dog.** Dog owners are more likely to be physically active, and having a dog may make you more likely to visit nature—especially if you have good off-leash hiking trails where you live.

- **Get closer to nature.** People who live and work closer to nature—including urban parks and green spaces—tend to be healthier overall than people who don't have access to nature. This is even true if all you do is look at nature: people with offices and homes that have views of nature tend to be healthier than those who look out on completely human-made environments.

"I LOST TOUCH WITH NATURE—AND MYSELF"

Rick, age twenty-eight, came to see me complaining of difficulty concentrating and memory issues, mental fatigue, depression, and malaise. "I used to have such a zest for life," he told me. "Now I just feel like I'm going through the motions."

Rick worked for a high-tech company in Silicon Valley—and that's about all he did. On most days he'd arrive at the office at 8:30 a.m. and wouldn't leave until after 9:00 p.m. He worked during the week-

(continued)

ends and on vacations, when he got around to taking them (which wasn't very often). I asked Rick about his childhood and what he loved to do. I noticed that almost everything he mentioned involved contact with nature: camping, going to the beach, surfing, snowboarding, and hiking in the mountains.

I suspected Rick was suffering from nature-deficit disorder, so I prescribed a regular program of getting outside and interacting with the natural world. At lunch, he drove to a hiking trail not far from his office and took a walk. He cut back on his work and started surfing again a few days a week. He enrolled in an outdoor tai chi class. And he scheduled a regular camping trip once every three months. Over the course of a year, Rick gradually regained his enthusiasm for life. "I don't dread getting out of bed like I used to. In fact, I look forward to my days now," he told me. "And the best part is, I'm getting even more done at work in less time."

A little bit of nature can go a long way!

WHY OUTDOOR EXERCISE BEATS INDOOR EXERCISE

Outdoor exercise provides more exposure to beneficial sunlight and more contact with nature. But there are additional advantages.

Running outdoors, for example, tends to affect your muscles differently than running inside on a treadmill; you flex your ankles more, and since you probably run up- and downhill at some point, you use different muscles in your legs. Outdoor exercise in general is often more strenuous than indoor exercise, in part because of wind resistance and changes in terrain. (Think of cycling, where wind resistance can cause significant drag and thus much higher energy expenditure.) There are also less tangible benefits of outdoor exercise. Compared with exercising indoors, outdoor exercise is associated with greater feelings of revitalization and positive engagement; decreases in tension, confusion, anger, and depression; and increased energy. Joggers who exercise in a natural, green setting with trees, foliage, and landscape views feel more restored than people who burn the same number of calories in gyms or other manmade settings. Those who exercise outdoors are also more likely to exercise longer and more often than those who exercise indoors. One study outfitted men and women over sixty-six years of age with a device that measured their activity levels for a week. Those who exercised outside got about thirty minutes more exercise during the week than those who walked or did other forms of exercise indoors. Exercise in natural (rather than man-made) environments appears to have benefits above and beyond simply exercising outdoors, especially for children. Research in Norway and Sweden compared preschool children who played on flat playgrounds to children who played for an equivalent amount of time on varied, natural terrain. At the end of the one-year study, the kids who played among the trees, rocks, and uneven natural surfaces tested better for balance, agility, and other markers of motor fitness. Here are some suggestions for boosting your outdoor exercise:

- Choose sports and hobbies that encourage outdoor activity, such as hiking, trail running, surfing, rock climbing, or snowboarding. If you swim or play tennis year-round, do it outside as much as possible.
- Consider a morning or an evening walk with your partner, dog, or children as a daily ritual. This will not only get you moving outside but also give you an opportunity to connect and play with those you love.
- Do your own yard work and gardening.
- Join an activity group that involves outdoor exercise, such as a running, cycling, or hiking club.
- Buy some high-quality all-weather gear so you won't be deterred from going outside when the weather is bad. You won't get the benefits of sunshine in these cases, but all of the other advantages of outdoor exercise still apply.

GO OUTSIDE: YOUR PERSONAL PALEO CURE

- Get approximately fifteen to twenty minutes of midday sun exposure without sunblock two to three days a week. Actual exposure time should vary based on skin tone, sun intensity, latitude, and time of year.
- Avoid sunburn by using safe, effective sunscreens, covering up with clothing and hats, or shading yourself with an umbrella or a canopy.
- Spend as much time in contact with nature as your schedule and lifestyle permit. Aim for, at a minimum, two excursions into nature (urban parks and green spaces included) each week.
- Put plants in your home and workplace. If you have outdoor space, plant a simple garden (a container garden is one easy option) and sit outside. If you have a choice, live in close proximity (and preferably in sight of) natural environments.
- Exercise outdoors whenever possible on varied terrain that includes hills, trails, rocks, and other natural features.

CHAPTER 17

Get Serious about Play

Play Quiz

Complete the quiz below and use the answer key to determine your play score.

	POINTS
I am a playful person.	1
I play with pets or children at least three times a week.	1
I play individual or group sports at least once a week.	2
I engage in playful/fun physical activity (e.g., surfing, snowboarding, ultimate Frisbee, and so on) at least once a week.	2
I play board games or other games at least once a week.	1
My work involves creativity and innovation.	1
I have a playful relationship with my spouse or partner.	1
I make time for play and consider it a priority.	2
I make a point of learning new skills and participating in activities that I think will be fun.	1
TOTAL	

Notes for this chapter may be found at ChrisKresser.com/ppcnotes/#ch17.

Answer key

Give yourself the correct number of points for all of the questions you answered yes to. Then use the chart below to determine your Play score.

TOTAL POINTS	WHAT YOUR POINTS MEAN	YOUR PERSONAL PALEO CURE
6+	You are probably getting adequate amounts of play.	Complete the *Paleo Cure* 3-Step program. No additional personalization is required.
3–5	You may benefit from more focus in this area.	Complete the *Paleo Cure* 3-Step program, and read this chapter for additional tips on how to bring even more play into your life.
0–2	You are likely not playing enough.	Complete both steps above. This should be a major focus for you, and ignoring this area may stand in the way of improvement elsewhere.

Imagine a life without play: no games, sports, movies, art, music, jokes, stories, daydreaming, flirting, make-believe, or roughhousing. Such a life would hardly be worth living. "If you think of all the things we do that are play-related and erase those," says play expert Dr. Stuart Brown, "it's pretty hard to keep going. Without play, there's a sense of dullness, lassitude and pessimism, which doesn't work well in the world we live in." We all start out playing naturally as kids; no one needs to teach us how to do it. It is effortless, spontaneous, and universal. As we grow older, though, we're often made to feel guilty for playing. Play is seen as a waste of time, and since "time is money," play is almost like throwing money down the drain. Yet despite these cultural attitudes, a growing body of evidence suggests that play is as fundamental to life as sleep, dreams, pleasure, and connection. Play is not simply a frivolous luxury; it's necessary for the development of empathy, social altruism, and other behaviors needed to handle stress. It keeps our minds and brains flexible, and it helps us adapt to a changing and unpredictable world.

WHY WE NEED PLAY

Play is part of our evolutionary heritage. It emerged and became more prevalent in warm-blooded animals with larger brains. In fact, the smarter an animal is, the more it plays. Dogs, snow leopards, dolphins, otters, killer whales, grizzly bears, and even ravens and ants devote time to play. They even have special play signals, such as a relaxed, open-mouth expression (the play face), that are recognized across species lines.

Why would this be? Evolution favors behavior that improves a species' chance of surviving and reproducing. On the surface, play appears to be a waste of time—and if there's anything nature doesn't tolerate, it's waste. But scientists now believe that play is "training for the unexpected": it encourages flexibility and variability in behavior and adaptation to a changing environment. And in an unpredictable world that presents constant challenges and obstacles, anything that helps a species adapt will also help it to survive and reproduce.

This may explain the findings of ethologist Robert Fagen, a professor at the University of Alaska, who spent fifteen years studying the behavior of bears in the wild. He discovered that the bears who played the most often throughout their childhood lived longer and healthier lives and thus left more offspring behind. Other studies of animals suggest that play may directly contribute to the growth of regions of the brain responsible for motor control, balance, and coordination. Professor John Byers, a zoologist at the University of Idaho, found a strong correlation between how often an animal plays and the growth of its cerebellum during childhood. Along the same lines, Canadian neuroscientist Sergio Pellis showed that rats that are deprived of play develop abnormalities in their brains. This research suggests that play is particularly crucial during the period of rapid brain development that occurs during childhood in both animals and humans. In adults, playfulness is associated with several positive behaviors, such as creativity, productivity, flexibility, optimism, empathy, social altruism, and the capacity to handle stress. It encourages cooperation, promotes problem solving, and fosters a sense of community and belonging. Perhaps above all, play helps us to face what play scholar Brian Sutton-Smith refers to as our existential dread—it opens us to possibilities and gives us hope for the future. This may explain why the human drive toward play exists even under horrific circumstances: children continued to play in concentration camps during the Holocaust.

However, play does diminish when basic needs are unmet or when children suffer long-term, chronic deprivation or abuse. The absence of play in these situations may have catastrophic consequences. Dr. Stuart Brown, a psychiatrist and author of the book *Play: How It Shapes the Brain, Opens the Imagination, and Invigorates the Soul*, studied a group of twenty-six young murderers in the Texas prison system. He found that 90 percent of the murderers he interviewed had been deprived of play or had major "play abnormalities" as children. Less than 10 percent of the nonviolent comparison group in the study had suffered play deprivation or abnormalities. In Dr. Brown's clinical psychiatry practice, playless lives were characterized by depression, over-control, driven ambition, envy, and, eventually, personal breakdown.

HOW TO BRING MORE PLAY INTO YOUR LIFE

Before we talk about how to bring more play back into our lives, we have to define what it is. It may seem like play is unnecessary—and perhaps even impossible—to define. But having a better understanding of what play is (and isn't) may help us see more opportunities for cultivating it in all aspects of our lives. According to Dr. Brown, play is:

- **Apparently purposeless.** Play is done for its own sake, not to achieve a goal.
- **Voluntary.** Play is not a requirement or an obligation.
- **Inherently attractive.** Play is fun and feels good.

- **Outside of time.** When fully engaged in play, we lose a sense of the passage of time.
- **Outside of self.** When fully engaged in play, we become less self-conscious. We don't worry about whether we look good or awkward or stupid.
- **Improvisational.** Play is spontaneous and doesn't lock us into a rigid way of doing things.
- **Mildly addictive.** Play makes us want to do more of it.

As you can see from this list, play isn't limited to games or sports. Art, music, and all forms of creative expression can be play. Cooking a meal for your family can be play. Even work can be play. Conversely, activities that are often considered play may not be experienced as play if they don't meet the criteria above. For example, if you're frustrated, miserable, and completely preoccupied with winning a round of golf or a tennis match, that's not play.

ARE VIDEO AND COMPUTER GAMES PLAY?

We live in an era where there seems to be less and less time for play — especially among children. Forty percent of elementary schools across the country have completely eliminated recess, in part to make time for an expanded academic curriculum. Many kids have a schedule that would put a busy CEO to shame, with little time for idle, creative, and unstructured play. And parents mourn that their kids don't play the way they themselves used to — spontaneously, out on the street, with whatever neighborhood kids happened to be around.

One form of play that *has* increased over the past two decades is playing computer and video games. According to a poll by the Kaiser Foundation, American children play an average of eight hours of video games per week, an increase of over 400 percent from 1999. A

(continued)

staggering 99 percent of American boys play video games, along with 94 percent of girls.

But are video games truly play? While they do satisfy many of the criteria of play, they lack the interpersonal nuance that can be achieved only by play that engages all five senses in the three-dimensional world. This doesn't mean video games should be avoided entirely; in fact, some studies have shown that playing video games can improve coordination, increase social behavior, and promote some kinds of learning. But it does suggest that they shouldn't be the sole means of play in a child's (or adult's) life.

With this in mind, here's a list of tips for encouraging more play in your life:

- **Take your play history.** Think about the things you loved to do as a child or when you had more play in your life. What got you excited? What gave you the most joy? What activities did you lose yourself in?
- **Make a list of play activities.** Using the results of your play history above, make a list of ways you love to play and put it somewhere you will see it every day. It's easy to get wrapped up in the hustle and bustle of life, and sometimes a quick glance at this list will be enough to remind you to do something playful.
- **Create opportunities for play.** Play is all about perspective. If you look for chances to play, they're everywhere: throw a ball for a dog, play hide-and-seek with your kids, improvise on the piano, have a board-game night, carry a sketchbook with you, or simply go on an aimless walk in the woods.
- **Embrace "beginner's mind."** In Zen practice, the term *beginner's mind* refers to an attitude of openness, curiosity, and humility and a lack of preconceived notions. This is an excellent mental state to cultivate for play, since fear of looking silly, awkward, or unskilled is one of the biggest obstacles to play for adults.

- **Follow your bliss—but don't mistake play for fun.** Play can be fun, but it can also be absorbing, challenging, and demanding. For example, if you've always dreamed of building your own sailboat and sailing it to Mexico, much of that process may not be fun, but it can still be play.
- **Make play a priority.** If you're busy with work, family, and other obligations, it can be difficult to find time for play. Schedule time for play just as you schedule time for other necessities in your life. If this seems daunting, start small—perhaps just thirty minutes a week. My guess is that after you experience the benefits of play, you'll naturally find time for more.

PLAY: YOUR PERSONAL PALEO CURE

- Think like a child—kids are the experts at play.
- Pick activities that bring you joy—repainting the bathroom may not sound like play, but if it meets the criteria (it feels good, you are fully engaged, you're doing it voluntarily, and so on) then go for it. Remember, one person's work can be another person's play.
- Look for opportunities to play everywhere.

REVIVE YOUR HEALTH

CHAPTER 18

Fine-Tuning Your Personal Paleo Cure

Now that you've developed your Personal Paleo Cure through beneficial changes to your diet and lifestyle, let's focus on five areas where you can fine-tune your code even further. You feel great now, but you'll feel (and look) even better once you zero in on personalized answers to these questions:

- **Macronutrient ratios:** How much carbohydrate, fat, and protein should you eat?
- **Calorie intake and meal frequency, timing, and size:** How often, and how much, should you eat?
- **High activity level:** What changes should athletes and highly active people make?
- **Superfoods:** Which foods are highest in essential nutrients? How can you further optimize your health and prevent disease?
- **Supplementation:** Which supplements should you take, and which should you avoid?

MACRONUTRIENT RATIOS

Macronutrients—protein, carbohydrate, and fat—are the nutrients that humans consume in the largest quantity and that make up the bulk of

---

Notes for this chapter may be found at ChrisKresser.com/ppcnotes/#ch18.

our caloric intake. In Step 1 we discussed macronutrient quality: which *types* of fat, protein, and carbohydrate are optimal for human health. In this section, we're going to discuss macronutrient ratios: *how much* protein, fat, and carbohydrate you should eat and in what proportion.

Despite various recommendations from mainstream health organizations, nutrition experts, and diet gurus advising you to go low-fat, low-carb, or high-protein (or some magic combination of all three), the truth is there's no one-size-fits-all approach when it comes to macronutrient ratios. We share a lot in common as human beings, but we're not robots; we have different genes, lifestyles, health issues, activity levels, and goals, and all of these factors will influence what an optimal macronutrient ratio is. And since these factors can change over time (for example, if you develop a chronic illness, significantly reduce your activity because of an injury, move to a new climate, or start training for an athletic competition), your ideal macronutrient ratio can also change over time—and even seasonally throughout the year. Learn how to listen to your own body and determine what it needs; don't just jump from one fashionable diet trend to the next.

For most people, the *quality* of macronutrients has a much more significant impact on health and well-being than the *quantity* or *ratio*. The fact that hunter-gatherers thrived on a variety of diets and macronutrient ratios supports this idea.

If the low-fat-diet gurus are correct, then you would expect the Inuit, Eskimos, and Masai, with their extremely high-fat diets (the Inuit get up to 90 percent of their calories from fat), to be obese and dropping dead left and right of heart attacks. If the low-carb gurus are correct, then you'd expect to see a lot of overweight and metabolically dysfunctional Tukisentans and Kitavans, whose diets are, on average, about 70 to 90 percent carbohydrates, or even higher! In fact, we see neither. All of these populations are virtually free of the modern diseases, like obesity, diabetes, heart disease, and autoimmune disorders, that are killing Americans every year. They also tend to be lean and muscular, and without having to spend hours on the StairMaster at the local gym.

What factors determine the ideal macronutrient ratio for you?

Humans can thrive on a wide range of macronutrient ratios; let's take a closer look at the factors that determine what specific mix of fat, carbohydrate, and protein is right for you:

- **Constitution (genetics, physiology, biology).** Modern studies have shown that some people have genes that predispose them to problems metabolizing glucose (sugar), while others have genes that make it more likely they will have problems burning fat. There is still much we don't understand about the contribution of genetics to diet and the relationship between genes and environmental factors.
- **Season.** During the summer, your body will naturally crave different foods than it does during the winter. It's true that our ancestors had access to certain foods only at certain times of the year. If they lived in Northern Europe, they weren't eating mangoes from Thailand in the winter.
- **Geography/climate.** If you've been to the tropics, you probably found yourself craving lighter foods with higher water content, like fruits and vegetables, more than you did at home. Likewise, in cold climates, you probably gravitate toward eating more protein- and fat-rich foods, like meat stews. There's a reason for this.
- **Health status.** Have you ever noticed that you crave different foods when you're coming down with a cold or the flu? The body has different needs in different physiological states. Women often crave more carbohydrates during pregnancy because the developing fetus has a need for glucose, and women naturally become somewhat insulin resistant as a result. People with thyroid problems may suffer on very low-carb diets, because insulin is required for proper thyroid-hormone conversion. As people age and become less active, they often find that they need less food, or

perhaps less of a particular macronutrient, than they did when they were younger.

- **Activity level.** A construction worker doing manual labor for eight hours a day or a high-level athlete in training will have different dietary and macronutrient needs than someone who works at a desk. This should go without saying, but, amazingly, it is often ignored in the discussion about macronutrients.

- **Goals.** If you're training for the next Mr. Olympia competition, you will very likely eat different foods than an obese person trying to lose weight.

Before we move on, keep these numbers in mind:

- 1 gram of carbohydrate has 4 calories.
- 1 gram of protein has 4 calories.
- 1 gram of fat has 9 calories.

You'll use these numbers to do some quick math as you calculate your own ratios.

Carbohydrates: Starting points for experimentation

In the United States, the average person gets about 45 to 60 percent of total calories from carbohydrates. For a moderately active man eating 2,600 calories a day, this works out to between 290 and 420 grams a day (using the numbers in the box above, that's approximately 1,200 to 1,700 calories from carbohydrates). For a moderately active woman eating 2,000 calories a day, it's about 225 to 325 grams a day (around 900 to 1,300 calories from carbohydrates). On a typical Personal Paleo diet that includes starchy vegetables, fruit, some dairy products, and perhaps white rice (if tolerated), carbohydrate intake tends to range between 15 and 30 percent of total calories a day. A low-carbohydrate Paleo diet ranges between 10 and 15 percent of total calories as carbohydrates, and a very low-carbohydrate Paleo diet would be anything lower than 10 percent. On a high-carbohydrate Paleo diet, carbohydrate intake would be somewhere between 30 and 45 percent (or higher) of total calories.

PALEO DIET	CARBOHYDRATES (% OF TOTAL CALORIES)
Very low-carb	<10
Low-carb	10–15
Moderate-carb	15–30
High-carb	30–45+

While many health experts include nonstarchy vegetables (such as green vegetables, carrots, peppers, and so on) when counting carbohydrates, I do not. Though these foods do contain carbohydrates (primarily glucose), they are difficult to break down, and our bodies actually expend glucose in the process of digesting these foods. Therefore, I count only carbohydrates from starchy plants (sweet potatoes, potatoes, taro, yuca, plantains, white rice, buckwheat, and so on), fruit, dairy products, and sweeteners.

Ultimately, the only way to determine your optimal macronutrient ratio is to experiment. Most of my patients do best with a standard, moderate-carbohydrate Paleo approach, with between 15 and 30 percent of total calories from carbohydrates per day, which I'll explain in a moment. First, however, here are some situations that may call for a carbohydrate intake that is either lower or higher than standard:

Low-carbohydrate: 10 to 15 percent of total calories (roughly 65 to 100 grams daily on a 2,600-calorie diet and 50 to 75 grams daily on a 2,000-calorie diet)

- Those who need to lose weight and have not tried low-carb before
- Anyone with metabolic problems, such as insulin or leptin resistance
- Those with high blood sugar (hyperglycemia) or low blood sugar (hypoglycemia, often seen as reactive hypoglycemia, which occurs after meals)

- Those with mood disturbances (though mood disturbances can sometimes be helped with higher carbohydrate intake, especially if sleep problems are involved)

Very low-carbohydrate: less than 10 percent of total calories (roughly less than 65 grams daily on a 2,600-calorie diet and less than 50 grams daily on a 2,000-calorie diet)

- Those who have significant amounts of weight to lose or metabolic issues and whose blood sugar responds very poorly to dietary carbohydrates
- Those with neurological or cognitive problems
- Those who have tried a low-carbohydrate diet with some success (who may find added benefit from trying a very low-carbohydrate diet)

High-carbohydrate: 30 to 45 percent or more of total calories (roughly 200 to 300 grams daily on a 2,600-calorie diet and 150 to 225 grams daily on a 2,000-calorie diet)

- Those who are highly active or training hard
- Those who are lean and have trouble maintaining their weight on low-carb diets

If none of the above applies to you, **begin with a moderate-carbohydrate Paleo diet** (that is, 15 to 30 percent of calories from carbohydrates). This amounts to roughly 100 to 200 grams per day on a 2,600-calorie diet (400 to 800 carbohydrate calories) or 75 to 150 grams per day on a 2,000-calorie diet (300 to 600 carbohydrate calories). (See the section below called "High Activity Level" for information on how many calories a day you should aim for if you're exercising regularly.)

Try eating at the lower end of the range for two weeks, and then the higher end of the range for the following two weeks. Performing this experiment is valuable, because you'll get a sense of how changing the ratio of carbs to fat affects you personally, and you can use that information to fine-tune your macronutrient intake, right down to the daily or even hourly level. For example, I've found that eating fewer carbohydrates helps me to focus mentally. By contrast, if I eat low-carb on a regular basis, my energy flags and I don't sleep well. So I will often eat a relatively low-carb breakfast and lunch, to support mental clarity throughout the day, and a higher-carb dinner, to support sleep and energy levels.

If you have any of the conditions I listed, try the low-carbohydrate or very low-carbohydrate approach as indicated. But remember, some people on low-carbohydrate diets find more benefit from adding carbohydrates back into their diet than from further reducing them. This is where your personal experience should guide you. Pay attention to all of the variables I listed above and adjust your ratios accordingly. As a general rule, as your activity level increases, you will want to increase your carbohydrate intake commensurately. If it's winter and you're living in a cold climate, you may find that eating extra fat helps keep you warm (although others get that result from eating more carbohydrates, possibly because of the effects of carbohydrate intake on thyroid hormone). In addition, following very low-carb diets over a long period may adversely affect the gut flora, leading to digestive symptoms like constipation or diarrhea, halitosis (bad breath), gas, bloating, and abdominal pain. If you experience these changes on a very low-carb diet, I'd suggest increasing your intake of fermentable fiber and fermented foods, and/or taking prebiotic and probiotic supplements. See chapter 10 and the bonus chapter on digestive disorders on my website for more information.

The point is this: You need to experiment. Nobody (including me) can tell you what your ideal ratio is. But by following these basic guidelines and keeping track of your symptoms, you should have no trouble figuring it out.

WHEN TO THINK TWICE ABOUT A VERY LOW-CARB DIET

There's no doubt that very low-carb diets are beneficial in certain situations. However, in some cases, they may actually be harmful. These include:

- **Hypothyroidism.** Some evidence suggests that very low-carb diets may contribute to poor thyroid function. Insulin is required to convert T4, the inactive form of thyroid hormone, into T3, the active form. Insulin levels are chronically low on a very low-carb diet, which in turn can lead to low levels of T3 and hypothyroid symptoms. This doesn't happen for everyone on a very low-carb diet, but I've seen it often in my practice. If you develop cold hands and feet, fatigue, difficulty concentrating and memory issues, hair loss, and other symptoms of poor thyroid function while on a very low-carb diet, try increasing your carbohydrate intake until the symptoms resolve.

- **Pregnancy.** Carbohydrate needs may be slightly higher during pregnancy due to the growing baby's need for glucose. I've noticed that most pregnant women tend to do better with moderate carbohydrate intake (about 15 to 30 percent of calories) than with low-carb or very low-carb diets. The exception would be women with type 1 or type 2 diabetes, who may need lower-carb approaches to avoid hyperglycemia, which can harm the growing baby.

- **Adrenal fatigue.** I've found that most of my patients with adrenal fatigue syndrome (described in more detail in the bonus chapter on this subject on my website) don't do well on a very low-carb diet.

- **Insomnia.** If you find yourself waking up frequently throughout the night, and you're on a very low-carb diet, try increasing your carbohydrate intake slightly. In some cases, this single change can resolve the insomnia.

- **High levels of physical activity.** If you're highly active and training hard, you're going to be burning a lot more fuel. While some athletes seem to do well on very low-carb diets, most do better with a significantly higher carbohydrate intake — as high as 50 to 60 percent of calories (roughly 325 to 400 grams per day on a 2,600-calorie diet and 250 to 300 grams on a 2,000-calorie diet) in some cases. See the section below on how to modify your diet if you're highly active.

As always, you'll have to experiment to see what works for you. But if you have hypothyroidism, are pregnant, or are training hard, I'd suggest beginning with a more moderate (about 100 to 200 grams per day) intake of carbohydrates.

SUMMARY OF CARBOHYDRATE INTAKE

GOAL/ POPULATION	CARB INTAKE (% OF TOTAL CALORIES)	CARB INTAKE (G/D ON A 2,600-CALORIE DIET)	CARB INTAKE (G/D ON A 2,000-CALORIE DIET)
Significant weight loss, severe blood-sugar issues, neurological and cognitive problems	<10	<65	<50
Weight loss, blood-sugar regulation, mood disturbances	10–15	65–100	50–75
General health and maintenance	15–30	100–200	75–150
Athletes, people who are highly active and/or lean with fast metabolism	30–45	200–300	150–225

Protein

Most people naturally eat the right amount of protein for their needs. Protein is such a crucial nutrient that the brain has specific mechanisms that increase your desire for it if you need more and decrease your desire for it if you're getting too much; these mechanisms are difficult to override through willpower alone. For this reason, my general recommendation is to simply eat as much protein as you crave. In most cases, this will be about 10 to 20 percent of total calories, or roughly 65 to 130 grams per day on a 2,600-calorie diet (260 to 520 protein calories) and 50 to 100 grams per day on a 2,000-calorie diet (200 to 300 protein calories).

This recommended range is supported by observing protein intakes (as a percentage of total calories) in healthy, preindustrial cultures around the world:

- Masai (Kenya and Northern Tanzania): 19 percent protein
- Kitava (Trobriand Islands, Papua New Guinea): 10 percent protein
- Tokelau (Pacific island territory of New Zealand): 12 percent protein
- Inuit (Arctic): 20 percent protein
- Kuna (Panama): 12 percent protein

Interestingly, it's also supported by observing what we consume here in the United States, where the average protein intake is 15 percent of calories. (As a comparison to another Western country, in Sweden, it is 12 percent.)

It's rarely a good idea to decrease protein intake below 10 percent of total calories. However, there are some situations where it may be advantageous to increase protein intake to 20 to 30 percent or even as high as 35 percent of total calories (that is, 150 to 175 grams per day on a 2,000-calorie diet), at least temporarily:

- **Weight loss.** Protein is one of the most satiating (that is, satisfying) macronutrients, and higher-protein diets can reduce appetite and calorie intake and increase metabolic rate, all of which contributes to weight loss.

- **Blood-sugar problems.** Higher protein intakes tend to have a stabilizing effect on blood sugar, whether it's high or low.
- **Muscle mass.** Protein is the nutrient required to build and rebuild muscle. Those who want to add or maintain muscle mass (endurance athletes, weightlifters, the elderly, or the chronically ill) should consume more protein.

Why stop at 35 percent? Studies suggest that the ability of humans to metabolize protein tops out at 35 percent of total calories. The body releases nitrogen in the process of metabolizing protein. Nitrogen forms toxic ammonia, which is then converted to urea, a safe, nontoxic compound. But conversion of ammonia to urea is limited when protein intake exceeds 35 percent of calories. Eating more protein than this for an extended period can lead to a toxic buildup of ammonia in the body, which may have serious consequences (including nausea, diarrhea, and death) if protein intake exceeds 45 percent of total calories consumed.

This threshold may be significantly lower in pregnant women. During pregnancy, the conversion of ammonia to urea appears to peak at a protein intake of 25 percent of total calories. Some studies suggest that protein intakes above this level may lead to poor pregnancy outcomes, such as decreased birth weight, and increased risk of disease and death for the baby. For these reasons, I recommend that pregnant women limit protein intake to 15 to 20 percent of calories, regardless of whether they are overweight or have blood-sugar problems.

There is some research surrounding protein restriction and longevity. To read more about these studies and the link between protein intake and increased life span, please see the notes for this chapter on my website.

		PROTEIN INTAKE (G/D ON A 2,600-CALORIE DIET)	PROTEIN INTAKE (G/D ON A 2,000-CALORIE DIET)
SUMMARY OF PROTEIN INTAKE			
GOAL/ POPULATION	**PROTEIN INTAKE (% OF TOTAL CALORIES)**		
Pregnancy	10–15	65–100	50–75
General health	10–20	65–130	50–100
Weight loss, blood-sugar regulation, gaining muscle mass	20–35*	130–230	100–175

*Once weight loss, blood-sugar regulation, and muscle-gain goals have been reached, I suggest decreasing protein intake into the general-health range listed above, or perhaps slightly higher (around 25 percent).

Fat

Once you've determined your optimal carbohydrate and protein intakes, the remainder of your calories will come from fat. This can range from as high as 80 to 85 percent on a very low-carb, relatively low-protein diet to as low as 10 to 15 percent on a high-protein, high-carb diet. Fortunately, as I mentioned above, studies of traditional diets indicate that humans can thrive and remain free of modern disease on a wide range of fat intakes — provided they have the right mix of fats (that is, mostly saturated and monounsaturated fats with a much smaller amount of polyunsaturated fat).

CALORIE INTAKE AND MEAL FREQUENCY, TIMING, AND SIZE

It's not just what we eat that affects our health but also how much and how often, though I don't think it's necessary for most people to count calories. Once you determine your Personal Paleo Cure and identify your optimal mix of protein, carbohydrate, and fat, you should simply eat to satisfy your appetite.

What if you're trying to lose weight? While it's true that eating fewer calories will lead to weight loss, it's also true that consciously restricting calories often fails as a weight-loss strategy. In the bonus chapter on weight loss on my website, I'll introduce an approach that leads to a spontaneous reduction (without conscious effort) in calorie intake.

Meal frequency and size are more variable. You'll hear some people claim that you should eat only one huge meal at night and fast for the entire day. Others will suggest eating six small meals throughout the day. And then you have the conventional approach of three squares a day. What about snacking? Again, some insist that snacking between meals will make you fat and should be strictly avoided. Others say there's no problem with snacking as long as you're eating the right kinds of foods.

My experience tells me that everybody (and every body!) is different. Some people do better with smaller meals spaced more frequently throughout the day (and/or snacking between meals), and others will do better with larger meals eaten less frequently with no snacks. The key, as always, is to choose an approach based on your health status and goals and to experiment and see what works for *you*.

With this in mind, I can give you some general guidelines:

- **If you're trying to lose weight or have high blood sugar, insulin resistance, or diabetes,** you'll probably have more success by not snacking between meals. Avoiding snacks may have a beneficial effect on the hormones that regulate fat storage. Some people with digestive problems feel better when they don't snack, because it gives the digestive system a chance to rest between meals.
- **If you have low blood sugar,** you'll likely feel better eating small meals every two to three hours throughout the day. This can prevent your blood sugar from dropping too low and making you crazy. And while some people with digestive problems do better when they don't snack, others do better eating frequent, small

311

meals, because they can't tolerate large amounts of food at one sitting. (See how individual this is?)

- **If you're generally healthy,** are not overweight, and don't have blood-sugar or immune problems, then three meals a day, with or without snacks (depending on your appetite), is a good approach. You may want to experiment with the other strategies above just to see if they make you feel better, but they're not necessary.

- **If you're fighting a chronic infection, have a weak immune system, are trying to optimize longevity, are overweight, or have high blood sugar and metabolic problems,** you may find that restricting your food intake to an eight-hour window each day (intermittent fasting) is helpful. See the section below for details.

Intermittent fasting

Intermittent fasting is a pattern of eating that alternates between periods of fasting and nonfasting. Studies suggest that intermittent fasting may be as effective (and easier to stick with) than voluntary calorie restricting for weight loss. It has also been shown to improve insulin sensitivity and other indicators of metabolic function, reduce inflammation and oxidative stress, decrease seizures, protect brain cells, and promote healthy brain function.

There are several theories about why intermittent fasting provides health benefits. One is that intermittent fasting causes positive stress. As you may recall from chapter 14, not all stress is harmful; when cells in the body are under mild stress, they adapt by enhancing their own ability to fight that stress and protect against disease. Another related theory is that intermittent fasting promotes a cellular cleanup and repair process called autophagy, which may protect against the degeneration of brain cells, infections, and cancer.

There are many ways to do intermittent fasting, but the method that I recommend involves restricting your food intake to an eight-hour window each day. For example, you would eat only between the hours of 12:00 p.m. and 8:00 p.m. During the fasting period, if you feel hungry or spaced out, you may have some coconut oil (by itself, or perhaps added to coffee—don't knock it until you try it!). This will not interfere with the benefits of the fast. During the feeding period, you simply eat as your hunger dictates; there's no need to purposely restrict calories, and you should not try to overeat to make up for the meal you skipped. You might have two meals only; two meals and a snack; or three meals. If you're aggressively trying to lose weight or you have very high blood sugar, eating two meals without a snack in between is probably the best strategy, but since you're already getting the benefits of a sixteen-hour fast, snacking during the feeding window of an intermittent fast is less likely to impede your progress than snacking while eating normally.

If you do well with the method I've described above and you want to further benefit from fasting, you can add an extended (forty-hour) fast once or twice a month (or as often as once a week, if you're highly motivated). This involves fasting for an additional twenty-four-hour period above and beyond your daily sixteen-hour fast. For example, on Tuesday you would eat between 12:00 p.m. and 8:00 p.m. as usual, but your next meal would come at 12:00 p.m. on Thursday rather than 12:00 p.m. on Wednesday.

You might discover that intermittent fasting every day is too much for you but that doing it three to four days a week is just right. This is what I find myself doing most of the time. I will typically skip breakfast about four days a week and eat normally on the other three days. I don't plan in advance; I let my schedule and my body tell me what to do. If I wake up feeling very hungry, and I have a long and active day ahead, I will probably eat breakfast. If I wake up feeling less hungry and I have a less active day planned, I might skip breakfast. (I'm aware of the research noting the link between skipping breakfast and overeating at lunch, but I am doing this in the context of intermittent fasting and finding what works for me; you should do the same.) The point is, there's no right or wrong way to do this—there's just the way that works best for your needs and goals.

While intermittent fasting is a good approach for many people, there are some situations where I don't recommend it:

- **Pregnancy.** While occasional intermittent fast days may be fine for some women during pregnancy (be sure to check with your doctor first), I don't recommend sixteen-hour fasts daily, nor do I recommend extended forty-hour fasts.
- **Adrenal fatigue.** In my clinical experience, intermittent fasting often worsens adrenal fatigue conditions. These patients usually do better with several small meals throughout the day or with three normal meals and snacks in between. See chapter 20 for more on adrenal fatigue syndrome.
- **Hypothyroidism.** While there's some evidence that suggests intermittent fasting can be helpful for hypothyroidism, most of my patients with this condition do better eating regular meals.
- **Eating disorders.** If you have a history of anorexia, bulimia, or any other eating disorder, please check with your health-care provider before embarking on an intermittent-fasting program.
- **Kids.** Growing children and young adults need to eat regular meals for physical and cognitive fuel and shouldn't go for long stretches without healthy foods.

High activity level

I often see patients who are competitive athletes, CrossFit enthusiasts, or just very active physically who are suffering from fatigue, hair loss, low libido, and other problems. Almost inevitably, they are on low-carb diets. Back in the 1980s, fat-phobia was the norm. Athletes who wanted to stay lean and competitive adopted the low-fat dogma just as most other health-conscious people did. Unfortunately, many found that dramatically restricting fat intake—particularly cutting out healthy traditional fats like butter, coconut oil, and lard—had a negative impact on their health. Rates of obesity, metabolic disease, and other problems continued to rise as unsuspecting people trying to do the right thing switched out their steak-and-eggs breakfasts for cold cereal, dry wheat toast, and orange juice. Then, in the mid-1990s, the pendulum swung back in the other direction as people realized the folly of avoiding dietary fat and the perils of processed carbohydrates. Suddenly low-carb diets were all the rage, and members of the athletic community, which is often on the forefront of nutritional changes, began to shun all carbohydrates (not just processed, refined carbs) with the same zeal with which they had previously shunned fat.

While some people are able to thrive for long periods, and even indefinitely, on a very low-carb diet, serious competitive athletes, martial artists, cyclists, runners, boxers, and high-intensity trainers like CrossFitters almost always begin to experience problems when they dramatically restrict carbohydrates. Why? Because intense physical activity is dependent on a steady supply of glucose to replace the muscle glycogen that is depleted during glucose-fueled activity. And studies have consistently shown that low-carbohydrate diets are not capable of maintaining optimal glycogen levels during intense exercise.

Lack of carbohydrate during this type of exercise causes glycogen depletion, which in turn leaves muscles unable to get the glucose they need to produce ATP (adenosine triphosphate), the fundamental energy unit of the cell. Glycogen depletion can be a good thing in certain circumstances, such as if you have diabetes or are trying to lose weight. But this is another example that there's no one-size-fits-all approach and demonstrates the key principle behind the Personal Paleo Cure. Just because something is appropriate for treating a disease or a specific problem doesn't mean it's appropriate for healthy people, especially serious athletes.

It's interesting to note that very low-carb diets (under 10 percent of total calories) never caught on among professional athletes whose livelihoods depend on consistently high performance. And while very low-carb diets were adopted by topflight bodybuilders for a short time, the trend has recently started moving in the other direction. A recent article in *Muscle Development* magazine chronicled this change, pointing out that Jay Cutler and Branch Warren, the number-one and number-two finishers in the 2009 Mr. Olympia, ate, respectively, 700 and 1,000 grams of carbohydrates per day! I'd say that's a pretty far cry from a low-carb diet.

Here's the bottom line: very low-carb diets are usually not a good idea for people who regularly perform strenuous exercise. That said, in keeping with the principle of this program, I don't want you to take my word for this. I want you to experiment and see what is true for you. Even the best theories are useless if they don't produce practical results. I'd recommend 25 percent of total calories from carbohydrates as an absolute minimum for anyone doing frequent, intense exercise. If you're training at a very high level, you may need much more than this. Keep in mind that a Mr. Olympia bodybuilder got up to 1,000 grams per day, which accounted for between 50 and 60 percent of his total caloric intake. Granted, few people are competing at that level, and few people will need that much; I mention it simply to illustrate the range.

Another important consideration when you're highly active is to make sure you're eating enough overall. I often see patients in my practice who are doing CrossFit or another intense physical activity and are simply not eating enough calories to sustain their activity level. This is a great formula for fat loss, but once your body fat reaches a low level, muscle will be broken down in order to provide the fuel your body needs to function properly.

With all of this in mind, here are some guidelines for highly active people (meaning those who are training at least three to five times a week at moderate to high intensity). The guidelines vary depending on whether the goal is fat loss, maintenance, or muscle gain.

GOAL	CARBOHYDRATE* (% OF TOTAL CALORIES)	CALORIES (PER LB. OF BODY WEIGHT)	PROTEIN (G/LB. OF BODY WEIGHT)
Fat loss	7–20	15–16	0.8–1.0
Maintenance	25–60	17–18	0.8–1.0
Muscle gain	25–60	19–21	1.0–1.25

*Remember, when I refer to grams of carbohydrates, I'm referring only to carbs from starchy vegetables, dairy products, and fruit, not from nonstarchy vegetables like broccoli and carrots.

Let's look at two examples of how this might work out in practice:

- A 125-pound lean female cyclist wants to increase muscle mass and performance. At 20 calories per pound of body weight, she'll require 2,500 calories a day to meet her goal. She should eat between 125 and 156 grams of protein per day (20 to 25 percent of total calories on her 2,500-calorie diet) and between 156 and 375 grams of carbohydrate per day (25 to 60 percent of total calories), depending on her activity level and individual preference/tolerance to carbs.

- A 230-pound male CrossFit athlete wants to lose 25 pounds and become more lean. At 15 calories per pound of body weight, he should have a target of 3,450 calories per day. He should eat between 184 and 230 grams of protein per day (21 to 27 percent of total calories on his 3,450-calorie diet) and between 60 and 170 grams of carbohydrates (7 to 20 percent of total calories), depending on activity level and individual preference/tolerance to carbs.

Carbohydrate timing

In addition to matching your overall carbohydrate intake with your activity level and goals, eating your carbs at specific times may provide additional benefit. After a workout is an ideal time to eat more carbohydrates, and carbohydrate intake should be higher on workout days than on nonworkout days. This will help with recovery and preserving (or adding) muscle mass, if that's your goal.

Some recent studies suggest that eating the majority (around 60 to 80 percent) of your carbohydrates at dinner leads to hormonal changes that promote fat loss and improve metabolic function. However, this can be difficult to do if you're eating a large amount of carbohydrates. For example, if you're eating three hundred grams of carbohydrate a day, and you aim for eating 60 percent of those at dinner, you'll have to eat three large baked potatoes! In practice, if you aim for eating a larger percentage of your carbohydrates after workouts, on workout days, and in the later part of the day, you'll get most of the benefit of carbohydrate timing.

SUPERFOODS

You hear a lot these days about superfoods that people promise will boost vitality, improve mood, increase libido, burn fat, lengthen your life, and turn you into a millionaire. Okay, maybe their proponents don't make that last claim exactly, but just about. I'm talking about protein powders, green drinks, energy bars, sports goo, bee pollen, maca root, acai berries, and all kinds of other stuff you've probably never heard of or have heard of but know nothing about.

In some cases, I think the sellers of these products make legitimate claims. Maca root does have a history of medicinal use (primarily to increase libido and improve sperm quality) in South America, where it is native. However, it contains glucosinolates, which in combination with a diet low in iodine can cause thyroid problems. It suppresses the function of the thyroid gland by interfering with iodine uptake, possibly leading to the development of a swelling of the thyroid gland, called a goiter.

This single example highlights one of the problems I have with most so-called superfoods. In general, they are:

- Powerful botanicals (herbal medicine) that can cause potentially serious side effects and complications when used improperly;
- Highly processed and refined isolated nutrients that don't share the beneficial qualities of the whole foods they were extracted from (protein powder falls into this category, in my opinion); or
- Surrounded by misinformation and misconceptions. For example, vegetarians and vegans have been led to believe that spirulina and brewer's yeast contain vitamin B_{12}, a nutrient that vegetarians and vegans are often deficient in. But spirulina and brewer's yeast contain B_{12} analogs called cobamides, which actually block the uptake and absorption of B_{12}.

You might not be surprised, then, to learn that I'm not generally a fan of these superfoods. Some of them, like protein powder and spirulina, probably won't hurt when used in moderate amounts in the context of an overall nutrient-dense diet. This is especially true for bodybuilders who are trying to put on significant amounts of muscle and are having trouble getting enough protein in their diets. However, I am a big fan of nature's own superfoods, and I believe they should be incorporated into every diet.

Another way of thinking of them is as nature's multivitamins. These are the foods that are densely packed with micronutrients that fuel our cellular machinery and keep us healthy and strong. I've mentioned these foods and their benefits throughout this book, but here's an all-in-one listing.

- Organ meats (nutrient dense)
- Eggs (including the yolk and its essential micronutrients)
- Cold-water, oily fish (salmon, mackerel, sardines, herring)
- Traditional fats (ghee, butter, and duck fat)
- Pastured-animal, full-fat dairy products (preferably raw)
- Bone broths (rich in all-important glycine)
- Tougher cuts of meat, skin, and cartilage (for the same reasons as bone broth)
- Dark, leafy greens (kale, collards, spinach, arugula, mustard greens, and more)
- Fermented foods (vegetables, dairy, and beverages like kombucha)
- Seaweed (loaded with minerals and nutrients that are difficult to obtain elsewhere in the diet)

SUPPLEMENT WISELY

The best way to obtain nutrients is from food. That's how we've naturally evolved to get them. Most nutrients require enzymes, synergistic cofactors, and organic-mineral activators to be properly absorbed. While these are naturally present in foods, they are often not included in synthetic vitamins with isolated nutrients.

That said, no matter how well we eat, some nutrients are difficult to obtain in significant quantities from food alone. For example, magnesium is found in many foods, but as soil quality has declined over the past several decades, so have magnesium levels in fresh produce. And with the exception of cold-water, fatty fish, food has never been a primary source of vitamin D; our ancestors produced it from exposure to sunlight. In addition, modern eating habits affect the amount of valuable nutrients we consume. Vitamin A (retinol) is present in high amounts only in organ meats, which our Paleolithic ancestors and many traditional cultures considered superior to muscle meats (which they are, from a nutritional perspective). However, organ meats have fallen out of favor, and few people eat them today.

The chart below lists the nutrients that are not abundant even in a typical Paleo diet, one that doesn't include organ meats, fish-liver oils, seaweed, and grass-fed-animal dairy, along with my recommendations for how to obtain them. Please see the website for a bonus chapter on supplementation with more detailed information about these nutrients as well as quizzes to help you determine which of them you may need to supplement. I also include specific, up-to-date brand recommendations for the supplements listed below.

NUTRIENT	RECOMMENDATION
Vitamin A	10,000–15,000 IU per day Best obtained from 1/2–1 tsp per day of high-vitamin cod-liver oil
Vitamin D	It is difficult to make a blanket recommendation for vitamin D because the optimal dose depends on so many factors. That said, 1/2–1 tsp per day of high-vitamin cod-liver oil is often sufficient to meet vitamin D needs, and it's an excellent choice since it also contains vitamin A, which works synergistically with vitamin D.

NUTRIENT	RECOMMENDATION
Magnesium	Most Americans are deficient in magnesium, and most people benefit from supplementing it because it's difficult to obtain from food. I suggest a dose of 300–500 mg/day in either malate or glycinate form.
Vitamin K_2	Vitamin K_2 improves bone health and protects against cardiovascular disease, among other benefits. Many people don't get enough of this important vitamin. You can meet vitamin K_2 needs by eating foods that are rich in it, such as natto, eggs and cheese from grass-fed cows, and fermented foods. See chapter 9 for a complete list. If you don't eat these foods, if you have low bone density, or if you are at risk for or have cardiovascular disease, I suggest taking 100–1,000 mcg/day of vitamin K_2 in MK-7 or MK-4 form. Doses as high as 45 mg/d have been used for osteoporosis, and vitamin K_2 appears to be safe and well tolerated even at that amount.
Iodine	Iodine is another important nutrient that can be difficult to obtain even in the context of a healthy diet. I suggest getting iodine from seaweeds (kelp, kombu, wakame, hijiki, arame, dulse), fish (especially cod, shrimp, and tuna), and dairy products if you tolerate them. See the bonus chapter on thyroid disorders on the website for a chart of iodine-rich foods. If these foods aren't an option for you, you should supplement with iodine at a dose of 800 mcg per day. Kelp tablets are a good option.

(continued)

NUTRIENT	RECOMMENDATION
Selenium	Selenium plays an important role in thyroid and immune health. Most people get enough selenium from food, but people with thyroid or immune-related issues may benefit from supplementation. The recommended dose is 200 mcg per day. This can be obtained by taking a selenium supplement or by eating two or three Brazil nuts a day. See the bonus chapter on thyroid disorders on the website for a chart of selenium-rich foods.
Vitamin C	A nutrient-dense Paleo diet with a wide spectrum of fruits and vegetables should provide sufficient levels of vitamin C. However, vitamin C deficiency is common: 34 percent of men and 27 percent of women don't get enough. If you're dealing with a chronic health challenge, fighting an infection, or just need immune support, I suggest supplementing with 500 to 1,000 mg/day of vitamin C. The liposomal form is best.

Five nutrients to be cautious with

We've talked about the four micronutrients I generally recommend supplementing—via superfoods like cod-liver oil or in man-made preparations—as well as other micronutrients people with specific health conditions or goals may wish to increase their intake of. But there are some micronutrients that I don't recommend unless you have a specific reason to do so; these are iron, calcium, beta-carotene, and folic acid.

- **Iron:** Essential for life, but too much causes inflammation and oxidative damage; excess iron can cause everything from blood-sugar problems to depression to fatigue to hypogonadism and hormonal imbalance.

- **Calcium:** Popular as a preventive measure against osteoporosis, but the newest research shows that calcium supplements don't reduce fracture rates in older women and may even increase the risk of hip fractures. Studies on the relationship between cardiovascular disease and calcium suggest that dietary intake of calcium protects against heart disease, but supplementation may increase the risk.

- **Vitamin E (alpha-tocopherol):** Some authorities recommend supplementing vitamin E to protect against heart disease, but studies show no real benefit and some studies have demonstrated potential harm.

- **Beta-carotene:** Can be converted into retinol (the active form of vitamin A) but it can also be converted into potentially harmful substances that increase the risk of oxidative damage and interfere with active vitamin A metabolism.

- **Folic acid:** By this, I mean the synthetic compound used in dietary supplements and food fortification; folate refers to the forms of the vitamin found in food and in natural folate supplements such as 5-methyl-tetrahydrofolate (5-MTHF). Folic acid can be converted to folate, but this conversion is limited in humans. High levels of unmetabolized folic acid in the blood can mask B_{12} deficiency; speed the progression of certain cancers; and depress immune function. Natural folate supplements like 5-MTHF do not have these effects and should be used instead of folic acid for protecting against neural-tube defects during pregnancy and in other situations where additional folate is indicated. See the bonus chapter on supplementation on the website for more on this topic.

For more information on how and why to exercise caution with these micronutrients, please visit ChrisKresser.com/PPC.

CHAPTER 19

Life-Hacking Your Personal Paleo Cure

Here are some final strategies for integrating Your Personal Paleo Cure into your life. Think of these techniques as ways to hack your code and therefore make it sustainable for years to come. You'll also find some information and support on what to do when you're not having as much success as you'd like.

STAYING FLEXIBLE: THE 80/20 RULE

There's no doubt in my mind that optimal nutrition is the key to health. Yet, as you know from working through Step 2 (and as I've said all along), there's more to health — and to life — than food. As you also learned in Step 2, social connection is a fundamental human need. Extreme dietary restriction can lead to social isolation, which in turn can cause illness and disease. I'd like to tell you a story that illustrates this.

When I began my medical studies, I interned for a holistic physician who specialized in treating people with chronic illness. We had a patient — I'll call him Sam — who was only twenty-four years old but was very sick. He was thin as a rail, with dark circles under his eyes, severe fatigue, terrible digestion, depression, skin problems, a dysfunctional immune system, and several other problems.

Notes for this chapter may be found at ChrisKresser.com/ppcnotes/#ch19.

Both the doctor I was working with and Sam were convinced his problems were food related, so he was on a very restrictive diet. But he just kept getting worse. The worse he felt, the more foods he removed from his diet. At one point, Sam was eating only steamed broccoli, quinoa, and lamb. That's it—nothing else. He stopped coming in for treatment after a while, and we lost track of him for a time. But about six months later he returned for a visit. He looked like a different person. He had gained about thirty pounds, and his color was good, his digestion improved, his mood lifted, his skin clear. It was an incredible transformation.

The doctor and I were of course dying to know what had happened. We asked him, "Was it diet?" Sam said, "Yep." "Well, which diet?" we asked. "The candida diet? Macrobiotics?" We listed several other popular diets. (This was fifteen years ago and I didn't know about the Paleo diet yet!)

He shook his head at each one. Finally, we said, "Tell us what it was, then!"

And here's what he told us. "It was the beer-and-pizza diet."

Sam made sure he went out to eat beer and pizza with his friends twice a week, and the rest of the week he ate a fairly healthful diet of foods he liked.

Previously, during his period of increasing food restriction, he had become more and more socially isolated. He couldn't eat out with friends. His girlfriend broke up with him because he never wanted to leave the house, eat out, or travel for fear of being exposed to toxic foods. And the more socially isolated he was, the more depressed he became. At some point, he decided that life wasn't really worth living the way he was living it.

Therefore, he didn't have anything to lose by abandoning his rigid diet and focusing instead on having fun, connecting with his friends, and eating the foods that brought him pleasure. It took only a few months of that to completely change his life. His health improved, he had friends again, he started a new relationship, and he found a new job that suited him much better than his old one.

I hope you understand that I'm not suggesting everyone should go out and eat beer and pizza twice a week. That's not the point. The point of this story is that there's more to life than food and that social engagement and pleasure are very important to health. There's a saying in Chinese medicine — the oldest continuous medical tradition in the world — that reflects this point: "It's better to eat the wrong food with the right attitude than the right food with the wrong attitude."

This is why I advise most people to follow something I call the 80/20 rule. It suggests that 80 percent of the time you should closely follow the guidelines I've outlined in this book, and 20 percent of the time you're free to loosen up and just eat what you want to eat. That might mean having beer and pizza once a week for you (although gluten-free pizza and beer would probably be better choices). Or it might mean going out for ice cream with your kids on Saturday nights. Or maybe it means grabbing something quick that isn't 100 percent Paleo when you're close to missing your flight.

In reality, most of my patients feel so much better when they follow their Personal Paleo Cure that the 80/20 rule becomes something more like the 95/5 rule, or even the 90/10 rule. Often the foods they thought they'd miss the most when they first started (like beer and pizza!) are no longer that appealing, or maybe the pleasure of eating them isn't worth the price that's paid the following day. The point of the 80/20 rule isn't the exact ratio; that's for you to determine based on your particular health circumstances, preferences, and goals. Instead, the purpose of the 80/20 rule is to make your approach to nutrition more flexible and adaptable, so that it simply becomes the way you eat rather than a diet that you follow.

This is one reason I don't like to refer to Paleo as a diet or refer to eating non-Paleo foods as cheating. Conceptualizing Paleo as a diet that you cheat on almost inevitably leads to additional stress (from struggling to perfectly adhere to the diet) or a yo-yo relationship with food. For example, before they started working with me, some of my patients had a history of doing Thirty-Day Resets interspersed with periods of almost completely returning to poor eating habits. Instead of transitioning to a more flexible approach after the Thirty-Day Reset, they tried to adhere to guidelines that were unnecessarily strict for them, which wasn't sustainable.

There may be something fundamental about human psychology at work here. I've noticed — and perhaps you have too — that most people don't like to be told what to do. This is true even when they're the ones telling themselves what to do! If you say to yourself, *I can never eat ice cream again,* that can create a dynamic where you eat ice cream just to set yourself free of that sense of overbearing control. The choice is often not completely conscious and may have little to do with actually craving that food. But what if you say, *I can have ice cream occasionally if I feel like it, but I choose not to eat it every day because I don't feel good when I do?* That shifts the dynamic. It's no longer about autonomy and control; it's about what makes you feel healthy and vibrant.

Unfortunately, the 80/20 rule doesn't always apply to those dealing with serious health challenges or allergies or intolerances to specific foods. It's never a good idea for someone with gluten intolerance or celiac disease, for example, to just throw caution to the wind and eat half a loaf of wheat bread. That could trigger an immune reaction lasting up to several weeks. Those who are allergic to certain foods or nutrients will have to avoid them 100 percent of the time; however, they may employ the 80/20 rule for other foods that aren't part of their Personal Paleo Cure but won't cause serious harm. Those with serious, chronic illness may be better off following a 90/10 or a 95/5 rule while still avoiding the most serious potential offenders, like gluten, refined sugar, or whatever it is that triggers a negative reaction. After all, the point of the 80/20 rule isn't to hurt yourself; it's to make you feel good.

TIPS FOR EATING IN RESTAURANTS

One of the biggest challenges to adopting a Paleo-type diet, especially at the start, is what to do when you're eating in a restaurant or traveling and trying to find good food. Enjoying a meal away from home should be a pleasurable and low-stress experience. Here are some ideas for how to make sure that it is:

- If you're eating out with friends, take control (in a friendly, helpful way!) and suggest a restaurant that you've researched and that you know will be safe for you—and enjoyable for everyone else.
- If you don't have control of where you're eating, go online and check out the menu so you aren't surprised when you get there. Call ahead and see if they can accommodate special requests or if they have special gluten-free options that may not be listed on the menu.
- If you're in an unfamiliar city, ask the concierge at your hotel or friends, family, and colleagues familiar with that city for suggestions. If you use it, social media can be a big help. Whenever I'm in a city I don't know well, I'll write a quick Tweet asking for restaurant recommendations, and I always get great responses.
- Search Google using keywords like *local*, *foodie*, *gluten-free*, *grass-fed*, *organic*, and *pasture-raised* together with *restaurants*. Those searches usually turn up some good prospects, including places that often feature locally grown produce and meats and wild fish. At such establishments, the waitstaff is also more likely to know what's in the food and more willing (and accustomed) to accommodate special requests.
- Use online review sites like Yelp, Chowhound, TripAdvisor, and Urbanspoon to read legitimate reviews of restaurants from people like you.
- Don't show up starving to a restaurant. That's a really good way to put yourself in a situation where you are likely to make bad choices (the 80/20 rule notwithstanding). Eat a healthy snack before you leave for the restaurant, especially if you're going to a place that won't have much you can eat.
- Be a pain in the butt. When you go out to restaurants, don't be afraid to be that person that asks the waiter a million questions. Yes, he might think you're a pain and it might be a little embar-

rassing if you're out on a date. But think of it this way: you'll probably never see the waiter again, and if your date is really annoyed by
your food intolerances, then is that someone you want to spend a
lot of time with? If you're gluten-intolerant, always ask if there is
gluten in a dish you're ordering, even when it seems like there isn't.
Restaurants use hidden ingredients all the time. And if the waiter
seems like he doesn't know, insist that he ask the chef.

- Avoid sauces. Sauces are likely to contain sugar, gluten, soy, and
  other ingredients you're trying to avoid. That's why eating out at
  Thai and Chinese places can be a bit of a challenge. If you're
  doing that as part of your 80/20 allowance, that's fine. But otherwise, it's best to stick with grilled, steamed, or roasted meats,
  steamed or baked vegetables, and simple starches like potatoes or
  white rice. They're less likely to have sauces — and you can ask for
  them on the side.
- Ask for the dressing on the side. Salad dressings, like sauces, often
  have a lot of undesirable ingredients in them. In particular, they
  tend to contain industrial seed oils. If you order a salad, which is
  otherwise a safe choice, ask for some olive oil and balsamic vinegar instead of the dressing that comes with it.

The charts below list some considerations for the different foods and
types of cuisines you're likely to encounter when you eat out.

FOOD	FOLLOW YOUR PERSONAL PALEO CURE
Meat, fish, poultry	Try to avoid sauces, as they often contain industrial seed oils, gluten, soy, and/or sugar; grilled, steamed, and poached are usually the safest cooking methods.
White rice	If you tolerate white rice, many Asian restaurants can serve a simple dish with meat, vegetables, and white rice.

(continued)

FOOD	FOLLOW YOUR PERSONAL PALEO CURE
Vegetables	Be careful with sauces, which may contain undesirable ingredients.
Starchy plants	Baked potatoes are a good choice and are available at steakhouses and other restaurants that serve American cuisine.
Salad	A salad with fish, beef, or chicken is available in some form at most restaurants; if in doubt on the dressing, ask for oil and vinegar on the side.

TYPE OF CUISINE	FOLLOW YOUR PERSONAL PALEO CURE
Mexican	Order a tostada and don't eat the tortilla, or order a fish, chicken, or beef plate with rice, vegetables, salsa, and guacamole.
Chinese/Thai/Korean/Vietnamese	Meat/fish, rice, vegetables, or rice-noodle soups with meat, fish, and vegetables; be careful with sauces.
Japanese/sushi	Bring your own wheat-free tamari to the restaurant and avoid soy sauce.
Italian	Italian food is one of the most challenging types of cuisine due to its heavy focus on pasta and bread. Choose a fish or meat dish with a vegetable or salad, and be careful to avoid cross-contamination.
Indian	Somewhat difficult because of sauces, but tandoori meat with rice and a vegetable curry might work; ask about gluten in food/sauces.
Ethiopian	Like Indian cuisine, Ethiopian can be tough because of the sauces. Choose meat and vegetable dishes without gluten, and avoid the *injera* (flat bread), which often contains wheat flour.

TYPE OF CUISINE	FOLLOW YOUR PERSONAL PALEO CURE
American/Continental	Often the safest choice; order grilled meat, vegetables, potatoes, and/or salad.
Seafood	Like American places, seafood restaurants are a good choice. Order fish, vegetables or salad, and a potato.
Barbecue	Barbecue can be tough for the same reason Indian and Ethiopian foods are: the sauces often contain sugar, gluten, and other undesirable ingredients. Ask for your meat smoked or with a dry rub instead of sauce.

For even more detailed tips on how to eat out safely, I recommend Robb Wolf's *Paleo Dining Out Guide*, a brief e-book with fantastic tips on planning ahead, choosing foods wisely, determining what's safe to order, asking the right questions of service staff, and more. See ChrisKresser .com/diningout for more information.

SMART SNACKING

Most typical snack foods—including so-called healthy snacks, like energy or granola bars, not to mention all the "healthy whole-grain" foods that jam the grocery-store aisles—are loaded with ingredients that you've eliminated from your diet. Fortunately, you can avoid eating those foods if you follow some simple advice.

- **Plan ahead.** Most people slip up because they haven't planned ahead. They get in the car and head out on a trip (whether it's a few hours of local errands or a true road trip) only to realize three hours later that they're starving and they forgot to bring food. They're stuck in a shopping mall or on an interstate highway and the only choices are the dreaded food court or the gas station's mini-mart. Avoid this by referring to the chart below and stocking up on some safe travel foods, and take them with you whether you'll be gone for a few hours or a few weeks.

- **Make big batches of snacks.** Let's say you're going to soak and dehydrate some nuts to have them around. Instead of doing just a few servings, why not do two pounds? That way you'll have nuts on hand for a couple of weeks—and they're one of the quickest and easiest snack foods available.
- **Eat before you go.** If possible, eat a substantial meal before you leave the house for an extended period. If you're starving when you leave the house, and you bring only a small snack, it's likely that you'll end up eating something you regret while you're out.

The following is a list of foods that are great for snacking and travel. See my website for a printable version of this chart and for information on where to obtain some of these foods.

FOOD	FOLLOW YOUR PERSONAL PALEO CURE
Grass-fed-beef jerky	Buy soy/gluten/sugar-free varieties locally or online.
Prepared meats	Salami, pepperoni, coppa, and other prepared meats, preferably from pasture-raised animals.
Smoked salmon	Make sure it's soy-free.
Nuts and seeds	Soaked and dehydrated to improve digestibility and absorption.
Raw vegetables or fruit with nut better	Macadamia, almond, and hazelnut butter are best.
Cheese	If you tolerate dairy products.
Hard-boiled/deviled eggs	Eat with cherry tomatoes and avocados for a hearty snack.

FOOD	FOLLOW YOUR PERSONAL PALEO CURE
Kale chips	Remove ribs from kale, cut into 1.5-inch pieces, brush with olive oil and sea salt, and bake at 175 degrees F until crisp (or use a dehydrator if you have one).
Plantain/taro/sweet potato chips	Slice thinly and roast at 400 degrees F in duck fat or lard for 10 to 13 minutes for best results.
Fruit smoothie	Make with coconut milk, almond milk, kefir, or yogurt as a base, depending on preference or tolerance.
Olives	Eat with nuts, cheese, or prepared meats.
Baba ghanoush	Not recommended if you are following the autoimmune version of the Paleo diet (eggplant is a nightshade).
Thin-sliced leftover meat	Enjoy with Paleo mustard or mayonnaise. See my website for recipes.
Canned salmon or tuna	Eat with avocado or shredded lettuce.
Lettuce wraps	Make with leftover meats, fish, avocado, shredded veggies, or other fixings.
Full-fat yogurt or kefir	If you tolerate dairy (cow or goat); consume alone or with fruit and/or nuts.

EATING PALEO ON A BUDGET

Making the switch from a standard American diet to a nutrient-dense Personal Paleo approach to eating can initially be a shock at the grocery-store checkout line. This is especially true for people accustomed to buying cheap grain products like bread and pasta, canned beans, and conventionally raised animal products. That first big trip to the store to prepare for your Thirty-Day Reset might produce a terrifying bill compared to what you're used to spending—and it might even be enough to deter some from sticking with their new, healthier diet.

Fortunately, if you plan a little and find some smart shopping techniques, there's no reason why eating Paleo should cost significantly more than your old way of eating. Granted, there may always be a slightly higher cost associated with eating high-quality real foods (isn't your health worth it?), but there are several ways to keep your grocery bills from getting out of control. Here are seven tips for eating Paleo on a budget.

(1) Buy ingredients, not products

It's cheaper to buy raw ingredients and cook food yourself than to buy prepackaged meals, snacks, and other food items. A lot of people who are new to Paleo tend to be overwhelmed at the grocery store and look for Paleo-friendly products like Larabars, nut milks, kale chips, beef jerky, and other items that can easily be made at home but are tempting to buy when you're just starting out. Also, some end up buying one or more of the many premade meals sold online or at CrossFit gyms that have been designed to be compliant with the Paleo diet but that often cost an arm and a leg.

The more food you cook from scratch, the more money you'll save. You'll find some fantastic recipes for meals and snacks in chapter 21, plus there are countless recipes online (at ChrisKresser.com and on other websites). Another major advantage to preparing your own food is that you know what all of the ingredients are, and you avoid mystery additives, preservatives, and artificial sweeteners.

(2) Buy in bulk and share

Buying in bulk (online or at your local store) can significantly reduce your food expenses, particularly for pantry goods like coconut oil, olive oil, ghee, canned tomatoes, and so on. To save money on grass-fed meat, try a cow share, where you and a group of health-minded friends purchase a whole cow. The more people involved, the lower the cost and the less need for extra freezer space. Joining a community-supported agriculture (CSA) farm allows you access to local produce for less than what you'd pay at most stores. (See page 149 for more information on CSAs.) Having Paleo potlucks with friends rather than going out to eat is a great way to save money on social dining occasions while still eating well. The more food you share with neighbors, friends, and extended family, the more money you'll save.

(3) Get down to basics

Buy ingredients that are versatile and can be used for a wide variety of dishes. Instead of buying expensive spices that you might use once, get the basics, like all-season salt, fresh garlic, onion powder, Italian/Mexican/Indian (fill in the ethnic food of your choice!) seasoning, curry paste, and anything else that can be used for a multitude of dishes. Choose a couple of go-to fats like olive oil, coconut oil, and butter and use them for all your dishes. Don't be afraid of frozen vegetables, as they're just as nutritious as fresh, can be used in many different dishes, and have a much longer shelf life than fresh veggies. For those who tolerate starches, white potatoes and sweet potatoes are cheap and filling and can be used at any meal. Avoid buying specialty items like gluten-free flours or other ingredients that sit in your pantry uneaten for months because you don't know what to use them for.

(4) Cook in bulk

Making large batches of meals (you can double many of the recipes you'll find in chapter 21) yields tasty leftovers that save both time and money. As those living on their own know, it gets expensive trying to buy single-serve food items, and food waste can be a huge problem when buying in bulk. That's why cooking large meals and saving the leftovers can be especially helpful for those cooking for just themselves or perhaps one other person. Try making multiple servings of an all-in-one meal like a soup or stew and freezing them for later in the week. Not only will you save cooking time but you'll also be able to use ingredients bought in bulk and not have to worry about spoilage if you can't eat all the meat or vegetables you've purchased.

(5) Choose your battles

Not everything you buy has to be organic, grass-fed, free-range, and local. There are many food items that are fine to buy from a conventional grocery store on a regular basis. While you always want to buy organic celery and strawberries, it might not be so important to look for organic onions or mangoes. See the Environmental Working Group's Dirty Dozen Plus and Clean Fifteen lists (see pages 142–143) for what to focus on. The same goes for animal products. While you would likely want to avoid conventionally raised chicken, pork, and animal-organ meats, you may be all right buying lamb, eggs, and some natural cheeses that aren't from 100 percent grass-fed and organic sources. Canned fish like salmon, skipjack tuna, sardines, and herring are far less expensive than fresh, wild fish and are extremely nutrient-dense choices. Of course, you should always get the highest-quality animal foods you can afford, but not everyone has access to ideal sources of meat. It's better to eat nonorganic eggs than organic cereal for breakfast, and it's better to have a dinner of conventionally raised beef and nonorganic asparagus than a plate of organic pasta. If you're unable to buy the best-quality meats and produce, it's a good idea to do your homework and figure out which items are worth the splurge and which might be all right to spend less money on.

(6) Cut out the extras

Write a list of those luxury items you buy—four-dollar coffees, bottled water, fancy ingredients you use once for an extravagant recipe, protein powders, and so forth—and cut them out. Yes, high-quality pastured-chicken eggs do cost two to three dollars more per dozen than conventional eggs, but simply forgoing your Starbucks Venti Mocha each day will easily make up the difference. Go through your food spending and see if you can identify what splurges are putting you in the red. Get rid of the nonessentials altogether or find a way to make them at home. Buy a good-quality reusable mug or water bottle and fill it up before you leave the house in the morning. Eat real food rather than expensive protein powders and supplements. Don't waste money on items that you can easily do without.

(7) Skip the filet mignon

A great way to save money on animal foods is by choosing cheaper cuts of meat, like brisket, chuck roast, and so on, and offal (such as liver and heart). These not only contain important nutrients that balance out those found in lean meats like steak and chicken breast (as we discussed in chapter 9) but also are some of the most tender and delicious cuts when wet/slow cooking methods are used. Many who can't afford other pastured-raised meat can afford these pastured-animal cuts. And it's especially important to buy organ meats that come from organic, grass-fed animals. These unpopular cuts are often just a few dollars a pound, and they deliver enormous nutritional benefits that will make a significant difference in your overall health.

HELP! THIS ISN'T WORKING!

If you're still having difficulty, don't worry. I know how frustrating that can be, but the truth is that making huge dietary and lifestyle changes can be hard, and sometimes it doesn't go so smoothly. This doesn't mean that the Personal Paleo Cure isn't a good choice for you; it just means you may need a little extra support.

To that end, I've created a Paleo troubleshooting guide, which you can download at ChrisKresser.com/PPC. It will help you break through the most common challenges that keep people from succeeding with Paleo, such as low energy and sugar cravings, digestive distress, and poor detox capacity.

GETTING THE SUPPORT YOU NEED TO SUCCEED

Having a strong network of social support is essential for long-term success when it comes to making big dietary and lifestyle changes. Developing a Personal Paleo Cure can be a challenge even when you do have family and friends behind you, but it's much harder if you're going it alone. Here are some ideas for how to build that support network.

Bringing the family onboard

If you live with family members, eating Paleo can be really tough if they're not eating that way—especially if you're not the one preparing the meals! Bringing your family on board is one of the best ways to ease your transition. But how do you do that? After all, not everyone in your family may be as enthusiastic about going Paleo as you are. Here are some tips:

- **Offer to take charge.** Change is hard. Sometimes the resistance to switching to Paleo is mostly about fear of the extra work involved in figuring out new recipes, new ingredients to buy at the store, and new ways of putting meals and snacks together. Even if you haven't historically been the primary meal planner and preparer, consider assuming this role—at least during the transition. Use the recipes and meal plans in chapter 21 and on my website to help you along.

- **Take it easy.** When you're living alone, it might be easy to radically change your diet on a dime. But when you're living with several family members, it's often more complicated. And sometimes, the more pressure you put on others to change, the more they'll resist. Consider starting with one Paleo meal a day (dinner is usually best). Once you've got that under your belt, you can move to lunch, then breakfast, then snacks. Before long, you'll be where you want to be, and you won't have alienated your family in the process.

- **Start with the biggies.** As an alternative to the one-meal-at-a-time approach, you might consider choosing one particular change at a time. For example, you could decide to eliminate sugar first, then gluten, then industrial seed oils (eliminating packaged/processed foods and eating out less), and then grains until you end up on a Personal Paleo Cure approach.

- **Find Paleo substitutes for your family's favorite meals.** Your family doesn't have to swear off pizza, pancakes, and other favorite foods forever; simply substitute them with delicious Paleo versions! See the recipes in this book and on my website.

If you have young kids, different strategies may apply. This is especially true if your child has a health problem you are trying to address with a Paleo approach. Here are some additional things to consider with young children:

- Depriving children of their favorite junk foods isn't child abuse—though they may certainly do their best to make you feel that way. I often hear parents say things like, "My kids would never give up their Kraft Mac and Cheese." Trust me—they won't starve if you stop feeding them this stuff. You may have some epic battles initially, but if you stand your ground, eventually they'll get hungry enough to eat what you've put in front of them. This may sound harsh, but when your child's health is at stake, it's actually the most loving action you can take.

- Kids don't need kid food; they need good food. Big Food has been wildly successful in convincing us that babies and kids need special foods (usually packaged, processed, and refined) that are different than what their parents eat. The reality is that kids need real, unprocessed food even more than adults do, because they're still growing and developing. The sooner you let go of the idea of kids' food, the better off you'll be. You won't have to prepare separate snacks and meals for your kids, and they'll naturally begin to eat the right foods—because they're what is available.

- Young kids don't have the same prejudices against foods as many adults do. For example, adults may think of cod-liver oil as gross, but a young toddler has no such preconception. When our daughter Sylvie was a toddler, she actually *asked for* unflavored fermented cod-liver oil after meals. And we couldn't keep her away from the raw sauerkraut!

I realize it can seem especially hard to make the transition with young kids. But know that thousands of parents have gone before you, and it's absolutely possible with a little perseverance and planning. And don't try to do it alone! Join the forum at ChrisKresser.com/PPC to get some support from parents who are on the other side.

Enlisting the support of your friends

Regardless of whether you live alone or with family, enlisting the support of your friends is another way to ease the transition to Paleo and increase your chances for success. Here are some tips for doing that:

- **Find a Paleo pal.** See if any of your friends are interested in doing the Thirty-Day Reset with you. That way, you'll have someone to share your challenges and successes with. And once your friend experiences the results, he or she is a lot more likely to stick with Paleo over the long term, which means you'll have at least one friend who's on your path.

- **Lead by example.** The best way to get your friends interested in Paleo is to "speak softly but carry a big stick." Proselytizing and being pushy usually just create resistance and may end up jeopardizing your friendship. But if they watch you drop thirty pounds in two months, see your skin clear up, and observe your energy level and mood improve dramatically, they'll start asking questions.

- **Educate them — gently.** If you sense that your friend is interested, rather than telling him all about Paleo yourself, consider giving him a book (like this one) as a gift. Sometimes the information is better received when it comes from a third party.

- **Find some new friends.** If the people you hang out with aren't really interested in improving their health, it's probably time for you to find some new friends that are. One of the best ways to do that is to join a gym, participate in group exercise or sports, or join a Paleo meet-up group in your local area. There are hundreds of these groups now around the world. See Paleo-Diet.meetup.com for a listing, or simply Google *Paleo Meet-up* and the name of your city.

Online Support

In addition to family and friends, tap into online support resources such as these:

ChrisKresser.com/PPC

Visit ChrisKresser.com/PPC to register for free bonus chapters, program-enhancing tools, resources, guides, and ongoing education and support to help you meet your health and wellness goals. There's also a forum where you can interact with people from around the world who are following the Personal Paleo Cure approach.

ChrisKresser.com

Check out my website and blog for regular articles on nutrition and health, recipes, book reviews, a lively discussion forum, recommended programs and products, and an online store with hand-picked supplements that I use every day in my clinical practice.

Revolution Health Radio

Don't miss my podcast, available on my website and iTunes, where I discuss my latest research, provide practical advice on how to use nutrition to prevent and reverse disease, interview expert guests on a wide range of health-related topics, and answer listener questions.

Other Paleo websites and forums

There are several fantastic websites and forums that cover various aspects of the Paleo approach. I've listed some of my favorites on my website.

Finding a Paleo-friendly health-care provider

Finding a health-care provider who understands and endorses the Paleo approach is another important step in making the transition successfully. Fortunately, that has become much easier now with two online directories of Paleo-oriented clinicians (physicians, naturopaths, chiropractors, acupuncturists, and so forth):

- The Paleo Physician's Network (PaleoPhysiciansNetwork.com)
- Primal Docs (PrimalDocs.com)

Both of these networks have practitioners listed in every state in the

United States and in many countries worldwide, and both are growing quickly, with new practitioners added on a weekly basis.

In addition to seeking out a Paleo-oriented clinician, I'd also suggest finding one that practices functional medicine. Functional medicine is neither conventional nor alternative medicine. It's a combination of the best elements of both, and it represents the future of medicine. For more information on the differences between functional and conventional medicine, see my website, where you'll also find a list of questions that you can ask your health-care provider to determine if he or she is Paleo-friendly.

CHAPTER 20

Personalize Your Paleo Code for Specific Health Conditions

Here are some basic nutritional and lifestyle strategies for ten of the most common health conditions people face today. At **ChrisKresser.com/ PPC,** you'll find a free bonus chapter for each health condition discussed below, with more background information and detailed recommendations for supplements (including dosage and brand recommendations) that may be beneficial. You'll also find an interactive quiz that will help you identify which of these bonus chapters you may benefit from reading, based on your particular symptoms.

WEIGHT LOSS

Diet

Start with the low-carbohydrate version of the Thirty-Day Reset that I recommended during Step 1. You can find specific instructions starting on page 42. If you've already tried this, follow the suggestions below:

- **Eat more protein.** Aim for as much as 35 percent of calories from protein until you reach your target weight.
- **Don't snack.** Snacking can lead to overeating and may cause hormonal shifts that aren't supportive of weight loss.
- **Go dairy-free.** Many of my patients find it easier to lose weight when they aren't eating dairy (with the exception of small amounts of butter and ghee).

- **Reduce calorie density** by adding extra vegetables (both non-starchy and starchy) to your meal.
- **Eat all of your food within an eight-hour period each day.** This is called intermittent fasting. See pages 312–313 to learn how to do it.

Lifestyle

Several lifestyle factors contribute to weight gain, including:

- Sitting too much and not moving enough
- Not getting enough sleep or poor sleep quality
- Too much exposure to artificial light at night
- Chronic stress and adrenal fatigue
- Poor gut health

Be sure to read chapters 10, 12, 13, and 14 in the book and the bonus chapters on adrenal fatigue and digestive conditions on the website for more information on these topics.

HIGH CHOLESTEROL AND HEART DISEASE

Diet

The basic Personal Paleo Cure diet I've suggested in this book is inherently a heart-healthy diet. That said, you can make your diet even more heart-healthy by getting enough of the following seven foods and macronutrients:

- **Cold-water, fatty fish and shellfish.** Aim for one pound (sixteen ounces) of fatty fish and/or oysters and mussels a week.
- **Monounsaturated fat.** Try adding a handful of macadamia nuts, a quarter or half an avocado, or a tablespoon of olive oil to your diet daily.
- **Antioxidant-rich foods.** "Eat the rainbow" by choosing a variety of colors of fruits and vegetables, and don't forget that animal products like organ meats, meats, eggs, and grass-fed-animal dairy are also rich in antioxidants.

- **Polyphenol-rich foods.** These include green tea, blueberries, extra-virgin olive oil, red wine, citrus fruits, hibiscus tea, dark chocolate, and turmeric and other herbs and spices.
- **Nuts.** Aim for a handful of tree nuts such as almonds, Brazil nuts, cashews, chestnuts, and filberts/hazelnuts each day. Be careful not to overeat nuts.
- **Fermented foods.** Add one to two tablespoons of raw sauerkraut or kimchi to each meal, and have half a cup of beet kvass or kombucha and half a cup of yogurt or kefir daily.
- **Soluble fiber.** Eat a wide range of fruits and vegetables every day, especially starchy tubers like sweet potatoes and yams, which are particularly high in soluble fiber.

Lifestyle

- **Meditation.** Chronic stress significantly increases the risk of heart disease, and stress-management practices such as meditation have been shown to reduce deaths from heart disease. See chapter 14 and the website for recommendations.
- **Sleep.** Chronic insomnia doubles the risk of heart attack and stroke. See chapter 13 for recommendations on improving sleep.
- **Physical activity.** Physical activity improves metabolic and cardiovascular function in several ways and extends life span. Remember, your goal should be not only to exercise more, but to sit less. See chapter 12 for recommendations.

HIGH BLOOD PRESSURE

Diet

- Strictly avoid refined sugar.
- Increase potassium intake. See the bonus chapter on high blood pressure for a chart of potassium-rich foods.

- Eat one pound (sixteen ounces) of cold-water, fatty fish and/or shellfish, like oysters and mussels, per week.
- Increase magnesium intake. Nuts, seeds, spinach, beet greens, and chocolate are the food sources highest in magnesium on a Personal Paleo Cure diet.
- Eat one silver-dollar-size serving of dark chocolate (greater than 80 percent cacao content) a day.
- Drink two to three cups of hibiscus tea each day.
- Add wakame (seaweed) to soups and stews, or rehydrate it and eat it on its own. Use caution if you're sensitive to sodium.

See the bonus chapter on blood pressure on the website for important information about salt. You might be surprised by what you learn!

Lifestyle

- **Weight loss.** Excess body fat can increase blood pressure, and reducing it can lower blood pressure. See above as well as the bonus chapter on weight loss on my website for specific recommendations.
- **Physical activity.** Endurance exercise, strength training, high-intensity interval training, and simple moving around more during the day (outside of a distinct exercise period) have all been shown to significantly reduce blood pressure. For specific recommendations on physical activity, see chapter 12.
- **Sleep.** Short sleep duration, poor sleep quality, and sleep apnea increase the risk that you'll develop high blood pressure. See chapter 13 for tips on improving your sleep.
- **Ultraviolet light (via sunshine or tanning beds).** Ultraviolet light increases the body's production of nitric oxide, which helps blood vessels to relax and lowers blood pressure. See chapter 16 for specific recommendations for ultraviolet-light exposure.

See the bonus chapter on the website for several other important lifestyle modifications for lowering blood pressure.

GERD, IBS, IBD, AND OTHER DIGESTIVE PROBLEMS

Diet

- Follow a low-FODMAP (fermentable oligosaccharides, disaccharides, monosaccharides, and polyols) diet. See the bonus chapter on digestive conditions on my website for a detailed description and printable cheat sheets.
- Reduce your consumption of nonstarchy vegetables high in insoluble fiber and prepare the ones you do eat with methods designed to make them more digestible (including fermentation). See page 174 for details.
- Consume one-half to two cups of bone broth per day, in soups, stocks, stews, or sauces. You can also drink it like tea.
- Eat plenty of fermentable fiber in the form of fruits and starchy vegetables such as potato, sweet potato, plantain, yuca, and taro. (If you have GERD, heartburn, or inflammatory bowel disease, you may need to limit these foods for a time.)
- Consume fermented foods like sauerkraut, kimchi, curtido (Salvadoran sauerkraut), beet kvass, kefir (dairy or water), and yogurt. Though milk (in kefir and yogurt) and cabbage (in sauerkraut and kimchi) are both high in FODMAPs, fermentation breaks them down and makes these foods tolerable for most people with digestive issues.
- Limit alcohol consumption to four to six drinks per week, or avoid it altogether if you have significant gut issues.

Lifestyle

- **Manage stress.** In plain language, stress wreaks havoc on the gut. See chapter 14 for recommendations on stress management.
- **Gut-directed hypnotherapy.** Gut-directed hypnotherapy is a form of self-hypnosis specifically designed to alleviate the symptoms of

IBS and other functional gut disorders. It is one of the single most effective treatments for IBS. See my website for a specific recommendation for a home-based, audio instruction program.

- **Sleep.** Disturbed sleep interferes with gut functions in several ways, and many IBS patients notice an increase in their symptoms when they don't sleep well. See chapter 13 for recommendations on improving sleep.

DIABETES AND OTHER BLOOD-SUGAR DISORDERS

Diet

- **Adjust carbohydrate intake.** Using a device called a glucometer to measure your blood sugar after meals, you can determine exactly how much carbohydrate is safe for you to eat. See the bonus chapter on blood-sugar disorders as well as the cheat sheet on blood-sugar testing on my website for detailed instructions.
- **Eat more protein.** Higher-protein diets seem to have a stabilizing effect on blood sugar, regardless of whether you have a tendency toward high or low blood sugar. Aim for between 25 and 30 percent of total calories from protein (160 to 195 grams per day on a 2,600-calorie diet, or 125 to 150 grams per day on a 2,000-calorie diet).
- **Eat fermented foods and fermentable fibers.** There's a strong connection between gut health and metabolic health. See chapter 10 and the bonus chapter on digestive conditions on my website for more info.
- **If your blood sugar is too high:** Avoid snacking and consider intermittent fasting (see pages 312–314 to learn how to do it).
- **If your blood sugar is too low:** Don't go more than two or three hours without eating; eat a high-protein breakfast (at least forty grams of protein) within thirty minutes of waking up; and eat a snack before bed. See the section below and the bonus chapter on

my website on adrenal fatigue syndrome for more detailed recommendations.

Lifestyle

- **Physical activity.** Getting adequate exercise and sitting less is crucial for regulating blood sugar. See chapter 12 for recommendations.
- **Sleep.** Sleep deprivation impairs metabolic function and blood-sugar control by several mechanisms. See page 238 for a recap of sleep recommendations.
- **Stress management.** Stress reduces blood-sugar control, promotes inflammation (a primary cause of blood sugar–related problems), and leads to low levels of cortisol (which can further disrupt blood-sugar control). See pages 254–255 for a recap of stress-management recommendations.

ANXIETY, DEPRESSION, AND COGNITIVE DISORDERS

Diet

- **Low-FODMAP diet.** See the bonus chapter on digestive conditions on my website for more info.
- **Glycine-rich foods.** Balance your intake of lean proteins (such as lean red meat, boneless, skinless chicken breasts, and so on) with more gelatinous cuts of meat (such as oxtail, shanks, brisket, and chuck roast), bone broth, and egg yolks.
- **Fermented foods.** See chapter 10 for more information, and visit my website for instructions on how to make fermented foods at home.
- **The GAPS (gut and psychology syndrome) diet.** The GAPS diet is a therapeutic approach to treating psychological and behavioral conditions by improving gut health. See my website for

an outline of the various stages of the diet, along with recommendations for books, websites, and how to find a GAPS-certified practitioner to work with.

Lifestyle

- **Sleep.** There are few things more important to maintaining brain function than sleep. See page 238 for a recap of sleep recommendations.
- **Stress management.** A regular stress-management program is a must for those suffering from brain disorders. See pages 254–255 for a recap of stress-management recommendations.
- **Physical activity.** Movement and exercise promote healthy brain function in several important ways. See page 224 for a recap of recommendations to increase your physical activity.
- **Nature.** Natural environments have restorative effects, reduce stress, and improve your outlook on life. See page 288 for a recap of recommendations for reconnecting with nature.
- **Light therapy.** Bright-light therapy involves sitting in front of or near a device that emits artificial light that mimics natural outdoor light. It is particularly effective for seasonal affective disorder but has also shown positive results for non-seasonal depression, postpartum depression, and bipolar disorder. See the bonus chapter and resources on my website for dosage and device recommendations.

THYROID DISORDERS

Diet

There are four primary dietary concerns for people with thyroid problems:

- Limiting intake of goitrogens, foods and chemicals that increase the need for iodine in small amounts and can damage the thyroid gland in large amounts.

- Ensuring adequate intake of iodine and selenium, which are crucial nutrients for thyroid function.
- Being aware of foods that have the potential to trigger an immune response (if you have one of the autoimmune forms of thyroid disease).
- Avoiding very low-carb and low-protein diets, which may decrease thyroid function by inhibiting the conversion of the less active form of thyroid hormone (T4) into the more active form (T3).

Please see the bonus chapter on thyroid disorders at the website for a detailed explanation of each of these topics, including a list of goitrogenic chemicals and foods, and foods highest in iodine and selenium.

Lifestyle

- **Stress management.** Chronic stress impairs thyroid function in numerous ways. See pages 254–255 for a recap of stress-management recommendations.
- **Gut health.** There's a strong — though not well known — connection between gut health and thyroid function. See chapter 10 and the bonus chapter on digestive conditions on my website for detailed information about healing your gut.
- **Ultraviolet light.** Ultraviolet light (via sun or UVA/UVB tanning beds) may help put the brakes on an overactive immune system. See chapter 16 for specific recommendations.

AUTOIMMUNE DISEASE

Diet

There are three approaches to addressing autoimmunity through diet:

- Remove foods that may trigger or exacerbate an immune response.

- Increase your intake of nutrients that promote optimal immune function.
- Increase your intake of foods that support a healthy gut microbiota.

Please see the bonus chapter on autoimmune disease on the website for a detailed discussion of each of these approaches.

Lifestyle

- **Physical activity.** Regular physical activity and exercise improve immune function via several different mechanisms. See chapter 12 for tips on how to increase your physical activity and sit less.
- **Acupuncture.** Acupuncture helps to bring the immune system back into balance. I recommend getting acupuncture two to three times a week for the first month and at least once a week thereafter. Please see my website for information about how to find a clinic near you.
- **Pleasure and connection.** Pleasure and connection release chemicals called endorphins that help to regulate the immune system. See chapter 15 for specific recommendations.
- **Ultraviolet light.** Exposure to sunlight (or UVA/UVB light in tanning beds) appears to be especially important for those with autoimmune disease. See chapter 16 for specific recommendations.

ADRENAL FATIGUE SYNDROME

You won't find adrenal fatigue syndrome (AFS) listed in medical textbooks, and if you ask your doctor about it, she'll probably just shrug or tell you to stop researching health conditions on the Internet. Yet there's no doubt in my mind that this is a legitimate, common, and potentially very serious condition. I see it every day in my work with patients, and I've experienced it myself. Please see the bonus chapter on adrenal fatigue syndrome at the website for more information on this condition.

Diet

- **Eat a moderate-carbohydrate diet.** I suggest between 15 and 30 percent of calories from carbohydrates. Start with 20 percent as a target, and experiment with slightly higher and lower to see what works best for you.
- **Eat adequate protein, especially in the morning.** Eat at least 15 percent of calories from protein, and start the day with a high-protein breakfast (greater than forty grams of protein).
- **Eat frequently throughout the day.** Try not to go more than two or three hours without eating. You can eat either five or six small meals spaced throughout the day or three regular meals with snacks in between. Snacks and meals should always have at least some protein and fat (never have carbohydrates alone).
- **Avoid excess dietary potassium.** Excess potassium can lower blood pressure, and many people with AFS already have low blood pressure to begin with. See the bonus chapter on blood pressure on my website for a list of high-potassium foods.
- **Ensure adequate sodium intake.** Sodium increases aldosterone, which is often low in AFS. If your adrenal fatigue is pronounced or if you have low blood pressure or strong salt cravings, I suggest starting each day with a full glass of water with one-half to one teaspoon of sea salt and using salt liberally on food, to taste. Monitor your blood pressure on occasion to make sure it remains in a healthy range.
- **Avoid caffeine and alcohol.** Both caffeine and alcohol place additional stress on the body. It's best to avoid caffeine entirely, and limit alcohol consumption to two or three drinks per week (or eliminate it entirely) until your adrenals recover.

Lifestyle

- **Get plenty of sleep and rest.** This is by far the most important recommendation for adrenal fatigue. See page 238 for a recap of recommendations for sleep.
- **Manage your stress.** Along with poor sleep, psychological and emotional stress are primary contributors to AFS, and managing stress is a crucial part of the recovery process. In fact, I have never seen someone fully recover from AFS without paying significant attention to stress management. See pages 254–255 for specific recommendations on stress management.
- **Moderate your physical activity.** Not enough physical activity can contribute to AFS, but overtraining is actually a more common cause. I see this particularly in my patients that are high-level athletes or CrossFit enthusiasts. See the section "Are You Overtraining?" in chapter 12 for more on this topic, including a list of signs and symptoms of overtraining.
- **Go outside.** Spending regular time outdoors in a natural environment is especially important for those with adrenal fatigue syndrome. See chapter 16 for specific recommendations.
- **Cultivate pleasure, have fun, and connect with others.** Pleasure, play, and social connection are all deeply nourishing and restorative on both a physical and an emotional level and can provide a powerful antidote to the symptoms of adrenal fatigue syndrome. See chapters 15 and 17 for specific recommendations.

SKIN DISORDERS

The skin is influenced by other organs in the body, and this is especially true of the brain and the gut; scientists coined the term *gut-brain-skin axis* to describe the interconnection of these three systems. See the bonus chapter on skin disorders at the website for important background information on the gut-brain-skin axis and for more detail on how to intervene when it is not functioning optimally.

Diet

I use one of two diets with my patients with skin conditions, depending on their particular presentations of signs and symptoms:

- Low-histamine diet
- Low-FODMAP diet

See the bonus chapter on skin conditions on my website to determine which is right for you and for more information on each of the diets. I also list several nutrients that are important for healthy skin. Fortunately, if you're following a Personal Paleo Cure approach, you'll naturally obtain adequate amounts of these nutrients.

Lifestyle

- **Stress management.** Stress is associated with numerous skin conditions, including psoriasis, dermatitis, alopecia, urticaria, vitiligo, acne, and exacerbations of the herpes simplex virus. See chapter 14 for specific recommendations and read the section on adrenal fatigue syndrome above for additional tips.
- **Physical activity.** If you have a skin problem along with symptoms of adrenal fatigue syndrome, I suggest doing more gentle forms of exercise, like walking, cycling, and yoga, along with strength training two to three times a week. Avoid strenuous workouts until your adrenals recover.
- **Sleep.** Chronic sleep deprivation promotes inflammation and disrupts hormones, both of which can trigger or exacerbate skin conditions. See chapter 13 for recommendations on improving sleep.
- **Ultraviolet light.** Ultraviolet light from sunlight or UVA/UVB tanning beds has been shown to improve certain skin conditions, such as psoriasis, vitiligo, acne, eczema, dermatitis, and lichen planus.

CHAPTER 21

Seven-Day Meal Plan and Recipes

I've provided a lot of guidance throughout the book about what to eat, what not to eat, and how to determine your own Personal Paleo Cure.

But all of this information really comes alive in the meal plan and recipes below, where you'll discover just how easy it is to eat delicious, satisfying, and healthy meals with this approach.

To get you started, I've provided a one-week meal plan with recipes. At **ChrisKresser.com/PPC,** you'll find an additional **three weeks** of meal plans and recipes. Finally, I've provided shopping lists for each week that you can print out and take to the store with you.

Although I list new recipes for each meal, I realize that it won't be possible for the vast majority of you to cook from scratch at every single meal. This is where leftovers and planning in advance come in. If you work outside the home, consider doubling the recipes the night before so you'll have enough to bring with you for lunch the next day. Another helpful strategy is setting aside a few hours on the weekend to prepare snacks, soup stocks, and/or larger meals that you can eat throughout the week. With a little bit of advance preparation, it's entirely possible to eat this way *without* spending hours in the kitchen each day!

Bon appétit!

SEVEN-DAY MEAL PLAN

Day 1

Breakfast:	Baked Eggs en Cocotte Florentine-Style
Lunch:	Butternut Squash Frittata with Salad
Snack:	Nori Chips
Dinner:	Beef Rendang
Side dish:	Roasted Carrots and Garlic

Day 2

Breakfast:	Poached Eggs with Swiss Chard
Lunch:	Hamburgers with Mushrooms Provençale-Style
Snack:	Nori Chips
Dinner:	Grilled Ahi Tuna Steaks with Chinese Five-Spice Powder
Side dish:	Cabbage, Bok Choy, and Shiitake Mushrooms

Day 3

Breakfast:	Green Smoothie
Lunch:	Cod with Coriander Red Pepper Sauce and Sautéed Broccoli
Snack:	Hard-Boiled Eggs with Avocado
Dinner:	Tom Kha Gai
Side dish:	Thai Basil Eggplant

Day 4

Breakfast:	Green Plantain Fritters with Sausage
Lunch:	Tuna, Ginger, and Avocado Salad
Snack:	Hard-Boiled Eggs with Avocado
Dinner:	Spanish Pork Loin Roast Adobado
Side dish:	Cauliflower Hash

Day 5

Breakfast:	Smoked Salmon with Scrambled Eggs and Asparagus
Lunch:	Greek Turkey Burgers with Zucchini Noodles
Snack:	Kale Chips
Dinner:	Chicken Tikka Masala
Side dish:	Green Salad with Shallot Vinaigrette

Day 6

Breakfast:	Taro and Bacon Hash
Lunch:	Chicken, Tarragon, and Grapefruit Salad
Snack:	Kale Chips
Dinner:	Rosemary Lamb Rib Chops
Side dish:	Yuca Fries

Day 7

Breakfast:	Cauliflower-Stuffed Acorn Squash
Lunch:	Salmon Fillets with Raspberry Vinaigrette Salad
Snack:	Guacamole with Carrot Chips
Dinner:	Rustic Meatball and Tomato Stew
Side dish:	Kale and Kabocha Squash Salad

Recipe notes:

- You'll see *traditional fat of choice* listed as an ingredient in several recipes. This means you're free to use any of the saturated or monounsaturated fats listed in chapter 5. If you're cooking at medium heat or above, I suggest choosing fats with a smoke point above 350°F. These include ghee, extra-light (not extra-virgin) olive oil, palm oil, expeller-pressed (not extra-virgin) coconut oil, macadamia oil, beef tallow, duck fat, and lard.

- If you're following the autoimmune or low-carb/high-blood-sugar version of the Thirty-Day Reset, please see ChrisKresser.com/PPC for specific meal plans for those approaches.
- You'll see nuts used in some of the recipes as a garnish or optional ingredient. In chapter 3 I explained that it's best to soak and then either roast or dehydrate nuts before eating them in order to make them more digestible and to improve the bioavailability of the nutrients they contain. However, when used in small quantities as part of a recipe, it's fine to simply use raw or roasted, unsoaked nuts to save time.
- I have purposely not included nutritional info for the recipes. As I mentioned in chapter 1, the Thirty-Day Reset is not about counting calories or macronutrients—it's about resetting your body with the nutrient-dense, whole foods humans have evolved to eat. That said, if you're following a low-carb version of the Thirty-Day Reset or you'd simply like to know how much protein, fat, or carbohydrate each recipe contains, you can enter the ingredients at NutritionData.com to find out.

BREAKFAST RECIPES

Baked Eggs en Cocotte Florentine-Style

For this recipe you'll need two 8-ounce ramekins, each of which fits two eggs plus some spinach.

Serves: 2
Prep time: 15 minutes
Cooking time: 15 minutes

    1 tablespoon traditional fat of choice
    ½ pound fresh spinach, whole leaves
    1 large garlic clove, peeled, crushed, and finely chopped

½ cup coconut milk

Pinch of nutmeg

Sea salt, to taste

Freshly ground black pepper, to taste

4 eggs

1 teaspoon snipped chives, to garnish

Preheat the oven to 350°F. Heat the fat in a sauté pan over medium-high heat. Add the spinach, garlic, coconut milk, nutmeg, salt, and pepper and cook at a medium-high heat until the spinach is wilted. Drain off the excess liquid. Arrange spinach mixture in the bottom of ramekins. Crack two of the eggs into a small bowl (in case there are bits of eggshell) and gently pour them into one of the ramekins. Repeat with the remaining two eggs. Bake in the oven until the eggs are cooked the way you like them. If your preference is soft-cooked eggs, 5 minutes should be enough. Serve garnished with chives.

Poached Eggs with Swiss Chard

To prepare chard, remove the leaves and coarsely chop. The stalk should be peeled (this is preferable with many stalk vegetables, such as celery, rhubarb, and so on) and chopped finely. Both stalks and leaves can then be cooked together.

Serves: 2

Prep time: 10 minutes

Cooking time: 15 minutes

Swiss chard

1 tablespoon traditional fat of choice

1 medium shallot, peeled and finely chopped

5 cups Swiss chard, chopped as described above

Sea salt, to taste

Freshly ground pepper, to taste

Pinch of nutmeg

Poached eggs

    1 tablespoon apple cider vinegar
    2 large eggs, as fresh as possible (fresh eggs are best for poaching)
    Juice of ½ lemon
    2 teaspoons finely chopped fresh tarragon to garnish (optional)

Swiss chard:

Heat the fat in a sauté pan over medium high heat, add the shallot, and cook until lightly browned, about 3 to 5 minutes. Add chard, salt, pepper, and nutmeg, and cook at medium-high heat until the chard has wilted. Drain off the excess liquid, divide between two plates, and keep warm.

Poached eggs:

Add the apple cider vinegar (this helps the eggs to set) to ½ inch of boiling water in a saucepan. Crack each egg into a small bowl. Reduce the boiling water to a simmer and pour the egg into the water while vigorously stirring around the outside of the egg with a chopstick or kebab skewer. This forces the egg to the center of the pot, helping to hold it together. After 4 minutes, remove the egg with a slotted spoon and place on top of a portion of warm chard. Repeat the process with the second egg. The white should be firm but the yolk should be some-what creamy, with a white film over it. Serve the chard and egg topped with a drizzle of lemon juice and a pinch of salt. Garnish with tarragon if using.

Green Smoothie

A quick, energizing, and delicious way to start the day. Note that raw spinach and kale contain compounds (such as goitrogens, nitriles, oxalates) that may impair thyroid function if consumed in excess. If you have a thyroid issue, I suggest lightly steaming the kale and spinach first and then cooling it before adding it to the smoothie. This will at least partially inactivate the potentially harmful compounds.

Serves: 1
Equipment: Blender
Prep time: 5 minutes

    1 cup unsweetened almond milk
    1 medium banana, or 1 cup of mango chunks
    ½ cup coconut milk
    ½ cup raw spinach
    ½ cup raw kale
    1 tablespoon almond butter (optional)

Blend all the ingredients in a blender until smooth.

Green Plantain Fritters with Sausage

These fritters (without the sausage) can also be served as a snack or side dish.

Serves: 2
Prep time: 15 minutes
Cooking time: 20 minutes

Fritters:

    2 strips bacon
    1 green plantain
    1 heaping teaspoon of lard (see note)
    Pinch sea salt

Sausage:

    12 ounces ground pork
    ½ teaspoon ground fennel seeds
    ¼ teaspoon sea salt
    Freshly ground black pepper, to taste
    1 heaping teaspoon of lard (see note)
    2 teaspoons chopped parsley for garnish

In a skillet, cook the bacon. When it is done, drain on a paper-towel-lined plate or rack. Leave the bacon fat in the skillet for the final step of the recipe and set aside.

Slice the plantain into four pieces: cut once across and once length-wise. Bring a pot of water to a low boil, add the plantain, and simmer for 5 minutes. Check for doneness by inserting a knife to see if it will go through easily. If not, simmer until tender. (The plantains could also be grilled, sautéed, or cooked by any other method.) When they are done, drain the plantains, place in a mixing bowl, and mash.

Chop the bacon into small pieces and add, along with a teaspoon of the lard, to the mashed plantain. Stir to create a batter. If the batter is dry or crumbly, add more lard bit by bit until it becomes moist enough to shape into fritters. Stir in pinch of salt, keeping in mind that the bacon adds some salt already.

Shape the batter into 4-inch-wide round patties of about 1 inch thick. (You should be able to make two fritters per plantain, using about 6 to 8 tablespoons of batter for each fritter, but you can make them as large or small as you wish.) Heat the skillet containing the bacon fat over low heat. Gently place the fritters in the skillet and allow to cook for 3 to 5 minutes per side. (The bacon fat will brown them nicely.)

Mix all the sausage ingredients together except the lard and parsley and shape into patties. Heat the lard in a skillet over medium heat and fry the patties over medium heat until thoroughly cooked, about 3 to 4 minutes on each side. Serve with the plantain fritters, and garnish with parsley.

Note: The lard can be prepared on the first day of Week 1 (see recipes in Basics).

Smoked Salmon with Scrambled Eggs and Asparagus

This Scandinavian-inspired dish can also be served cold with sliced cucumber on the side.

Serves: 2
Prep time: 10 minutes
Cooking time: 15 minutes

> 10 green asparagus stalks, tough ends snapped off and discarded
> Sea salt, to taste

3 eggs

6 tablespoons full-fat coconut milk

Freshly ground pepper, to taste

2 tablespoons lard

4 ounces smoked salmon, sliced

2 teaspoons fresh chives, chopped for garnish

Blanch the asparagus in slightly salted boiling water for 5 minutes and refresh in cold water. Beat the eggs with coconut milk and pepper. Heat the lard in a saucepan over low heat, add the egg mixture, and cook for 3 to 4 minutes until just set, occasionally scraping the mixture from the bottom of the pan. Arrange the scrambled eggs on top of the asparagus, then place the smoked salmon on top of the eggs, and garnish with chopped chives.

Note: When making scrambled eggs or omelets, season with salt *after* cooking, otherwise the eggs will be rubbery. Also, remember that the smoked salmon is already quite salty.

Taro and Bacon Hash

Taro is usually available in Asian markets or in the ethnic sections of grocery stores. Make sure to peel away the purple layer, if present. If taro is not available, substitute 4 cups celery root (celeriac) or parsnips (cubed and parboiled the same way).

Serves: 2

Prep time: 10 minutes

Cooking time: 15 minutes

4 cups taro, peeled and cut into small cubes

1 tablespoon lard

8 strips bacon, cut into ½-inch pieces

1 medium onion, roughly chopped

Sea salt, to taste

Freshly ground black pepper, to taste

2 teaspoons apple cider vinegar (optional)

2 teaspoons chopped parsley, to garnish

Parboil the taro for 3 minutes in lightly salted, boiling water. Drain and let cool. Heat the lard in a sauté pan over medium heat, add the bacon, and fry until crisp. Add the onions and cook until browned, about 5 to 7 minutes. Add the taro, salt, and pepper and sauté until crisp, about 8 to 10 minutes. Drizzle with vinegar (if using). Serve garnished with parsley.

Cauliflower-Stuffed Acorn Squash

This can be prepared the day before and reheated. Shiitake mushrooms are a great touch but you can use any mushroom variety or a mix.

Serves: 8
Prep time: 15 minutes
Cooking time: 30 to 45 minutes

- 4 acorn squash, halved and seeds removed
- 1 head cauliflower, cut into florets
- 1/3 cup chicken stock
- 1 yellow onion, finely chopped
- 4 stalks celery, finely chopped
- 2 tablespoons traditional fat of choice
- 2 heaping cups coarsely chopped mushrooms of choice
- 1 tablespoon cinnamon
- 2 teaspoons ground ginger
- 1/2 teaspoon nutmeg
- 1/4 teaspoon ground cloves
- 1/4 teaspoon ground cardamom

Preheat the oven to 375 degrees. Place the acorn squash halves cut-side down in a baking dish (or two dishes if necessary) and cook for 30 to 45 minutes, until done. Meanwhile, rice the cauliflower: pulse the small florets in a food processor. Place the cauliflower, now in small pieces, in a pot with the chicken stock, cover, and steam over medium-low heat until softened, about 5 minutes. While the cauliflower is cooking, heat the fat in a sauté pan over medium heat and sauté the onion and celery until translucent, about 10 minutes. Add the mushrooms and continue cooking for an additional 5 to 10 minutes. Add the spices. Cook, stirring for a few additional minutes, allowing the flavors to mix.

Remove the acorn squash from the oven and set aside until cool enough to handle. Scoop a small amount around the edge of each acorn squash to make the opening a little bigger. Take the scooped squash and mix it into the cauliflower mixture; this gives the stuffing a nice orange color. Fill the acorn-squash halves with the cauliflower stuffing until heaping.

Feel free to add ½ cup of chopped nuts of your choice to the cauliflower mix for some extra crunch.

LUNCH RECIPES

Butternut Squash Frittata with Salad

This works for lunch, but also for breakfast or dinner.

Serves: 6
Prep time: 20 minutes
Cooking time: 20 minutes

Butternut Squash Frittata:

- 1 tablespoon traditional fat of choice
- ½ red onion, chopped
- 1 teaspoon sea salt, divided
- ½ teaspoon freshly ground black pepper, divided
- 1 medium butternut squash, peeled and cut into 1-inch cubes (you'll need about 6 cups total)
- 7 large eggs
- ⅓ cup full-fat coconut milk
- ¼ cup chopped parsley

Salad:

- Enough salad greens for 6 servings
- ¾ cup shallot vinaigrette (see recipe on page 392)

Preheat the oven to 375°F. Heat the fat in a cast-iron (or ovenproof) skillet over medium heat, add the onion, ½ teaspoon of the salt, and ¼ teaspoon of the pepper, and cook until onions are translucent, about 5 minutes. Add the squash cubes and continue to cook, stirring lightly, until the squash is cooked through but retains its shape, about 10 minutes (do not let it turn mushy). Set aside.

In a large bowl, whisk the eggs, coconut milk, parsley, and remaining ½ teaspoon salt and ¼ teaspoon pepper. Pour the eggs into the skillet with the squash and place it in the oven. Bake until the eggs are just set, about 10 minutes. If the top is not browned, place the skillet under the broiler for 1 or 2 additional minutes. Cool briefly, cut into wedges, and serve, accompanied by the salad greens tossed with shallot vinaigrette.

Hamburgers with Mushrooms Provençale-Style

In cooking, Provençale traditionally means a dish made with tomatoes, basil, thyme, and other herbs, but it can also refer to a rich mix of garlic, parsley, and extra-virgin olive oil. Use any mix of mushrooms you like.

Serves: 2
Prep time: 5 minutes
Cooking time: 15 minutes

    1 pound ground beef, preferably grass-fed
    1 tablespoon lard
    ½ lb. mixed mushrooms
    ½ teaspoon sea salt
    Freshly ground black pepper, to taste
    Juice of 1 lemon
    4 large garlic cloves, peeled, crushed, and finely chopped
    1 tablespoon extra-virgin olive oil
    4 tablespoons chopped parsley, plus 2 teaspoons for garnish

Shape two hamburger patties from the ground beef. Heat the lard in a sauté pan over medium heat, and sauté the hamburgers for 4 to 5 minutes on each side. Remove and keep warm. Add the mushrooms, salt, and pepper to the skillet and sauté until browned, stirring in the lemon juice while cooking. Add the garlic, extra-virgin olive oil, and parsley and cook for 3 more minutes. Serve the hamburgers topped with the cooked mushrooms and garnished with parsley.

Cod with Coriander
Red Pepper Sauce and Sautéed Broccoli

A simple-to-prepare entrée with the subtle, flavorful mix of coriander seeds and ginger.

Serves: 2
Prep time: 15 minutes
Cooking time: 30 minutes

Sautéed Broccoli:

> 1 head broccoli, florets only, broken into 1½-inch pieces
> Sea salt, to taste

Cod with Coriander Red Pepper Sauce:

> 1 tablespoon traditional fat of choice
> 1 cup chopped red onion (about half a large onion)
> 2 teaspoons minced fresh ginger, peeled
> 3 large garlic cloves, peeled and minced or pressed
> 1 large red bell pepper, seeded and chopped
> 2 teaspoons coriander seeds, freshly ground with a mortar and pestle or in a spice grinder (or 2 teaspoons ground coriander)
> 2 6- to 8-ounce cod fillets
> Sea salt and freshly ground black pepper
> 1 bay leaf, optional
> 1 tablespoon freshly squeezed lime juice
> 2 tablespoons minced fresh cilantro for garnish, optional

Blanch the broccoli in boiling, salted water for 5 minutes and then refresh with cold water. Drain and set aside.

In a sauté pan, heat half of the fat over medium-low heat. Add the onion and gently cook for 5 minutes. Add the ginger and cook for about 3 minutes more. Stir in the garlic and cook 1 minute more. Add the red pepper and coriander and cook until the pepper is softened, about 10 minutes.

Meanwhile, season the cod with salt and pepper and lay the fillets in a pan. Cover with water and add a bay leaf if using. Bring to a boil, then reduce the heat to low and cover the pan. Allow the cod fillets to simmer for 8 minutes. They should be fork tender. Remove from the cooking liquid with a slotted spoon and keep warm.

Heat the remaining fat in another sauté pan over medium heat (you can use the same pan you cooked the cod in, if you wish), add the broccoli, and cook for 5 minutes. Remove from heat. When the red pepper sauce is cooked through, turn off the heat and stir in the lime juice. Plate the cod fillets with the broccoli. Divide the sauce between the two plates; garnish with cilantro, and season with salt, if desired.

Tuna, Ginger, and Avocado Salad

A refreshing, easy, and quick salad.

Serves: 2
Prep time: 10 minutes

    1 6-ounce can tuna packed in water, drained
    2 avocados, peeled, pitted, and roughly chopped
    1 teaspoon grated fresh ginger, peeled
    1 small shallot, finely minced
    1 tablespoon freshly squeezed lime juice
    ¼ cup Paleo Mayonnaise (see recipe on pages 391–392)
    Sea salt, to taste
    Freshly ground black pepper, to taste
    Enough mixed salad greens for 2 servings
    2 teaspoons chopped cilantro, to garnish

Gently fold together all the ingredients except the mixed greens and cilantro in a bowl. Serve the tuna with mixed greens on the side and garnish with cilantro.

Greek Turkey Burgers with Zucchini Noodles

Greek flavors combine to provide a nice twist to burgers.

Serves: 4
Prep time: 20 minutes
Cooking time: 15 minutes

Zucchini Noodles:

  6 zucchini, julienned lengthwise into "noodles" about ⅛-inch thick
  1 tablespoon traditional fat of choice
  1 tablespoon sea salt

Greek Turkey Burgers:

  1 pound ground turkey
  ¼ cup minced red onion
  1 large garlic clove, peeled and minced
  ¼ cup kalamata olives, pitted and chopped
  2 tablespoons sun-dried tomatoes packed in oil, chopped
  1 egg
  2 tablespoons finely chopped fresh parsley
  Pinch of sea salt
  1 tablespoon traditional fat of choice (if cooking on stovetop)

Toss the zucchini noodles in coarse salt, let drain 20 minutes in a colander, and then plunge into a pot of boiling water for no more than 1 minute. Remove the noodles, refresh in cold water, and set aside.

In a large mixing bowl, combine the turkey, onion, garlic, olives, sun-dried tomatoes, egg, and parsley, and salt well. Shape into four patties. If grilling, grill the burgers for about 6 minutes on each side. If cooking on a stovetop, heat the fat in a large skillet over medium heat and cook 6 minutes on each side. Three minutes before the burgers are done, heat the fat of choice in a skillet over high heat and sauté the zucchini noodles for no more than 2 minutes. Serve the burgers accompanied by the noodles.

Chicken, Tarragon, and Grapefruit Salad

Tarragon goes famously with chicken, fish, salads, and sauces. Fresh herbs are always preferable, but if you have to substitute dried, use half the amount called for in the recipe. (In this recipe, use two tablespoons fresh tarragon or one tablespoon dried; fresh herbs in a salad, however, are much better.) If you can find a pomelo—an Asian citrus fruit similar to grapefruit—use that in place of the grapefruit for an extra-special taste.

Serves: 2
Prep time: 10 minutes (marinate 1 to 2 hours)
Cooking time: 20 minutes

- 2 6-ounce boneless chicken breasts
- 3 tablespoons sea salt
- ½ cup extra-virgin olive oil
- 2 tablespoons apple cider vinegar
- ½ teaspoon sea salt
- Freshly ground black pepper, to taste
- 1 medium shallot, minced
- 2 teaspoons Dijon mustard
- 1 medium head romaine, washed and roughly chopped
- 1 small red onion, halved and thinly sliced
- 1 large red grapefruit, peeled and segmented
- ¼ cup black olives, pitted and halved (optional but recommended)
- 2 heaping tablespoons finely chopped fresh tarragon or 1 heaping tablespoon dried, plus tarragon sprigs to garnish

Marinate the chicken breasts for 1 to 2 hours in brine (3 tablespoons of sea salt dissolved in 1 quart of water). This can be done in advance and helps to keep the breasts moist during cooking. Grill the breasts on low heat, 10 minutes on each side, and then thinly slice them lengthwise. In a small bowl, combine the olive oil with the apple cider vinegar, salt, pepper, shallot, and Dijon mustard to make a vinaigrette. Arrange the romaine on a plate, and top with the sliced red onion, grapefruit, chicken, and black olives. Pour over the vinaigrette and garnish with the tarragon sprigs.

Salmon Fillets with Raspberry Vinaigrette Salad

Adding sautéed salmon fillets to this light but satisfying salad transforms it into a complete meal. Note: This recipe makes enough vinaigrette for 6 to 8 servings. Store the extra dressing in an airtight container in the refrigerator for up to 1 week.

Serves: 2
Prep time: 15 minutes
Cooking time: 15 minutes

Raspberry Vinaigrette Salad:

- 3 ounces raspberries (about 15 berries)
- 1½ tablespoons balsamic vinegar
- ¼ teaspoon Dijon mustard or mustard powder
- ¼ cup extra-light olive oil (extra-virgin is fine if that's all you have on hand)
- 2 teaspoons fresh thyme leaves
- 8 cups mixed salad greens
- ¼ cup or more toasted and crumbled pecans or walnuts (or ½ cup crispy, cooked bacon pieces)
- Any other vegetables or salad toppings you'd like to add—we like shredded carrots and quartered, hard-boiled eggs

Salmon Fillets:

- 2 6- to 8-ounce salmon fillets
- Freshly ground black pepper, to taste
- Sea salt, to taste
- 1 tablespoon traditional fat of choice

To make the dressing, blend the raspberries, balsamic vinegar, and mustard in a blender. Transfer to a small mixing bowl. Whisk in the olive oil and thyme. Set aside.

Season the salmon fillets with salt and pepper. Heat the fat in a sauté pan over medium-high heat, add the salmon fillets, and cook for 5 minutes on each side.

Meanwhile, in a large salad bowl, toss the greens and nuts (or bacon pieces), 4 tablespoons of the dressing, and any other salad ingredients you want to include. Serve the salmon fillets accompanied by salad.

DINNERS

Beef Rendang

This slow-cooked, Indonesian-inspired stew uses ingredients easily found in the market and has a quick prep time. Look for dried kaffir lime leaves in the spice section at your grocery store if you can't locate fresh (Thai Kitchen is one brand). Lemongrass can usually be found in the fresh-vegetables section.

Serves: 2 to 4
Prep time: 15 minutes
Cooking time: About 4 hours, largely unattended

- 6 shallots or 1½ red onions, roughly chopped
- 4 large garlic cloves, peeled, crushed, and roughly chopped
- 1½ tablespoons minced fresh ginger, peeled
- 2 red chilies, seeded and roughly chopped
- 5 cloves
- 3 kaffir lime leaves, fresh or dried
- 2 pounds beef stew cubes
- 1½ cups full-fat coconut milk
- 1 teaspoon turmeric
- 1 teaspoon ground coriander
- 1 teaspoon ground cumin
- ½ teaspoon ground cinnamon
- ¼ teaspoon ground nutmeg
- ¼ teaspoon sea salt, or to taste
- 3 stalks lemongrass

Preheat the oven to 300°F. To a food processor or blender, add the shallots or red onions, garlic, ginger, chilies, and dried kaffir lime leaves, if using. (If using fresh lime leaves, set aside, as they will be added later.)

Pulse until combined into a purée and set aside. (You can also do this by hand using a mortar and pestle.)

In an oven-safe pot with lid, add the beef and coconut milk. Stir in the spice purée. Then stir in the turmeric, coriander, cumin, cinnamon, nutmeg, and salt.

Prepare the lemongrass stalks: Peel off the tough outer layer and discard. Cut off the stem end and the green tops to end up with about a 10-inch piece of lemongrass. Place the stalks on the cutting board and bang on them with a kitchen tool (such as a potato masher or pestle) to release the flavor. Place them in the stew whole (you will remove them later, as you would bay leaves). If you are using fresh kaffir lime leaves, similarly bruise them using a mortar and pestle and add them in this step (to remove with the lemongrass later).

Heat the stew, uncovered, on the stovetop over medium heat until it comes to a simmer. Cover and place the pot in the oven. Cook for 3 hours, stirring once or twice. Carefully bring the pot back to the stovetop and uncover. Remove the lemongrass (and fresh kaffir, if using) with tongs and discard. Bring the stew to a simmer over low heat. Cook, stirring often, until the meat is tender and the sauce has reduced by half, about 45 minutes. Stir constantly toward the end of the cooking process.

Grilled Ahi Tuna Steaks with Chinese Five-Spice Powder

You can find Chinese five-spice powder in Asian markets or in any well-stocked spice section.

Serves: 2
Prep time: 5 minutes (marinate ½ hour)
Cooking time: 10 minutes for the tuna and 25 minutes for the Cabbage, Bok Choy, and Shiitake Mushrooms side dish (see pages 381–382 for recipe)

  1½ tablespoons Chinese five-spice powder
  2 tablespoons coconut oil
  1 teaspoon sea salt

Juice of 1 lemon

2 8-ounce ahi tuna steaks, 1-inch thick

1 tablespoon chopped cilantro, to garnish

Mix spice powder, oil, salt, and lemon to make a paste and rub on both sides of the tuna steaks. Allow to marinate for 30 minutes. Grill the steaks for 5 minutes on each side at a medium heat. (You can also broil them.) Arrange the tuna steaks on top of the accompanying Cabbage, Bok Choy, and Shiitake Mushrooms side dish (see pages 381–382). Garnish with fresh, chopped cilantro.

Tom Kha Gai

Made with real bone broth and coconut milk, Tom Kha Gai, a creamy, flavorful, savory soup, is surprisingly nutrient dense. Move over chicken noodle soup— when it comes to brothy comfort foods ideal for colds and sore throats, this Thai coconut soup is the champion.

Serves: 4

Prep time: 5 minutes

Cooking time: 15 minutes

3 cups Paleo Chicken Stock (see recipe on pages 390–391)

3 cups coconut milk

2 to 3 stalks lemongrass

4 kaffir lime leaves, fresh or dried, ripped into four pieces each

2 or more Thai bird chilies or other chili of choice, stems removed and pods lightly crushed (optional)

4 cups cooked and shredded chicken

1 to 2 cups thinly sliced shiitake or oyster mushrooms (or any other mushrooms)

½ teaspoon sea salt

2 tablespoons fish sauce (I like Red Boat brand)

Juice of 1 lime

1 green onion, thinly sliced

1 tablespoon chopped cilantro

Bring the stock to a boil, reduce to a simmer, skim off any foam that rises to the top, and add all the ingredients except the fish sauce, lime juice, green onion, and cilantro. Reduce the heat to a simmer and cook for about 5 minutes. Season to taste with fish sauce. Remove the kaffir lime leaves, lemongrass, and chilies and ladle into soup bowls or mugs. Garnish with lime juice, green onions, and cilantro.

Spanish Pork Loin Roast Adobado

This savory pork dish is irresistible!

Serves: 4

Prep time: 15 minutes (marinate 8 to 24 hours)

Cooking time: 1 to 1½ hours depending on size of roast

  1 tablespoon paprika

  6 large garlic cloves, peeled, crushed, and roughly chopped

  1 teaspoon ground cumin

  1 teaspoon dried thyme or 2 teaspoons chopped fresh thyme

  2 teaspoons dried oregano

  ½ teaspoon sea salt

  ½ cup apple cider vinegar

  Freshly ground black pepper, to taste

  1 2- to 3-pound boneless pork loin roast

  4 teaspoons chopped fresh parsley

Combine the paprika, garlic, cumin, thyme, oregano, salt, vinegar, and black pepper in a bowl and whisk together. Place the pork in a nonreactive dish/bowl just large enough for it and coat the meat thoroughly on all sides with the marinade. Cover the bowl and refrigerate for 8 to 24 hours.

Bring the pork to room temperature for about 20 minutes before cooking and preheat the oven to 350°F. Place the pork fat-side up in a roasting pan with rack (if you don't have a rack, it's also fine to put it directly on the pan). If your roast does not have any fat on it, dab 3 tablespoons of lard or other fat on top of the roast. Cook until the internal temperature reaches

145°F. Cooking times will vary depending on the size of your roast. For a 1½- to 2-pound roast, check after 45 minutes; check a 2½- to 3-pound roast after 60 minutes. When it's done, if the top isn't browned, place under the broiler for a minute or two. Remove from the oven and allow the roast to rest in the pan for 10 minutes. Transfer to a cutting board and slice into thick or thin slices, as you prefer. Garnish with fresh parsley.

Chicken Tikka Masala

Tikka means that the food is cut into small pieces and then marinated and usually cooked on skewers. It's then added to the sauce (the masala). Note that I use bamboo skewers in this recipe. Soak them in water for 30 minutes to 1 hour just before using.

Serves: 4
Prep time: 20 minutes (marinate 1 to 3 hours)
Cooking time: 25 minutes

For the marinade:

    1 cup full-fat coconut milk
    2 teaspoons garam masala
    2 teaspoons ground coriander
    1 tablespoon paprika
    2 tablespoons minced fresh ginger, peeled
    4 large garlic cloves, peeled and minced or pressed
    4 boneless, skinless chicken breasts, cut into 1½-inch chunks

For the sauce:

    2 tablespoons coconut oil
    1 onion, minced
    2 garlic cloves, peeled and minced or pressed
    2 teaspoons minced ginger, peeled
    1 chili (such as serrano or jalapeño), seeded and minced
    1 teaspoon paprika
    1 teaspoon coriander

1 tablespoon tomato paste

2 cups puréed or fresh, finely diced tomatoes

½ cup coconut cream (skimmed from the top of coconut milk or, if you can find it, coconut cream concentrate from Tropical Traditions)

½ tablespoon garam masala

Sea salt, to taste

¼ cup chopped cilantro

Prepare the marinade: In a bowl, combine all the marinade ingredients. Pour over the chicken to coat well. Cover and refrigerate for 1 to 3 hours.

When ready to cook recipe, soak 8 bamboo or wooden skewers (if using) for 30 minutes to 1 hour.

Prepare the sauce: Heat the coconut oil in a large pan over medium heat. Add the onion and cook until softened, about 5 minutes. Add the garlic, ginger, chili, paprika, coriander, and tomato paste and stir well for a minute. Add the puréed tomatoes. Reduce the heat to medium low, cover the pan, and simmer for about 15 minutes, stirring occasionally.

While the sauce simmers, preheat the broiler (or prepare the grill). Thread the marinated chicken onto skewers, or simply arrange in a single layer in a broiler pan, if broiling. Grill or broil, turning occasionally. Look for a light char, about 6 to 8 minutes per side.

Purée the sauce by transferring it to a blender or food processor, or use an immersion blender. Return the sauce to the pan. Add the coconut cream to the sauce and mix it in well.

Remove the chicken from the skewers. Stir the pieces into the sauce and allow to cook for 5 to 8 minutes in the sauce. Stir in the garam masala. Salt to taste and serve garnished with the cilantro.

Rosemary Lamb Rib Chops

Frenched lamb rib chops are also referred to as lamb lollipop chops because of the rib bone that is attached to this small chop. Because this recipe calls for only half a pound of lamb, spring for the pastured, organic lamb if you can find it.

Serves: 2
Prep time: 5 minutes (marinate 1 to 3 hours)
Cooking time: 10 minutes

> 2 tablespoons traditional fat of choice
> 4 garlic cloves, minced or pressed
> 1 tablespoon minced fresh rosemary
> Freshly ground black pepper, to taste
> ½ pound (about 6) Frenched lamb rib chops
> Sea salt, to taste

Combine melted fat, garlic, rosemary, and pepper in a bowl and add the lamb chops, taking care to make sure the meat is well coated with marinade. Marinate for 1 to 3 hours. Grill, broil, or pan-fry the chops. I use the following method: Preheat a cast-iron skillet to medium heat. Sprinkle the chops with salt on both sides. Once the pan is hot (you should hear a sizzle when the meat is dropped in), pan-sear for about 3 to 4 minutes per side, until a golden-brown crust develops. Transfer the chops to a plate and allow them to rest for 5 minutes before serving.

Rustic Meatball and Tomato Stew

Rustic in this recipe means that you want to keep the tomatoes, celery, and carrots as whole as possible, to retain their shape and visual appeal.

Serves: 4
Prep time: 15 minutes
Cooking time: 1 hour

For the Meatballs:

> 1½ pounds ground beef (preferably from grass-fed animals)
> 1 onion, peeled and finely chopped
> 2 large garlic cloves, peeled, crushed, and finely chopped
> 1 teaspoon fennel seeds, coarsely ground, or 1 teaspoon powdered
>   fennel

2 eggs

Freshly ground black pepper, to taste

1 teaspoon sea salt, or to taste

5 tablespoons extra-virgin olive oil

For the Stew:

1 onion, peeled and cut into 8 wedges

4 garlic cloves, crushed and coarsely chopped

2 cups beef bone broth (see recipe on pages 388–389)

4 medium carrots, peeled and sliced on the bias into 2-inch pieces

2 large celery stalks, sliced on the bias into 2-inch pieces

1/4 teaspoon red chili flakes (optional)

1 teaspoon sea salt, or to taste

Freshly ground black pepper, to taste

2 8-ounce cans of whole plum tomatoes, drained

1 tablespoon balsamic vinegar

4 tablespoons chopped fresh basil, for garnish

The meatballs:

Combine all the ingredients but only 2 tablespoons of the olive oil in a bowl and mix well. Heat the remaining 3 tablespoons oil in a pan and fry a small portion of the mixture to taste to test for salt; add salt if necessary. Shape into golf-ball-size meatballs and fry until well browned on all sides and firm, about 10 minutes. Remember that the meatballs will be simmered in the stew later, so at this stage, don't overcook. Remove the meatballs and set aside. Do not clean the pan.

The stew:

In the same pan, briefly fry the onion and garlic over low heat, about 10 minutes. Add the bone broth, bring it to a boil, and add all the other ingredients except the tomatoes, vinegar, and basil. Cover and let the stew simmer until the carrots and celery are tender, about 5 to 7 minutes. Add the meatballs, tomatoes, and vinegar and simmer uncovered for 15 minutes. Taste for salt and serve in soup bowls, garnished with the chopped basil.

SIDE DISHES

Roasted Carrots and Garlic

I like to use duck fat for maximum taste, but any traditional fat will do. Whatever fat you choose, warm it to a liquid state before tossing it with the carrots.

Serves: 4

Prep time: 10 minutes

Cooking time: 35 minutes

- 1½ pounds carrots, peeled and quartered
- 1 head garlic, separated into individual cloves and peeled (about 20 cloves)
- Sea salt, to taste
- 2 tablespoons traditional fat of choice plus extra if needed (duck fat is preferred)
- 2 tablespoons chopped fresh rosemary

Preheat the oven to 400°F. Place the carrots in a roasting pan in a single layer. Spread the garlic cloves around the pan. Sprinkle with salt and add the fat, then toss the carrots and garlic to coat. Roast 15 minutes, then remove pan and stir. If the vegetables seem dry, add a little additional fat. Roast 15 more minutes, then check for doneness. The garlic should be browning slightly and the carrots should be fork tender. Stir again, and sprinkle with rosemary. Roast an additional 5 minutes, remove from the oven, let cool slightly, and serve.

Cabbage, Bok Choy, and Shiitake Mushrooms

Umeboshi plum vinegar from Japan (available in Asian markets as well as many grocery stores, since it's now widely used in the United States) adds a great touch to this dish, but you can use any vinegar of your choice. Use as much or as little garlic as you'd like.

Serves: 4
Prep time: 10 minutes
Cooking time: 25 minutes

  3 tablespoons coconut oil
  3 to 6 garlic cloves (to taste), pressed
  2 tablespoons minced fresh ginger, peeled
  4 packed cups roughly chopped cabbage (1-inch chunks)
  8 ounces sliced shiitake mushrooms (about 4 cups)
  3 cups sliced bok choy (1/4-inch slices)
  1 teaspoon umeboshi plum vinegar
  Sea salt and freshly ground black pepper, to taste

Heat the coconut oil in a large pot over medium-low heat. Add the garlic and ginger and stir until fragrant, about 2 minutes. Add the cabbage and mushrooms. Cook for 10 minutes, stirring frequently. Reduce the heat to low, add the bok choy, and cook 15 more minutes, continuing to stir until done. Turn off the heat and stir in the vinegar. Season to taste with salt and pepper. Remove the vegetables with a slotted spoon to drain off the liquid, and serve.

Thai Basil Eggplant

The Thai basil and chili pepper in this recipe give the eggplant an exotic twist. In Thailand, the eggplants are green and long, unlike the big purplish eggplants found in the United States. You may be able to locate Thai eggplant and Thai basil in an Asian market, but if not, you may use regular eggplant and basil.

Serves: 4
Prep time: 5 minutes
Cooking time: 10 minutes

  2½ lbs. eggplant (about 2 medium regular eggplants)
  1 tablespoon coconut oil
  1 chili pepper, seeded and sliced thin, or a pinch of red chili flakes
  2 garlic cloves, chopped

2 tablespoons fish sauce (I like Red Boat brand)

1 cup loosely packed Thai basil leaves (or regular fresh basil)

Cut the eggplants into chunky 1½-inch irregular shapes for easy turning in the pan. In a steamer basket, steam the eggplant for about 5 minutes, until softened. Heat a pan or wok over medium heat. Add the oil, chili pepper or flakes, and garlic. Stir until the garlic turns golden brown; cook no more than 5 minutes or it'll burn. Add the steamed eggplant and cook for a few minutes, stirring, to blend the flavors. Stir in the fish sauce and cook until heated through. Add the basil and turn off the heat immediately so that the basil retains its color.

Cauliflower Hash

This side dish is a hearty accompaniment to roast meats and chicken.

Serves: 4
Prep time: 5 minutes
Cooking time: 25 minutes

1 large head cauliflower

1 onion, peeled and finely chopped

2 bay leaves

2 garlic cloves

2 teaspoons fresh thyme

4 cloves

3 tablespoons bacon drippings or traditional fat of choice

½ teaspoon sea salt, or to taste

Freshly ground black pepper, to taste

3 tablespoons chopped parsley, to garnish

Cut off the bottom of the cauliflower to remove any green leaves and remove the stem and tough bottom core. Place the cauliflower bottom-side up in a large pot and add enough water to cover. Add the onion, bay leaves, garlic, thyme, and cloves, bring to a boil, then reduce the heat and simmer for 10 minutes. Remove the cauliflower, drain, cool, and coarsely chop. The cauliflower should have a crumbly consistency. Heat the bacon drippings or traditional fat of choice in a sauté pan over medium-high heat, add the cauliflower bits, and cook, stirring occasionally, for 10 minutes. Season to taste with salt and pepper, and serve garnished with chopped parsley.

Green Salad with Shallot Vinaigrette

This salad uses romaine lettuce, which retains its crispness, but any lettuce or mixed salad greens will do. Always make sure your salad greens (and herbs) are well dried—a salad spinner is a good and inexpensive investment.

Serves: 2
Prep time: 5 minutes

- 1 small head romaine, leaves washed, dried, and torn into pieces as desired
- ½ cup shallot vinaigrette (see recipe on page 392)

In a large salad bowl, add the vinaigrette first, then the romaine, and gently toss.

Yuca Fries

These "fries" are extra good sprinkled with paprika or chili powder before roasting. Note: Each yuca root has a tough, stringy bit in its center. This will turn up in some of the fries, so watch out for it. I used to boil the yuca in halves and remove this stringy part before cutting into fry shapes, but I found that it was easier to just avoid it while eating the fries.

Serves: 4
Prep time: 10 minutes
Cooking time: 30 minutes

- 2 medium yuca (cassava) roots, each about 6 to 8 inches long
- 3 to 4 tablespoons duck fat, lard, or tallow (warmed until it's in a liquid state)
- Sea salt and freshly ground black pepper, to taste

Bring about 3 quarts of water to a boil. Peel the yuca and cut it into the shape of fries, about 3 inches long and 1½ inches thick. (Don't cut them thinner than this or they'll get too dry and tough when you roast them.) Boil the yuca fries for 30 minutes until soft but not falling apart. Meanwhile, preheat the oven to 475°F. Drain the fries and put them in a mixing bowl. Pour liquefied fat over fries and mix to distribute evenly. Spread the fries on a baking sheet and season generously with salt and pepper. Place the baking sheet on a lower rack in the oven and roast for about 15 minutes. Remove from the oven and flip the fries. Roast for another 5 to 7 minutes or until golden brown.

Kale and Kabocha Squash Salad

I love kale and squash in any recipe, but the lemony bacon dressing here really makes their flavors pop.

Serves: 2 to 3
Prep time: 10 minutes
Cooking time: 1 hour

> 1½-pound kabocha squash, peeled, seeded, and cut into ½-inch to 1-inch cubes
> 5 strips bacon, chopped
> 4 packed cups finely sliced kale
> 3 tablespoons freshly squeezed lemon juice
> 1 tablespoon finely sliced fresh chives
> 1 tablespoon finely chopped fresh sage
> ½ to ¾ cup toasted walnuts or pecans
> Sea salt and freshly ground black pepper, to taste

Preheat the oven to 350°F. In a baking dish, roast the squash cubes with the chopped bacon for 1 hour, stirring well every 15 minutes. In a large mixing bowl, combine the salt and kale. With impeccably clean hands, strongly massage the salt into the kale for 1 minute. Add 2 table-spoons of the lemon juice and continue massaging the kale leaves for

1 additional minute. Set aside until ready to assemble the salad. When the squash is tender and the bacon crispy, remove the pan and carefully drain off the bacon fat into a small mixing bowl. Whisk the fat (there should be about 3 tablespoons) with the remaining tablespoon of lemon juice.

There will be a lot of liquid in the bottom of the kale. Squeeze it out and put the drained kale in a salad bowl. Add the squash, bacon, chives, sage, and walnuts. Toss with the lemon-bacon dressing, season with salt and pepper to taste, and serve.

SNACKS

Nori Chips

You'll save money making your own nori chips instead of paying for prepackaged versions — plus, it's really easy.

Serves: Enough snacks for two days
Prep time: 5 minutes
Cooking time: 15 minutes

- 9 nori sheets, untoasted or toasted
- 2 tablespoons extra-virgin olive oil
- Sea salt, to taste
- Optional spices of your choice such as onion powder, garlic powder, or sesame seeds

Preheat the oven to 350°F. Cut the nori sheets into squares with a knife or kitchen shears, or cut into smaller pieces if you prefer (for easy storage). Place the nori on a baking sheet in a single layer. Lightly brush the nori on one side with oil using a pastry brush or your fingers. Sprinkle the oiled side of the nori with salt and the powdered spice of your choice. Bake for about 15 minutes, until the nori chips become dry and crispy and just begin to pucker a bit. Let them cool and serve or store in an airtight container for up to 5 days.

Hard-Boiled Eggs with Avocado

Salt and pepper bring out the flavors in this satisfying combination.

Serves: Enough snacks for two days
Prep time: 5 minutes
Cooking time: 12 minutes

> 6 hard-boiled eggs
> 3 ripe avocados, pitted and sliced
> Sea salt and freshly ground black pepper, to taste

Cut the eggs in half and serve sprinkled with salt and pepper with avocado slices on the side.

Kale Chips

A nutrient-rich snack — the goal is to make the kale chips as crisp as possible.

Serves: Enough for two days of snacks
Prep time: 5 minutes
Cooking time: 12 to 15 minutes

> 2 large bunches kale, washed, stemmed, and patted dry
> 4 tablespoons traditional fat of choice, melted
> 3 tablespoons apple cider vinegar
> Sea salt, to taste
> Freshly ground black pepper, to taste

Preheat the oven to 300°F. Cut the kale leaves into large uniform pieces. In a mixing bowl combine the kale, melted fat, and vinegar until the kale is well coated. Season with salt and freshly ground pepper. Spread the kale on a baking tray (you may have to do this in two batches) and bake for 12 to 15 minutes, tossing the kale chips at least once to help dry them out. Remove from the oven and let cool. Serve or store in an airtight container for up to 5 days.

Guacamole with Carrot Chips

An easy snack that can be prepared up to two days in advance.

Serves: Enough for two days of snacks
Prep time: 10 minutes

4 ripe avocados
2 tablespoons lemon juice
1 tablespoon very finely minced onion
¼ cup coconut cream
½ teaspoon sea salt
Freshly ground black pepper, to taste
2 pounds carrots, peeled

Cut the avocados in half, remove the pits, and scoop them out. (If you have unripe avocados, place them in a paper bag with half an apple for 2 to 3 days to ripen.) Combine all the ingredients except the carrots in a bowl and mash.

Slice the carrots on the bias into chips. Serve the guacamole with the carrot chips on the side.

To store guacamole, cover with plastic wrap to keep it from turning gray (oxidizing), lightly pressing the wrap onto the surface of the guacamole to "seal" it. The guacamole can be stored in the refrigerator, but eat it quickly because it will stay fresh for only 2 or 3 days. The carrot chips can be stored in a bowl of water, covered, in the refrigerator for up to 1 day.

BASICS

Beef Bone Broth/Stock

This stock should be rich. The best bones to use are marrow bones combined with any other beef bones such as knuckle bones. Any scraps of meat cooked or uncooked can also be added.

Yield: About 4 quarts
Prep time: 10 minutes
Cooking time: 3½ hours

- 4 pounds beef bones (preferably marrow and knuckle bones)
- 2 onions, peeled and halved
- 4 carrots, peeled and cut into large pieces
- 2 bay leaves (preferably fresh, but dried will also work)
- 2 teaspoons fresh thyme
- 4 cloves
- 4 celery ribs, chopped
- 1 cup parsley

Preheat the oven to 400°F. Place the bones, onions, and carrots in a roasting pan and roast for 15 minutes or until very well browned. Add ½ inch of water to the pan so drippings don't burn and stick to the bottom. Add everything from the roasting pan (scraping the bottom), 6 quarts of water, and all the remaining ingredients to a stockpot. Bring stockpot to a boil, reduce to low heat, and simmer, covered, for 3 hours. Strain the stock. When the stock is completely cold, pour it into 1-quart mason jars and refrigerate for later use. It should last about a week in the refrigerator; you can also freeze it in bulk or individual portions in freezer-safe plastic bags.

Lard

Home-rendered lard is easy to make, particularly after you make one or two practice batches. You'll use this traditional fat in many Paleo recipes so it's worth learning how to prepare it yourself. The trick is not to burn the lard. If made on the first day of the week, this recipe will yield more than enough for the full seven-day meal plan.

Yield: About 1 quart
Prep time: 5 minutes
Cooking time: 1 hour plus

- 5 pounds pork back fat, cut into 1-inch cubes

Heat the pork fat in a large stockpot over medium-low heat and stir frequently for about an hour. If you use too low a heat setting, little will happen during the cooking. However, too high a heat setting will cause sticking and burning. Aim for medium low and stir frequently; this is a slow-cooking process. Eventually, a quarter inch of rendered liquid fat will gather at the bottom of the pan and you will see the cubes start to change in color from pink to tan. Keep stirring to prevent sticking and to keep the heat even throughout the pieces. Soon the liquid will begin to accumulate to cover the cubes. Once all the cubes are submerged, stirring is no longer necessary for even cooking, but it may be necessary to prevent sticking. The fat should never smoke or come close to smoking. When the cubes have lost much of their original size and are light brown (not burned), they have turned into cracklings and you are ready to strain the lard. You can dry the cracklings on a paper towel and eat them, of course! Using care—the lard is very hot—strain the mixture through a fine-mesh strainer into a 1-quart glass jar. It should be the color of apple juice. Once the lard has cooled, cover and store in the refrigerator. When it is refrigerated and solidifies, it should be white in color. If the lard is a brown color when solid, it means the lard has burned and should not be used. It will keep for several weeks in the refrigerator.

Paleo Chicken Stock

Chicken stock is used for everything from soups to sauces, stews, and sautéed dishes. It goes well not only with poultry but also with pork, veal, and eggs. The ingredients and preparation are simple but it takes time. Be patient and let it simmer for several hours to bring out the full flavor of the ingredients. Adding chicken heads and/or feet to the stock makes it more gelatinous and beneficial for gut health, but it is not required.

Yield: About 4 quarts
Prep time: 15 minutes
Cooking time: 3 hours (largely unattended)

   1 3- to 4-pound chicken (preferably an old stewing hen), cut into pieces
   4½ quarts water

2 onions, peeled and halved

4 carrots, peeled and cut into large chunks

2 fresh bay leaves

4 sprigs fresh thyme or 1 tablespoon dried thyme

4 celery ribs, cut into large pieces

4 cloves

1 bunch fresh parsley

2 chicken heads and/or 2 chicken feet

Add all the ingredients to a large stockpot, bring to a boil, reduce the heat, and simmer, covered, for 3 hours. While still warm, strain the stock through a sieve. A wet cheesecloth can then be used to strain out all the fine particles. When the stock is at room temperature, the pot can be placed in a refrigerator for a few hours. This will cause the fat to harden on the surface. The fat can then be skimmed off and used for cooking, and it will keep for up to 1 week if refrigerated in a tightly sealed jar.

Paleo Mayonnaise

An essential base for many cold sauces, mayonnaise should always be served cold. Very fresh pastured/organic eggs are a must for this recipe. The oil should have a neutral taste, which is why olive oil is not recommended for basic mayonnaise.

Yield: 2 cups
Prep time: 10 minutes

2 pastured/organic-chicken egg yolks

1½ cups avocado or macadamia nut oil

1 tablespoon Dijon mustard

½ teaspoon sea salt

⅛ teaspoon white pepper

2 tablespoons freshly squeezed lemon juice

All the ingredients and equipment must be at room temperature. Combine the egg yolks, mustard, salt, pepper, and lemon juice together in a ceramic or steel bowl (do not use glass or plastic) and whisk until smooth. (You may use a blender but the container must be steel; a bowl is actually preferable.) While whisking, begin adding the oil in a very thin stream at first. When the mixture starts to cling to the sides of the bowl, then and only then add the remaining oil in a slow stream, whisking the whole time. A tip: Place a folded wet dish towel beneath the bowl to prevent it from moving while you're whisking. Fresh mayonnaise can be kept in a bowl covered with cling film in the refrigerator for up to 3 days.

Shallot Vinaigrette

Shallots are actually more aromatic than both garlic and onions, so a little goes a long way. The quantity of vinegar used is very much a question of personal taste, so add it in stages, keeping in mind the Dijon mustard has vinegar in it as well. You don't need to use extra-virgin olive oil in this recipe, as the taste of the shallots is the priority here.

Yield: 1 quart
Prep time: 10 minutes

> 3 cups olive oil
> 2 shallots, roughly minced
> 3 tablespoons Dijon mustard
> 1½ teaspoon sea salt
> Freshly ground black pepper, to taste
> 1 cup apple cider vinegar

In a bowl, whisk all the ingredients except the vinegar together. Add the vinegar slowly, occasionally tasting for acidity. Pour the vinaigrette into a glass container with a lid and refrigerate. Vinaigrette will keep for at least 3 weeks. Before use, give it a good shake, as the oil and vinegar tend to separate.

Acknowledgments

Writing a book is a monumental task, and not something I could have done on my own. It emerged out of a thriving community of readers, patients, colleagues, teachers, friends, family, and other supporters, both past and present. Though my name is on the cover, this book was truly a collaborative effort.

I am grateful for the contribution of pioneering scientists, physicians, and bloggers whose work continually inspired and enlightened me. This book wouldn't have been possible without their willingness to challenge mainstream dogma and blaze new trails. I especially want to thank Dr. Chris Masterjohn, Dr. Stephan Guyenet, Dan Pardi, Dr. Mat Lalonde, Robb Wolf, Dr. Kurt Harris, and Dr. Emily Deans for their input and feedback on the manuscript and their ongoing advocacy, support, and friendship.

My patients continue to be my greatest teachers. Thank you for putting your trust in me, and allowing me to bear witness to your healing journey.

To the fantastic team (Diane, Shannon, Keith, Jon, Kelsey, Laura, Aidan, Andrew, Jordan, Steve, and many more) behind my private practice and ChrisKresser.com: thank you for all of the ways you have supported this endeavor, both seen and unseen, and for your help in making the world a healthier place, one person at a time.

I'd like to thank the incredible group of people that helped transform this book from an idea into reality. Betsy Rapoport's keen insight and belief in my vision were instrumental in developing the proposal and initial structure of the book. Becky Cabaza helped me wrangle 165,000 words into a polished final draft. My editor, Tracy Behar, took a chance on a new author and was a source of constant support and encouragement. Carolyn O'Keefe, Miriam Parker, and countless others at Little, Brown were tireless advocates of the book and worked hard to ensure its success; I couldn't have asked for a better first experience with a publisher. My agent, Richard Pine, shepherded the book through each stage of the publishing process with wisdom, clarity, and candor.

Finally, my deepest gratitude goes to my family and friends for their unconditional love, selfless support, and enduring belief in me. I wish there were room to name you all; you know who you are, and I am thankful for your presence in my life.

I can't finish without mentioning four very special people specifically. Mom and Dad, you provided the foundation that made all of this possible, and have always been there when I needed you. Elanne and Sylvie, the joy and light of my life, thank you for putting up with the long hours, hectic schedule, and time away. Sharing my life with you both is the most precious gift I could have ever imagined, and you've made me the luckiest man in the world.

Index

About the Author

CHRIS KRESSER, M.S., L.Ac, is a practitioner of integrative and functional medicine and the creator of ChrisKresser.com, one of the most respected natural-health sites in the world. He is widely known for his in-depth research uncovering myths and misconceptions in modern medicine and providing natural-health solutions with proven results. He developed the Personal Paleo Cure based on more than ten years of research, his own recovery from a debilitating, decade-long illness, and his clinical work with patients. Chris maintains a private practice in Berkeley, California, where he lives with his wife and daughter.